IMAGING OF THE BREAST – TECHNICAL ASPECTS AND CLINICAL IMPLICATION

Edited by **Laszlo Tabar**

Imaging of the Breast – Technical Aspects and Clinical Implication
Edited by Laszlo Tabar

Published by InTech

Janeza Trdine 9, 51000 Rijeka, Croatia

Publishing Process Manager Bojan Rafaj

Technical Editor Teodora Smiljanic

Cover Designer InTech Design Team

Additional hard copies can be obtained from orders@intechopen.com

Imaging of the Breast – Technical Aspects and Clinical Implication,
Edited by Laszlo Tabar
p. cm.
ISBN 978-953-51-0284-7

For EU product safety concerns:
IN TECH d.o.o., Prolaz Marije Krucifikse Kozulić 3, 51000 Rijeka, Croatia,
info@intechopen.com or visit our website at intechopen.com.

Meet the editor

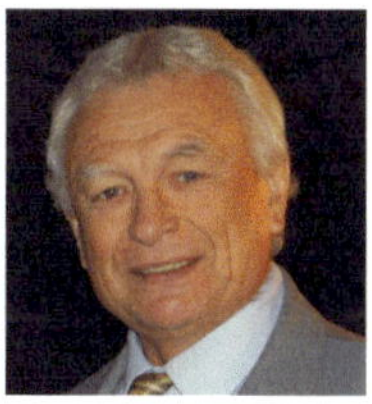

Professor Laszlo Tabar, M.D, is a radiologist who has devoted his career to the early diagnosis of breast cancer. He was a leader in the first successful mammography screening trial and has gained a reputation as a clinician, researcher and teacher of the art and science of the early detection of breast cancer. He has co-authored more that 150 peer-reviewed articles and book chapters, as well as five textbooks on breast cancer diagnosis and screening. He has directed more than 400 continuing medical education courses around the world teaching technologists, radiologists and other members of the multidisciplinary diagnostic team the principles and practice of the early detection of breast cancer.

Contents

Preface

Early detection of breast cancer combined with targeted therapy offers the best outcome for breast cancer patients. The development of low-dose screen-film mammography made the early detection of breast cancer a reality. This technology was successfully implemented in the population-based screening trials, which proved that the early detection of breast cancer through mammography screening can prevent at least 40% of the deaths from breast cancer in participating women. Additionally, these smaller and less advanced cancers do not need as extensive therapy as the larger, palpable cancers.

The heterogeneity of benign and malignant breast diseases has necessitated the development of supplementary imaging methods for their improved detection and differential diagnosis. The optimum preoperative diagnosis and mapping of the full disease extent has become an important prerequisite for adequate management of the disease. This volume deal with a wide range of new technical innovations for improving breast cancer detection, diagnosis and therapy. There is a special focus on improvements in mammographic image quality, image analysis, magnetic resonance imaging of the breast and molecular imaging. A chapter on targeted therapy explores the option of less radical postoperative therapy for women with early, screen-detected breast cancers.

Laszlo Tabar, M.D., F.A.C.R.
Department of Mammography
Falun Central Hospital
Falun,
Sweden

Part 1

New, Innovative Breast Imaging Modalities

1

Magnetic Resonance Imaging of the Breast

Marc Lobbes and Carla Boetes
Maastricht University Medical Center
The Netherlands

1. Introduction

Magnetic resonance imaging (MRI) of the breast was first performed in the late 1980s. At first, differentiation between benign and malignant breast lesions was primarily based on their differences in T1 and T2 relaxations times (Rausch et al., 2006). Due to the large overlap in T1 and T2 relaxation times in benign and malignant breast lesions, it became apparent that contrast administration was mandatory for reliable breast MRI. Heywang et al. demonstrated that breast carcinomas showed significant enhancement within 5 minutes after contrast administration (Heywang et al., 1989).

Since then, increasing field strengths, dedicated breast coil designs, and improvements in sequence protocols have led to a large improvement in diagnostic accuracy of breast MRI. Currently, the sensitivity of contrast-enhanced MRI for detecting breast cancer reaches 88%, with a specificity of 68%. The positive predictive value is reported to be 72%, with a negative predictive value of 85% (Bluemke et al., 2004). The reported sensitivity and specificity may vary in different publications due to differences in study populations, and technical and diagnostic criteria used. Reported sensitivities therefore vary from 83-100%, with reported specificities varying from 29-100% (Rausch et al., 2006).

These numbers are superior to mammography and ultrasound, and are independent of factors such as tumor histology, breast density, and hormonal therapy use. They also show that breast MRI is highly accurate for detecting breast cancer. However, due to the rather limited specificity, false-positive results are frequently observed, requiring additional imaging or (MR guided) biopsy, in turn causing patient anxiety and discomfort.

In this chapter, the technical aspects and proper indications of breast MRI are discussed. In addition, a systematic approach to the image interpretation of breast MRI is proposed.

2. Performing magnetic resonance imaging of the breast

2.1 Patient handling

Before performing breast MRI, it is important to instruct the patient thoroughly. It is important to inform the patient that lying comfortly and motionless is important for succesfull imaging of the breast. They should be instructed that administration of the contrast agent can result in various physical sensations, which may cause patient anxiety (and motion) when not properly instructed.

A dedicated breast coil should be used for breast MRI. These coils usually consist of a multichannel coil (nowadays up to 32-channel) with two loops in which the breasts are placed while the patient is lying in prone position. The breasts should be placed as deep as possible in the coil loops, with the nipples pointing downward if possible. To further reduce motion artefacts, the breasts can be gently fixated using cushions. Excessive compression should be avoided, as this might influence breast perfusion, and thus contrast enhancement pharmacokinetics.

In premenopausal women, the enhancement of the fibroglandular tissue after contrast administration is dependent of the menstrual cycle. MR imaging of the breast in the wrong phase of the menstrual cycle can result in strong glandular enhancement, complicating the interpretation of the images. Elective breast MRI is ideally performed in the first phase of the menstrual cycle, i.e. days 3-14, with day 1 being the first day of menstruation (Delille et al., 2005). In patients with proven breast cancer who undergo breast MRI as part of their preoperative staging, MRI should be performed at the earliest opportunity. In these cases, rapid presurgical patient work-up is preferred over optimal MR image quality.

2.2 Technical aspects

2.2.1 Field strengths

Increasing field strengths are associated with increased signal-to-noise (SNR) ratios. In order to acquire sufficient spatial resolution for accurate assessment of lesion morphology, it is generally accepted that field strengths of more than 1.5 Tesla are recommended for breast MRI (Weinstein et al., 2010). Theoretically, a higher field strength (e.g. 3 Tesla) increases the SNR for breast MRI. At a similar temporal resolution, this increased SNR might be used to increase spatial resolution, and thus improve lesion morphology evaluation and diagnostic accuracy.

In a proof-of-concept study, Kuhl et al. compared the accuracy of both 1.5 and 3.0 Tesla breast MRI in the same patients. Although the study population was small (n=37, total of 53 breast lesions, both malignant and benign), they demonstrated that the overall image quality scores for the dynamic contrast-enhanced series were higher ($p<0.01$). They also demonstrated that at 3.0 Tesla, the differential diagnosis of enhancing lesions was possible with a higher diagnostic confidence, as reflected by a larger area under the ROC-curve (Kuhl et al., 2006).

In another proof-of-concept study by Pinker et al., contrast-enhanced breast MRI was performed on a 3 Tesla MRI scanner in 34 patients (having 55 breast lesions). Their imaging protocol enabled accurate detection and assessment of breast lesions, with a sensitivity of 100% (95% confidence interval 90.6-100.0%. The specificity was 72.2%, with a 95% confidence interval of 49.1-87.5% (Pinker et al., 2009). Although these preliminary results are promising, there is no strong evidence to date of the superiority of 3.0 over 1.5 Tesla breast MR imaging.

2.2.2 Imaging planes

In the past, breast MR imaging was usually performed in a sagittal plane. The advantage of this imaging plane was that a relatively small field-of-view could be selected to cover the breast, resulting in an improved spatial resolution. However, simultaneous contralateral breast cancer can be detected in 3% of the cases (Lehman et al., 2007), indicating that bilateral breast imaging is strongly recommended. Bilateral sagittal imaging of the breast can lead to decrease of SNR and spatial resolution (Kuhl, 2007). Therefore, current bilateral imaging protocols use the transverse or coronal plane. Coronal imaging of the breast tends to give more respiratory motion artifacts. Also, nipple and chest wall involvement is more difficult to detect on coronal images. Therefore, the transverse imaging plane is preferred when bilateral breast imaging is performed (Kuhl, 2007).

2.2.3 Spatial and temporal resolution

Breast MRI needs to be performed with adequate spatial resolution in order to assess lesion morphology accurately. It is widely adopted that an optimal breast MRI should have a minimum size threshold for detection of lesions of 5 mm. Therefore, a voxel size of at least 2.5 mm in any direction should be used (Mann et al., 2008). However, higher in-plane spatial resolution results in more accurate lesion morphology assessment. Therefore, the minimal in-plane spatial resolution as recommended by the American College of Radiology is ≤ 1 mm (Weinstein et al., 2010).

2.2.4 Temporal resolution and contrast-enhanced dynamic T1 weighted imaging sequences

Gadolinium (Gd, atom number 64) is a chemical that belongs to the element category of the lanthanides. Due to it's paramagnetic properties, it is often used as an intravenous contrast agent in MRI. However, free Gd-atoms are highly toxic and as a result, gadolinium-based contrast agents consist of a chelated Gd-complex to render it non-toxic. Gd-based contrast agents lower T1, T2, and T2* relaxation times. Since the decrease is highest for T1 relaxation times, contrast-enhanced MR imaging sequences are mostly T1-weighted.

The contrast agent is administered intravenously with an automated injector to ensure a continuous inflow of contrast. Although the optimal dose is unknown, a dose of 0.1-0.2 mmol per kilogram of body weight and a flow rate of 3 mL/second is generally accepted (Kuhl, 2007, Rausch et al., 2006). The administration is followed by a saline flush to ensure complete administration of the dose.

After intravenous administration, the contrast agent leaks through immature ('leaky') microvessels that were formed by tumor angiogenesis (Carmeliet et al., 2000, Hashizume et al., 2000, Jansen et al., 2009). As a result, breast lesions tend to demonstrate a peak enhancement between 90-120 seconds. In order to assess the pharmacokinetic enhancement curves (see paragraph 4 on 'Image interpretation'), a minimum of three different time points should be included: first, a non enhanced scan; second, a scan which captures the peak enhancement of the lesion, and third, a scan with shows the delayed enhancement characteristics of the lesion. In order to capture the peak enhancement of the lesion, temporal resolution of the acquisitions performed should be in the order of 60-120 seconds, but they should not compromise the in-plane spatial resolution (which must be used for lesion morphology). In order to acquire a reliable measurement of the delayed enhancement characteristics, it is recommended to continue imaging until approximately 8 minutes after contrast administration (Weinstein et al., 2010).

2.2.5 T2-weighted imaging sequences

This sequence is often used as 'problem solver' sequence, since it provides additional relevant information on different breast lesions, narrowing down the differential diagnostic considerations.

For example, breast cysts (when inflammed) can show rim enhancement after administration of contrast agent. In these cases, signal intensity of the cyst is often slightly increased on the non-enhanced T1-weighted image due to the proteinacious content of the cyst. Due to the high water content and, consequently, the longer T2 relaxation times, cysts show a very high signal intensity on T2-weighted images, and can thus be distinguished (in combination with their sharp margins) from malignant breast lesions (Figure 1).

In 1999, Kuhl et al. demonstrated the additional value of T2-weighted imaging in breast MRI by examining 205 benign and malignant tumors. By means of visual assessment of the lesion appearance on T2-weighted fast spin echo images, they were able to distinguish between fibroadenomas and breast cancers, with a respective (age-dependent) sensitivity, specificity, positive predictive value, and negative predictive value for patients over 50 years of age of 89%, 62%, 85%, and 68% (Kuhl et al., 1999a).

In another recent study, Baltzer et al. evaluated 316 patients, of which 65 showed nonmass like enhancement on breast MRI. BI-RADS predictors could not discriminate between benign and malignant lesions with respect to nonmass like enhancement. However, the signal intensity of T2-weighted images and the presence of cysts improved the diagnostic accuracy, with a sensitivity of 91% and a specificity of 65% (Baltzer et al., 2011).

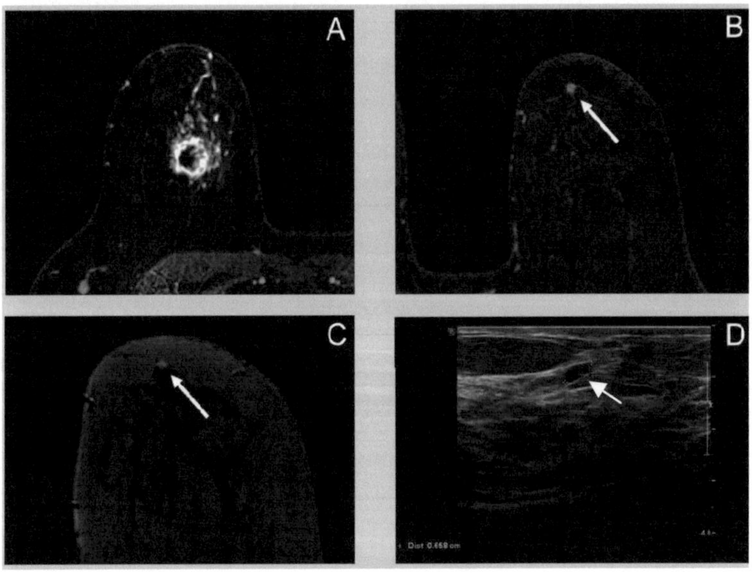

Fig. 1. Example of the added value of T2-weighted breast imaging. (A) shows the primary metaplastic tumor in the right breast. At MRI, a suspicious lesion was observed in the contralateral breast (B), with a corresponding high signal intensity on T2-weighted imaging (C). Second look ultrasound demonstrated a small simple cyst at this site, which was subsequently aspirated (D).

However, both benign and malignant breast lesions may show increased signal intensity on T2-weighted images. In a review of the histopathologic findings in such a group of lesions, Santamaria et al. stated that MR signal hyperintensity is most likely to be associated with the following conditions: extensive necrosis, (micro)cysts, fatty or sebaceous components, mucinous stroma, loose myxoid stroma, edema or hemorrhage (Santamaria et al., 2010). But also other benign entities, such as myxoid fibroadenomas, oil cysts, and intramammary lymph nodes are known to show an increased signal intensity on these sequences (Kuhl, 2007). In addition, some malignant lesions might also demonstrate an increased signal intensity on T2-weighted images, especially mucinous carcinomas due to their mucinous content (Santamaria et al., 2010).

3. Indications for breast MRI

Breast MRI can be used for a variety of diagnostic problems. Proper indications for performing breast MRI (as supported by the European Society of Breast Cancer Specialists and the European Society of Breast Imaging) are: inconclusive findings in conventional imaging, preoperative staging, unknown primary cancer, evaluation of therapy response in neoadjuvant chemotherapy, imaging of the breast after conservative therapy, screening of the high risk patient, breast implant imaging, and MR-guided interventions, such as biopsy and lesion localization (Mann et al., 2008, Sardanelli et al., 2010, Yeh, 2010).

3.1 Inconclusive findings in conventional imaging

In a study by Berg et al., 177 malignant lesions in 121 breast were evaluated with mammography, ultrasound, and MRI. They showed that the sensitivity for detecting tumors decreased from 100% in fatty breasts, to only 45% in extremely dense breasts. The sensitivity of mammography was highest for invasive ductal carcinoma (89%), versus 55% for ductal carcinoma in situ, and only 34% for invasive lobular carcinoma. Ultrasound demonstrated a higher sensitivity for both invasive ductal (94%) and invasive lobular carcinoma (86%). Sensitivity for detecting ductal carcinoma in situ was worse for ultrasound (47%), presumably owing to the fine microcalcifications associated with ductal carcinoma in situ, which are much better visualized on mammography. However, MRI was superior to all other modalities and for all tumor types: it detected 95% of the cases of invasive ductal carcinoma, 96% of the cases of invasive lobular carcinoma, and 89% of the cases of ductal carcinoma in situ (Berg et al., 2004). Due to this superior ability to detect breast cancer, MRI can be used as a problem-solving modality, when inconclusive findings in conventional imaging are encountered. For example, patients can be reffered from the mammography screening programm with abnormalities owing to a presumable superposition of fibroglandular tissue. These patients can undergo a single breast MRI to exclude possible underlying malignancies. Also, if there are discrepancies between clinical examination, mammography, and/or ultrasound, MRI can serve as a powerful problem-solving entity.

This was demonstrated by Moy et al., who retrospectively reviewed all MRI examinations (n=115) of the breast that were performed for inconclusive findings at mammography. They found no suspicious correlate on MRI in 87% of the cases. In the remaining 15 cases (13%), 6 malignancies were found. However, 18 incidental lesions were also observed on these examinations (Moy et al., 2009). Similar results were observed by Yau et al., who reviewed

3001 MRI exams and found 204 MRI exams that were performed for 'problem solving'. Of these 204 exams, 42 were graded as BI-RADS category 4 or 5 (see also paragraph 4.4). Malignant lesions were found in 14 cases, whereas benign findings or follow-up imaging encompassed the remaining 28 cases. 162 exams were graded as BI-RADS category 0, 1, 2, or 3. In this group, biopsy was performed in 28 cases, revealing 1 malignant lesions. In the remaining 134 cases, no biopsy was performed within the following 12 months (Yau et al., 2011). Both studies concluded that MRI is a valuable tool for evaluation of inconclusive mammography findings, but patient selection criteria should be strict because of the high incidence of incidental lesions seen on MRI.

3.2 Preoperative staging

The assessment of tumor size and additional tumor foci is essential for establishing the proper surgical and post-surgical treatment of each individual patient.

Recently, Uetmatsu et al. compared the ability to assess breast cancer extension for mammography, ultrasound, breast MRI, and even multidetector row computed tomography (MDCT). In this study of 210 breast tumors, they showed that the accuracy for establish the tumor extent (compared to histopathological results) was highest for breast MRI: 76%. The accuracy of establishing the tumor extent was lower for the other modalities: MDCT 71%, ultrasound 56%, and mammography 52%. However, they showed that MRI and ultrasound had a substantial risk of overestimating the tumor size. With respect to ductal carcinoma in situ extent, their study showed that the accuracy of breast MRI was also highest: 89% (followed by MDCT (72%), ultrasound (61%), and mammography (22%)). They concluded that breast MRI had the highest accuracy for assessing the true breast cancer extent, but emphasize that there is a risk of overestimation, which should be considered in pre-surgical planning (Uematsu et al. 2008). In line with these results, the superiority of assessing the proper breast tumor extension was also demonstrated by several other studies (Mann et al., 2008, 2008b).

Also, MRI can be helpful for detecting additional tumor foci (Figure 2). In a study of 969 patients by Lehman et al., simultaneous contralateral breast cancer was detected by breast MRI in 3% of the cases (Lehman et al., 2007).

Tumor multifocality or multicentricity can also be accurately assessed by MRI (Figure 3). For instance, this was demonstrated by Drew et al. in their study of 334 women, with 178 confirmed cancer cases. With preoperative breast MRI, multifocal or multicentric breast cancers was suggested in 38% of the cases. In this particular group, histology eventually demonstrated multifocality or multicentricity in 74% of the cases. Unifocal breast cancer was found in 22% of the cases, benign breast disease in 4%. Their observations resulted in a sensitivity of breast MRI for detecting multifocal/multicentric cancer of 100%, with corresponding specificity, positive predictive value, and negative predictive value of 86%, 73%, and 100%, respectively (Drew et al., 1999).

Although these results seem promising, the effectiveness of performing pre-operative breast MRI was not evaluated until recently. In 2010, the COMICE trial, by Turnbull et al., randomly assigned a total of 1623 patients to undergo either pre-operative breast MRI (n=816) or no breast MRI (n=807). They demonstrated that next to the conventional triple

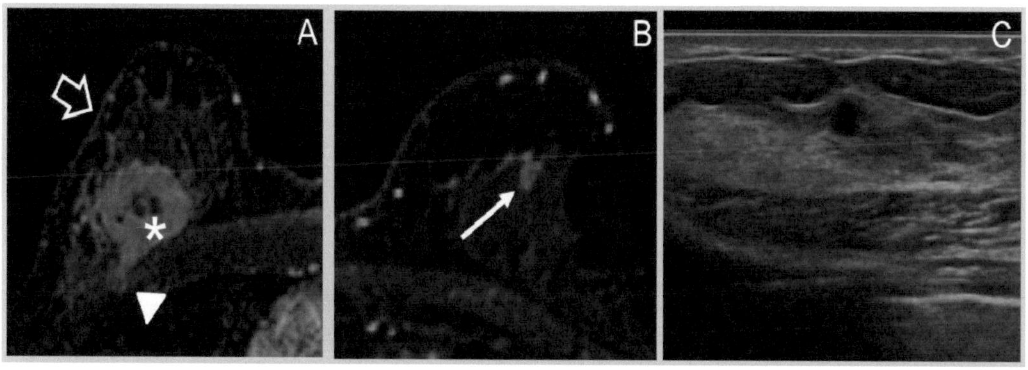

Fig. 2. Detection of contralateral breast cancer by breast MRI. (A) shows the primary index tumor in the right breast, presenting as an irregular mass with rim enhancement. The tumor shows a surrounding area of nonmass-like enhancement, with skin enhancement (open arrow) and pectoral muscle ingrowth (arrow head). (B) shows an additional small enhancing mass in the left breast (arrow), which corresponded with a small hypoechoic mass on second look targeted ultrasound (C). Histologic biopsy of this small mass revealed invasive ductal carcinoma, similar to the primary mass in the right breast.

assessment performed in breast cancer, addition of a pre-operative breast MRI did not result in a significantly reduced re-operation rate (odds ratio 0.96, 95% confidence interval 0.75-1.24, p=0.77, Turnbull et al., 2010).

In another (randomized controlled) trial of 418 patients (the MONET trial), Peters et al. allocated 207 patients to preoperative stageing with MRI, and 21 patients to the control group (no preoperative MRI). They found that the number of re-excisions performed because of positive resection margins after primary breast conserving therapy was increased in the MRI group: 34% in the MRI group versus 12% in the control group (p=0.008). The number of conversions to mastectomy were similar (Peters et al., 2011).

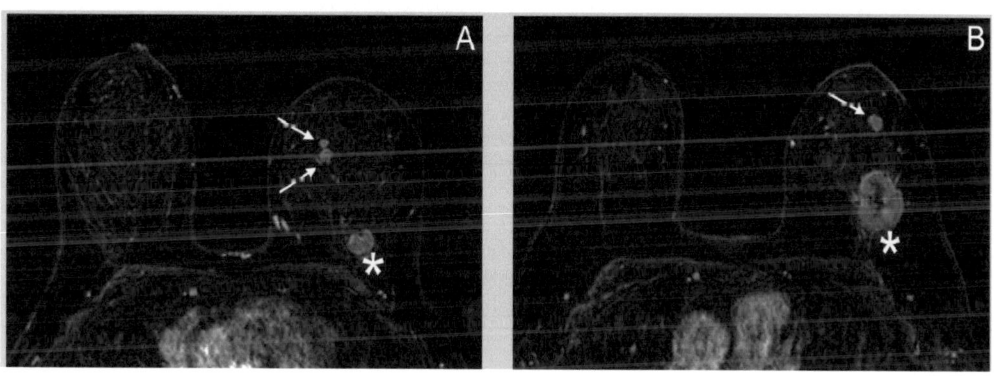

Fig. 3. Detection of tumor multifocality and/or multicentricity by breast MRI. (A) shows the index tumor in the lateral side of the left breast (*), with additional tumor deposits in the medial part of the breast (arrows), resulting in a multifocal, multicentric malignancy. (B) shows the index tumor in the lateral side of the left breast (*), with an additional tumor deposit in the same quadrant (arrow), resulting in a multifocal malignancy. Both cancers proved to be invasive ductal carcinomas at biopsy.

However, both studies have some limitations. For example, the COMICE trial recruited patients from 45 centres, resulting in a large variation of radiologic experience when evaluating the breast MRI exams. The MONET trial only evaluated non-palpable breast tumors and a subanalysis of their results showed that the volume of the lumpectomy specimen was significantly larger in the control group than in the group which was assigned to preoperative breast MRI.

3.3 Unknown primary cancer

This indication refers to the group of patients who are diagnosed with metastases, but in who a primary tumor cannot be identified. Schorn et al. demonstrated that MRI was helpful in patients with an unknown primary cancer and a negative mammography and ultrasound of the breasts. Breast cancer was detected by MRI in almost 50% of the cases. However, it should be mentioned that this study only consisted of 14 patients (Schorn et al. 1999). When looking only at axillary lymph node metastasis, Orel et al. demonstrated in a study of 38 patients that breast MRI could detect the previously unknow breast cancer in even 86% of the cases (Orel et al. 1999). Therefore, in patients diagnosed with metastasis and negative mammography and ultrasound, breast MRI should be strongly considered.

3.4 Evaluation of therapy respons in neoadjuvant chemotherapy

In a study by Yeh et al., 31 women who underwent neoadjuvant therapy for palpable breast cancer were included. Agreements with the therapy respons rate as measured by clinical examination, mammography, ultrasound, and breast MRI (as compared with pathology results) were 19%, 26%, 35%, and 71%, respectively. Of these four modalities, MRI agreed with the pathology results significantly more often: $p<0.002$ for all three comparisons with MRI (Yeh et al., 2005).

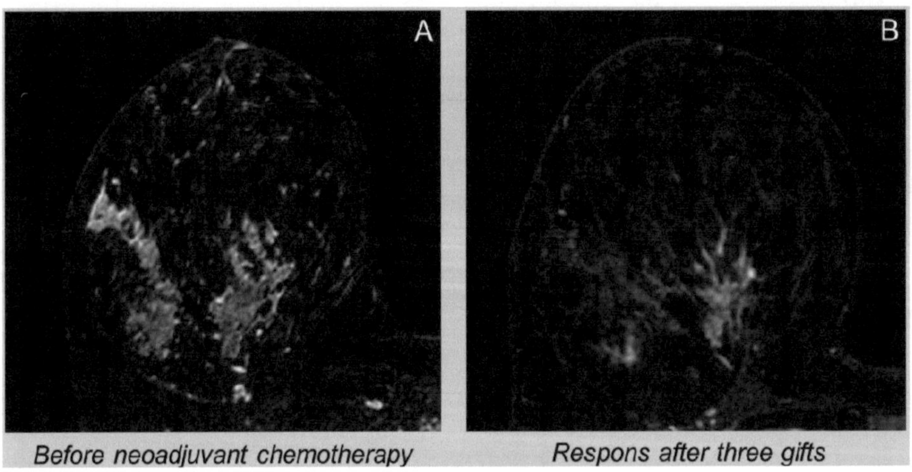

Fig. 4. Evaluation of tumor respons after neoadjuvant chemotherapy. (A) shows the initial (large) tumor (invasive lobular carcinoma at biopsy) in the right breast, presenting as a large area of regional nonmass like enhancement. (B) shows significant reduction in tumor size and enhancing volume after three gifts of chemotherapy. Thus, adequate chemotherapy respons was proven and continued in this patient.

In another study, Shin et al. prospectively included 43 patients with locally advanced or inflammatory breast cancer who underwent neoadjuvant therapy. The assessment of therapy respons was evaluated for clinical examination, mammography, ultrasound, and breast MRI. The intraclass correlation coefficients between predicted tumor size (as assessed by the different modalities) and the pathologically determined tumor size were calculated. The values were highest for breast MRI (0.97), followed by ultrasound (0.78), mammography (0.69), and clinical examination (0.65). Agreement between the prediction of final therapy respons and the respons assessed by pathology were expressed as the Kappa-value and were highest for MRI (0.82), followed by ultrasound (0.50), mammography (0.44), and clinical examination (0.43, Shin et al., 2010).

These results show that breast MRI is the most suitable imaging modality to assess chemotherapy respons (Figure 4). In addition, it is significantly more accurate in assessing the respons than non-imaging techniques, such as clinical examination.

3.5 Imaging of the breast after conservative therapy

There are three important reasons to perform breast MRI after breast conserving therapy: 1) an evaluation tool for detecting residual disease after positive tumor margins, 2) evaluation when recurrence is suspected, and 3) screening for patients that underwent breast conservative therapy in the past (Mann et al., 2008).

Due to the strong enhancement of the breast tissue immediately after surgery (which can last for more than a year), the interpretation of breast MR images for residual disease is hampered (Orel et al., 1997). Lee et al. concluded that the evaluation of MRI for residual disease in patients with close or positive margins is limited due to overlap in the appearances of benign and malignant lesions (Lee et al., 2004). Image interpretation can also be hampered by post-radiation enhancement of the breast, which is known to occur up to three months after the last irradiation of the breast. Nonetheless, Morakkabati et al. demonstrated that the detection and characterization of breast lesions can be performed with comparible diagnostic accuracies in irradiated breasts (when compared with non-irradiated breasts, Morakkabati et al., 2003).

Finally, the risk of local recurrence is dependent on the age of the patient at the time of the diagnosis (Mann et al., 2008). Even with additional booster radiation therapy, these patients still have a life-time risk of developing breast cancer of probably more than 20%, which is equal to the life time risk for breast MRI screening for the high risk patient, as discussed in paragraph 3.6. Therefore, annual MRI screening can be considered for patients that underwent breast conservative surgery for primary breast cancer, but large trials are needed to confirm this assumption.

3.6 Screening of the high risk patient

The first non-randomised studies to determine the additional value of breast MRI to conventional mammography in women who were BRCA1 or -2 gene mutation carriers, or who had a lifetime risk of at least 20-25% for developing breast cancer were published in the 1990s. Based on these studies initiated in the Netherlands, the United Kingdom, the United States, Canada, Italy, and Germany, the American Cancer Society (ACS) and European Society of Breast Imaging (EUSOBI) recommended annual MR evaluation of the breasts for all women with a lifetime risk for breast cancer of more than 20-25% (Saslow et al., 2007, Mann et al., 2008). These women include known BRCA gene mutation carriers, first-degree untested relatives of a BRCA gene mutation carrier, women with radiation to the chest wall between ages 10 and 30 years, Li-Fraumeni syndrome and first degree relatives, and Cowden syndrome with first degree relatives (Boetes, 2010).

3.7 Breast implant imaging

Past publications have shown that breast MRI can be an excellent modality to assess breast implant integrity. The sensitivity of MRI for detecting implant rupture can be as high as 80 to 90%, with a specificity of over 90% (Brown et al., 2000, Cher et al., 2001, Hölmich et al., 2005). However, specific sequences have to be used to optimize the visualisation of silicone and to provide concurrent suppression of water signal. Depending on the reason the study was requested, these prothesis-specific sequences can replace, or can be added to the previously discussed dynamic, contrast-enhanced breast MR imaging protocol. It is the authors' opinion, however, that a more eloborate description on the technical aspects and interpretation of images in breast implant imaging is beyond the scope of this chapter. An instructive pictorial essay on breast implant rupture was recently published by Colombo et al. (Colombo et al., 2011).

3.8 MR guided interventions

Despite the high sensitivity of breast MRI, it's specificity is relatively low. In practice, this leads to many false-positive findings, which require additional tissue sampling to exclude malignancy. In 2009, an interdisciplinary European committee established a consensus on the uses and technique of MR-guided vacuum-assisted breast biopsies (Heywang-Köbrunner et al., 2009). Although an elaborate discussion on the indications and techniques of MR guided breast interventions is beyond the scope of this chapter, the authors wish to emphasize some essential recommendations of this consensus meeting

Before performing any kind of MR guided breast intervention, a full imaging work-up should be completed. It must be absolutely certain that the culprit lesion can only be visualized by breast MRI. Patients should not have any kind of contra-indication for MRI or contrast administration. Relative contra-indications are lesions close to the chest wall who are estimated to be unfeasible or unsafe, patients with coagulation disorders, and patients with breast implants. When these criteria are met, MR guided biopsy of a breast lesion should be performed using a vacuum-assisted breast biopsy system (core needle biopsies are not recommended). Minimum probe size should be 11 Gauge, and the average number of cores taken should be 24 or more (or an equivalent volume if a larger probe is used). The intervention does not stop with acquiring the samples: proper correlation between histopathologic results and MR findings should be performed, preferably in a multidisciplinary setting. If the correlation is uncertain, re-biopsy or short-term follow-up should be considered (Heywang-Köbrunner et al., 2009).

4. Image interpretation

According to the Breast Imaging Reporting and Data System (BI-RADS), the interpretation of breast MR images should start with the analysis of the type of enhancement observed.

Three categories of enhancement can be observed: focal, mass-, and nonmass-like enhancement (Figure 5, Molleran et al., 2010).

Subsequently, shapes and margins of the lesions should be assessed in the case of masslike enhancement. In the case of nonmass-like enhancement, it should be assessed whether this enhancement pattern is linear, ductal, regional, or segmental. In addition, the reader should assess if the nonmass-like enhancement is clumped, in other words beaded or cobblestonelike.

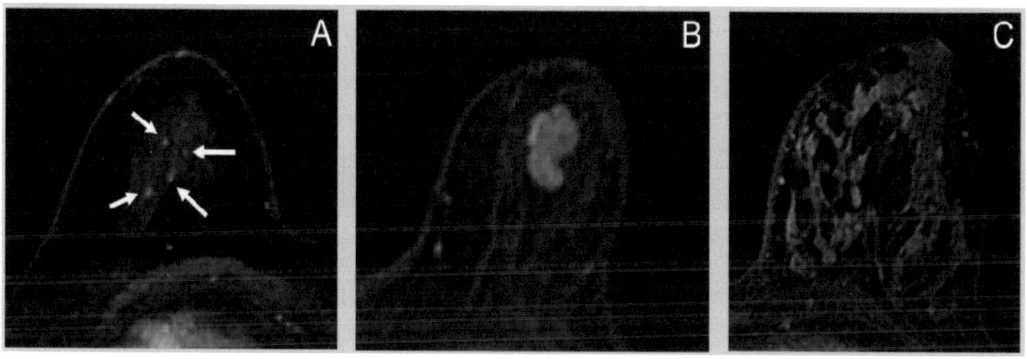

Fig. 5. Examples of focus (A), mass (B), and segmental (clumped) nonmass-like enhancement (C).

Finally, the enhancement characteristics of the lesion should be assessed by looking at both the internal enhancement characteristics and the signal intensity time curves. Internal enhancement characteristics can be described as homogeneous, heterogeneous, rim enhancement, or dark internal septations (American College of Radiology, 2003). Lesions can demonstrate slow, intermediate, or rapid contrast enhancement in the initial enhancement phase. In general, this initial enhancement phase can be followed by three different types of enhancement curves in the delayed phase: persistent enhancement, plateau phase, or wash-out. The enhancement characteristics of lesions can be indicative for their benign or malignant character.

By combining the findings of these different analyses, the radiologist estimates the likelihood of a lesion being benign or malignant. This estimation can be expressed in the final conclusion of the report as the BI-RADS classification, and should be the basis for management recommendations (i.e. biopsy or follow-up).

4.1 Focal, mass-, and nonmass-like enhancement

Focal enhancement can be described as small (less than 5 mm) area of enhancement that cannot be specified otherwise. A mass is a lesion that is visible in three dimensions and which occupies a space. Masses can be round, oval, lobulated, or irregular, and may have smooth, irregular, or spiculated margins. Nonmass-like enhancement is an area of enhancement that does not belong to a three dimensional mass or that has no distinct mass characteristics (American College of Radiology, 2003, Erguvan-Dogan et al., 2006). Nonmass-like enhancement patterns can be divided in linear, ductal, segmental, and regional enhancement (Figures 5 and 6).

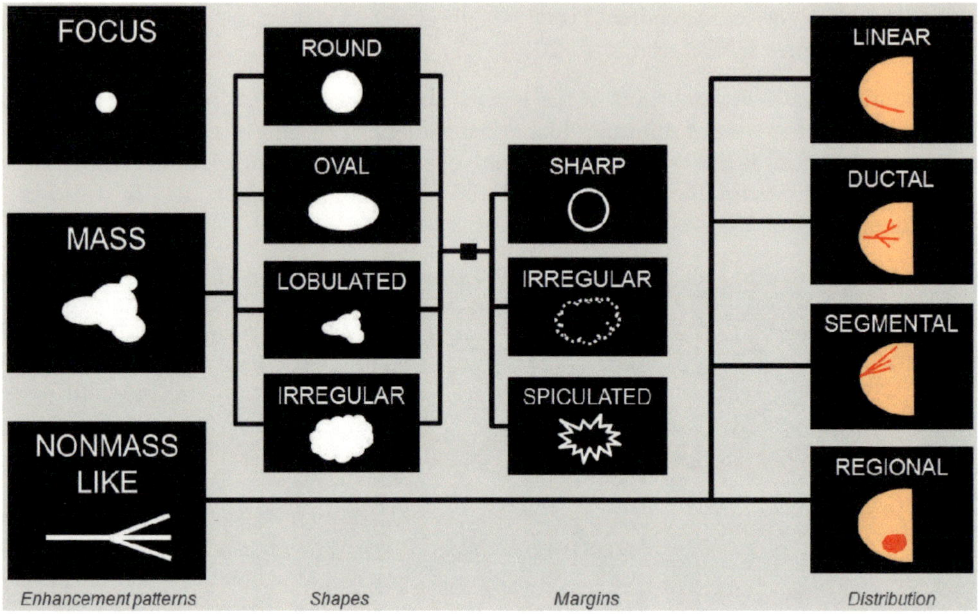

Fig. 6. Proper terminology (according to the BI-RADS lexicon) for enhancement patterns, shapes, margins, and nonmass-like enhancement distributions.

Linear nonmass-like enhancement is defined according to the BI-RADS lexicon of the American College of Radiology as 'enhancement in a line that is not definitely in a duct'. Ductal enhancement can be defined as 'enhancement in a line that points towards the nipple, and may have branching, conforming to a duct'. Segmental enhancement can be defined as 'a triangular region or cone of enhancement, with the apex pointing towards the nipple'. Finally, regional enhancement can be defined as 'enhancement in a large volume of tissue not conforming to a ductal distribution' (American College of Radiology, 2003).

Jansen et al. recently investigated the pathology and kinetics of mass, nonmass, and focal enhancement in a retrospective study using dynamic contrast-enhanced breast MRI. They analyzed a total of 852 breast lesions (histologically proven) in 697 patients. Of the lesions demonstrating mass-like enhancement (n=552), 71.7% proved to be malignant. Of the lesions demonstrating nonmass-like enhancement (n=261), 81.2% proved to be malignant. The remaining lesions demonstrated focal enhancement (n=30), which were usually benign (76.9%). Malignant mass- and nonmass-like enhancing lesions differed significantly in their pathology ($p<0.0001$), with mass-like enhancing lesions usually consisting of invasive ductal carcinoma and nonmass-like enhancement usually consisting of ductal carcinoma in situ. Similarly, benign mass- and nonmass-like enhancing lesions differed significantly in their pathology ($p<0.002$), with the former usually consisting of fibroadenomas and the latter usually presenting fibrocystic changes. Finally, the predominant pathology of focal enhancing lesions was fibrocystic changes (Jansen et al., 2011).

4.2 Morphologic descriptors in masslike- and nonmass-like enhancement

Margins of masses can be described as smooth (or sharp), irregular, or spiculated. Similar to mammography, some morphologic features of a lesion are more associated with malignancy than others (Liberman et al., 1998). Past studies showed that spiculated margins, irregular shapes, and linear/ductal nonmass-like enhancement had the highest positive predictive values for malignancy (Nunes et al., 1997, 2001). However, these studies included patients with mammographic or palpable findings, creating a potential bias in the study population.

Therefore, Liberman et al. performed a retrospective review of 100 consecutive solitary MR imaging-detected lesions. For mass-like enhancement, margins and shape were evaluated. With respect to lesion margins, spiculated margins had the highest positive predictive value for malignancy (80%), much higher than irregular (22%) and smooth (17%) margins. With respect to lesion shapes, irregular shapes had the highest positive predictive value for malignancy (32%), lobular shapes had a positive predictive value for malignancy of only 13% (Liberman et al., 2002).

In the same study, the pattern of nonmass-like enhancement was evaluated. With respect to linear or ductal enhancement, clumped enhancement (or beadlike enhancement) had a positive predictive value for malignancy of 31%. Smooth linear enhancement was not observed in malignant lesions. Clumped regional enhancement had a positive predictive value of 67%, whereas clumped segmental enhancement had a positive predictive value of 67% too (Liberman et al., 2002).

In addition, Siegmann et al. looked at lesion size as a additional descriptor for the assessment of malignancy. They showed in a study of 51 lesions (in 45 patients) that lesions with a diameter of more than 10 mm have a higher positive predictive value (45.5%) than lesions smaller than 10 mm (27.6%, Siegmann et al., 2002).

To summarize, features that have the highest positive predictive value for malignancy are spiculated (ill-defined) margins and irregular shapes (based on morphology alone and in the case of masslike enhancement). For nonmass-like enhancement, features that have the highest positive predicitive value are clumped linear, segmental or regional enhancement. Lesions larger than 10 mm have a higher positive predictive value for being malignant than lesions $\leq$ 10 mm (Tse et al., 2007).

4.3 Kinetic analysis of the signal intensity time curves

Lesion enhancement is described as homogeneous, heterogeneous, rim enhancement, or enhancement with dark internal septations (American College of Radiology, 2003, Figure 7).

In a landmark paper by Kuhl et al., the value of signal intensity time curves was evaluated with respect to the differential diagnosis of enhancing breast lesions. A total of 266 breast lesions (101 malignant, 165 benign) were examined using a dynamic contrast-enhanced breast imaging protocol. The relative enhancement of breast lesions was assessed by drawing a region-of-interest in the lesion itself. The enhancement was then calculated according to the following formula:

$$\text{Relative signal enhancement (\%)} = (SI_{post} - SI_{pre}) / SI_{pre} \times 100$$

In this formula, SI_{pre} and SI_{post} represent pre-contrast and post-contrast signal intensities, respectively. By calculating the signal intensity time curves, it was demonstrated that enhancement patterns can be divided into two phases: early enhancement (from contrast administration to approximately two minutes post-contrast, or when the curve starts to change), followed by the delayed enhancement.

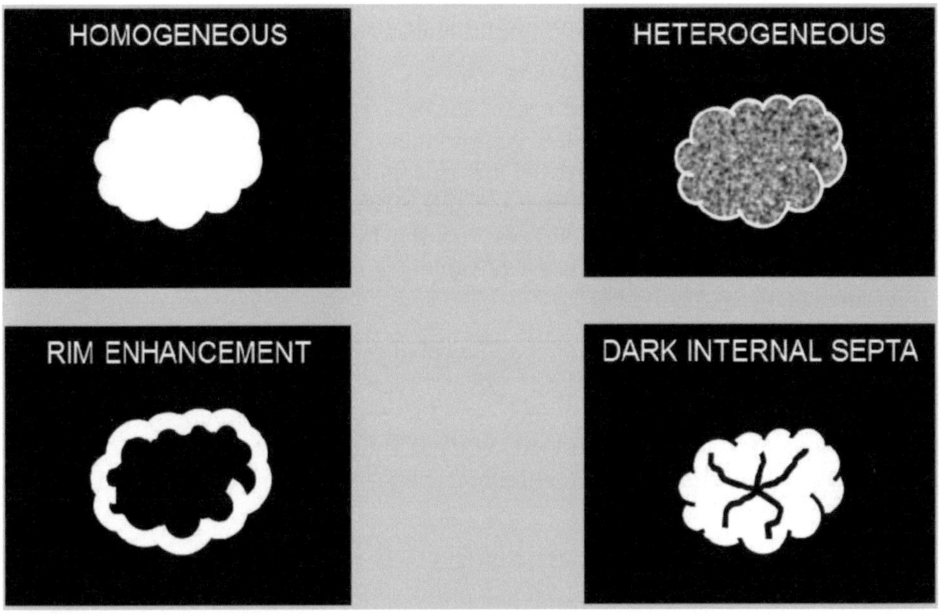

Fig. 7. Proper terminology (according to the BI-RADS lexicon for lesions enhancement patterns) homogeneous, heterogeneous, rim enhancement, and enhancement with dark internal septa.

For the early enhancement phase, it was assumed that benign lesions had a (slow) enhancement of 60% or less. Indeterminate lesions were assumed to have an (intermediate) enhancement of more than 60%, but less than 80%. Finally, malignant lesions were assumed to have a (strong) enhancement of more than 80%. For these assumptions, the diagnostic accuracies in this study were: sensitivity 91%, specificity 37%, positive predictive value 47%, negative predictive value 87%, diagnostic accuracy 58%. Mean peak enhancement was significantly higher for malignant lesions than for benign lesions: mean enhancement 104% versus 72%, $p<0.001$ (Kuhl et al., 1999b).

For the delayed phase, three different type of signal intensity curves were defined. A type I curve was characterized by a persistent increase in signal intensity over time. A type II curve was characterized by a plateau in signal intensity values over time. Finally, a type III curve was characterized by a so-called washout, i.e. the signal intensity decreases in time after the initial upslope in the early enhancement phase (Figure 8).

For benign lesions, a type I curve was observed in 83.0% of the cases. A type II curve was observed in 11.5% of the cases, whereas a type III curve was hardly seen in benign lesions: 5.5% of the cases. For malignant lesions, a type III curve was most frequently observed: 57.4% of the cases. A type II curve was observed in 33.6% of the cases, whereas a type I curve was infrequently seen in these cases: 8.9%. The assessment of the signal intensity time curves had an excellent interreader agreement with a Kappa-value of 0.849, $p<0.001$ (Kuhl et al., 1999b).

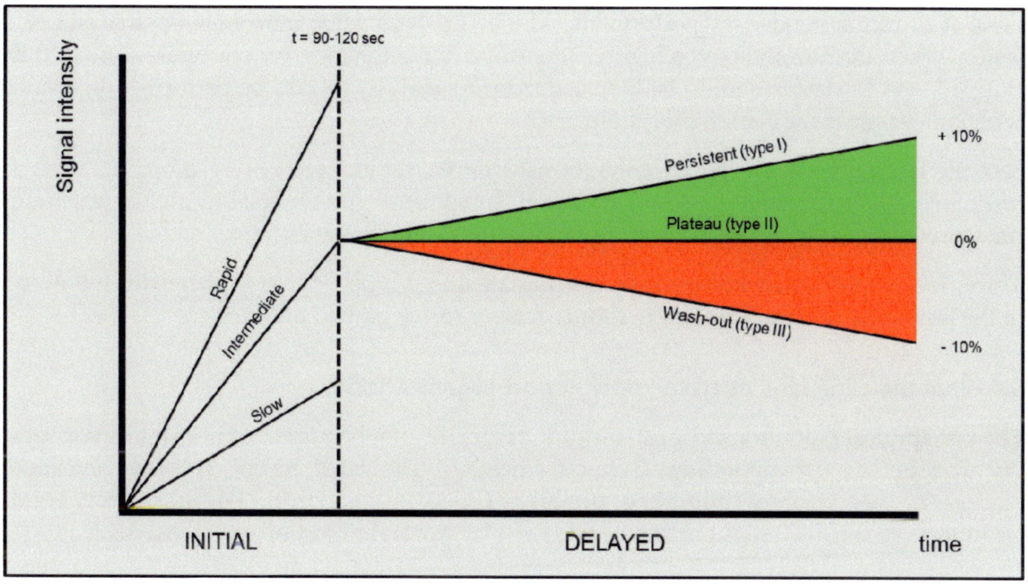

Fig. 8. Possible enhancement characteristics that can be observed in dynamic contrast-enhanced breast MRI.

In the past, Jansen et al. demonstrated that analysis of the signal intensity time curve can help distinguish between benign and malignant mass lesions effectively, but the analysis is not that useful in discriminating between benign and malignant nonmass-like lesions. Although their pilotstudy only consisted of a total of 108 breast lesions with 70 observed masses, 44 of which were malignant and 26 benign. There were 38 nonmass-like lesions observed, of which 31 were malignant and 7 benign. Despite these relatively small numbers, they showed that analysis of the signal intensity time curve was helpful in distinguishing between benign and malignant masses on MRI. However, it could not be used to accurately distinguish between benign and malignant nonmass-like lesions. Therefore, they suggested that analysis of the signal intensity time curves of nonmass-like enhancement is not very useful and that morphology analysis should be favored (Jansen et al., 2008).

In summary, it is advised by the BI-RADS MRI lexicon that the signal intensity curve of a lesion should be described qualitatively. A proper region-of-interest should at least contain 3 pixels and if this enhancement of the lesion is heterogeneous, the most suspicious enhancement curve should be mentioned in the final report. Initial enhancement can be slow, moderate, or rapid, while the delayed enhancement can show a persistent, plateau, or wash-out curve (American College of Radiology, 2003). A strong early enhancement is suggestive of malignancy, whereas a slow signal intensity increase is suggestive of a benign entity. More importantly, type I signal intensity curves are suggestive of benign breast lesions, whereas type III curves are suggestive of malignancy. The indeterminate type II curve scan be observed in both benign and malignant breast lesions, albeit slightly more suggestive of malignancy (in a ratio of 2:3, Kuhl et al., 1999b).

It should be emphasized that kinetic analysis of contrast enhancement is no substitute for morphology analysis. It should be used as an aid in further narrowing the differential diagnosis. With this respect, several recommendations can be made:

First, it is recommended to perform the kinetic analysis after morphologic analysis of a lesion. When the morphology is highly suggestive of malignancy, kinetic analysis should be skipped, and the lesion should be biopsied. Kinetic analysis should be performed in lesions with indeterminate or benign morphologies.

Second, lesions with a type III enhancement curve should always be biopsied, even if morphology is suggestive of a benign lesion. In contrast, the absence of a clear wash-out phase in the signal intensity time curve cannot rule out malignancy.

Third, when lesion morphology is indeterminate and a type I curve is observed, follow-up of the lesion might be considered to reduce false-positive biopsy findings.

4.4 What the clinicians need to know: report organization

The pre-surgical planning and post-surgical treatment is dependent not only on tumor type, but also on it's corresponding TNM-classification. The most recent TNM-classification, edition 7, was recently published in 2010. (Edge et al., 2010). For a proper TNM-classification, several issues need to be adressed in the final report of any breast MRI.

For a proper T-classification of breast cancer, the maximum diameter of the culprit mass should be mentioned in the report, including any suspicious nonmass-like enhancement that can be associated with an extensive intraductal component. In addition, the relationship of the tumor to the skin, pectoral muscle and thoracic wall must be accurately described. Enhancement of the pectoral muscle or skin is one of the most reliable signs for the assesment of tumor invasion in these structures. Although inflammatory breast cancer is clinical diagnosis, it can be suggested in MRI when strong enhancement of the breast is observed, together with diffuse skin thickening and enhancement.

Many authors have tried to developed accurate criteria for the assessment of axillary lymph node status on MRI. In a study of 65 patients, Kvistad et al. demonstrated a significant correlation between flow kinetics and axillary lymph node status (Kvistad et al., 2000). Murray et al. demonstrated a correlation between nodal enhancement and nodal area and axillary lymph node status in a study encompassing 47 patients (Murray et al., 2002). More recently, Mortellaro et al. stated in their study of 56 patients that the presence of any axillary lymph node without a fatty hilum and the number of nodes without a fatty hilum correlated significantly with axillary lymph node positivity for metastases (Mortellaro et al., 2009). In summary, study results on MRI of axillary lymph node status vary in study design, study population, and outcome. Until now, there are no reliable criteria for the evaluation of axillary lymph node positivity. However, it is the authors' opinion that analysis of the axillae is an important part of the total breast MRI evaluation. Patients with suspicious axillary lymph nodes on MRI should be considered for (re)evaluation with (second look) ultrasound.

With respect to a proper M-classification, it should be emphasized that other imaging modalities, such as (PET-)CT, need to be performed. However, extramammary findings on breast MRI should be noted and reported. In a retrospective review of 1535 breast MRI examinations, Rinaldi et al. observed 285 patients with extramammary (incidental) findings. Most incidental findings occured in the liver (51.9%). Other sites were lung (11.2%), bone (7%), and mediastinum (4.2%). Pleural or pericardial effusions were observed in 15.4% of the cases. Of all these incidental findings, 20.4% proved to be malignant (Rinaldi et al. 2011). Therefore, the occurence of extramammary findings is a non-negligible phenomenon.

Finally, the radiologst should construct a comprehensible report of all findings observed on breast MRI. By analyzing morphology, enhancement, and signal intensity time curves, the probability of malignancy should be estimated. The maximum diameter of suspicious lesions should be provided, together with their location within the breast and their relationship with the skin, pectoral muscle, or thoracic wall. Together with an assessment of the axillary lymph node morphology and incidental extra-mammary findings, the radiologist should finish the report with the appropriate BI-RADS classification and possible management recommendations (Americal College of Radiology, 2003):

BI-RADS 1:	Additional imaging is needed (i.e. failure of equipment, severe artefacts)
BI-RADS 1:	Normal, there is nothing to comment on
BI-RADS 2:	Benign findings
BI-RADS 3:	Probably benign findings; the probability of malignancy is less than 2%. Short-term follow-up is recommended
BI-RADS 4:	Suspicious findings; the probability of malignancy is 2-95%. Biopsy should be considered
BI-RADS 5:	Highly suggestive of malignancy; the probability of malignancy is higher than 95%. Appropriate action should be taken
BI-RADS 6:	Proven malignancy (through histopathologic results)

In conclusion, dynamic, contrast-enhanced breast MRI can be a powerful adjuvant imaging modality for the detection of breast cancer. It can be of help when inconclusive findings are encountered on conventional imaging or in the case of an unknown primary cancer. The evaluation of neoadjuvant chemotherapy respons can be evaluated with breast MRI, and it can aid in the assessment of the postoperative breast. Breast MRI is advised in screening certain populations with high risk of developing breast cancer, breast implants can be accurately analyzed with MRI, and it can aid in MR guided breast interventions. One of the most important indications of breast MRI is preoperative planning, and it's superiority compared to other breast imaging modalities to evaluate disease extent, multifocality or multicentricity, and the presence of (occult) contralateral malignancy. However, due to it's limited specificity, false-positive findings are frequently observed. Therefore, patient selection should be performed with care and the proper indications for breast MRI should be observed.

This chapter is dedicated to professor Carla Boetes (1949 2011).

5. References

American College of Radiology (2003). *Breast imaging reporting and data system (BI-RADS)* (4th edition). American College of Radiology, Reston, USA.

Baltzer et al. (2011). Nonmass lesions in magnetic resonance imaging of the breast: additional T2-weighted images improve diagnostic accuracy. *J Comput Assist Tomogr*. Vol. 35, No. 3, May/June 2011, pp. 361- 366.

Berg et al. (2004). Diagnostic accuracy of mammography, clinical examination, US, and MR imaging in preoperative assessment of breast cancer. *Radiology*. Vol. 233, No. 3, December 2004, pp. 830-849.

Bluemke et al. (2004). Magnetic resonance imaging of the breast prior to biopsy. *JAMA*. Vol. 292, No. 22, December 2004, pp. 2735-2742.

Boetes (2011). Update on screening breast MRI in high-risk women. Obstet Gynecol Clin N Am. Vol. 38, No. 1, March 2011, pp. 149-158.

Brown et al. (2000). Prevalence of rupture of silicone gel breast implants revealed on MR imaging in a populationof women in Birmingham, Alabama. *AJR Am J Roentgenol*. Vol. 175, No. 4, October 2000, pp. 1057-1064.

Carmeliet et al. (2000). Angiogenesis in cancer and other diseases. *Nature*. Vol. 407, No. 6801, September 2000, pp. 249-257.

Cher et al. (2001). MRI for detecting silicone breast implant rupture: meta-analysis and implications. *Ann Plast Surg*. Vol. 47, No. 4, October 2001, pp. 367-380.

Colombo et al. (2011). Prosthetic breast implant rupture: imaging-pictorial essay. Aesthetic Plast Surg. April 2011, Epub ahead of print.

Delille et al. (2005). Physiologic changes in breast magnetic resonance imaging during the menstrual cycle: perfusion imaging, signal enhancement, and influence of the T1 relaxation time of breast tissue. *Breast J*. Vol. 11, No. 4, July-August 2005, pp. 236-241.

Drew et al. (1999). Dynamic contrast enhanced magnetic resonance imaging of the breast is superior to triple assessment for the pre-operative detection of multifocal breast cancer. *Ann Surg Oncol*. Vol. 6, No. 6, September 1999, pp. 599-603.

Erguvan-Dogan et al. (2006). BI-RADS MRI: a primer. *AJR Am J Roentgenol*. Vol. 187, No. 2, August 2006, pp. W152-160.

Hashizume et al. (2000). Opening between defective endothelial cells explain tumour vessel leakiness. *Am J Path*. Vol. 156, No. 4, April 2000, pp. 1363-1380.

Heywang et al. (1989). MR imaging of the breast with Gd-DTPA: use and limitations. *Radiology*. Vol. 171, No. 1, April 1989, pp. 95-103.

Heywang-Köbrunner et al. (2009). Interdisciplinary consensus on the uses and technique of MR-guided vacuum-assisted biopsy (VAB): results of a European consensus meeting. *Eur J Radiol*. Vol. 72, No. 2, November 2009, pp. 289-294.

Hölmich et al. (2005). The diagnosis of breast implant rupture: MRI findings compared with findings at explantation. *Eur J Radiol*. Vol. 53, No. 2, February 2005, pp. 213-225.

Jansen et al. (2008). DCEMRI of breast lesions: is kinetic analysis equally effective for both mass and nonmass-like enhancement? *Med Phys*. Vol. 35, No. 7, July 2008, pp. 3102-3109.

Jansen et al. (2009). Ductal carcinoma in situ: X-ray fluorescence microscopy and dynamic contrast-enhanced MR imaging reveals gadoliniumm uptake within neoplastic mammary ducts in a murine model. *Radiology*. Vol. 253, No. 1, January 2009, pp. 399-406.

Jansen et al. (2011). The diverse pathology and kinetics of mass, nonmass, and focus enhancement on MR imaging of the breast. *J Magn Reson Imaging*. Vol. 33., No. 6, June 2011, pp. 1382-1389.

Kuhl et al. (1999). Do T2-weighted pulse sequences help with the differential diagnosis of enhancing lesions in dynamic breast MRI? *J Magn Reson Imaging*. Vol. 9, No. 2, February 1999, pp. 187-196.

Kuhl et al. (1999). Dynamic breast MR imaging: are signal intensity time course data useful for differential diagnosis of enhancing lesions? *Radiology*. Vol. 211, No. 1, April 1999, pp. 101-110.

Kuhl et al. (2006). Contrast-enhanced MR imaging of the breast at 3.0 and 1.5 Tesla in the same patients: initial experience. *Radiology*. Vol. 239, No. 3, June 2006, pp. 666-676.

Kuhl (2007). The current status of breast MR imaging, part 1: Choice of technique, image interpretation, diagnostic accuracy, and transfer to clinical practice. *Radiology*. Vol. 244, No. 2, August 2007, pp. 356-378.

Kvistad et al. (2000). Axillary lymph node metastases in breast cancer: preoperative detection with dynamic contrast-enhanced MRI. *Eur Radiol*. Vol. 10, No. 9, pp. 1464-1471.

Lee et al. (2004). MRI before reexcision surgery in patients with breast cancer. *AJR Am J Roentgenol*. Vol. 182, No. 2, February 2004, pp. 473-480.

Lehman et al. (2007). MRI evaluation of the contralateral breast in women with recently diagnosed breast cancer. *N Engl J Med*. Vol. 356, No. 13, March 2007, pp. 1295-1303.

Liberman et al. (1998). The Breast Imaging Reporting and Data System: positive predictive value of mammographic features and final assessment categories. *AJR Am J Roentgenol*. Vol. 171, No. 1, July 1998, pp. 35-40.

Liberman et al. (2002). Breast lesions detected on MR imaging: features and positive predictive value. *AJR Am J Roentgenol*. Vol. 179, No. 1, July 2002, pp. 171-178.

Mann et al. (2008). The value of MRI compared to mammography in the assessment of tumour extent in invasive lobular carcinoma of the breast. *Eur J Surg Oncol*. Vol. 34, No. 2, February 2008, pp. 135-142.

Mann et al. (2008). Breast MRI: guidelines from the European Society of Breast Imaging. *Eur Radiol*. Vol. 18, No. 7, July 2008, pp. 1307-1318.

Molleran et al. (2010). The BI-RADS breast magnetic resonance imaging lexicon. *Magn Reson Imaging Clin N Am*. Vol. 18, No. 2, May 2010, pp. 171-185.

Morakkabati et al. (2003). Breast MR imaging during or soon after radiation therapy. *Radiology*. Vol. 229, No. 3, December 2003, pp. 893-901.

Morris. (2010). Should we dispense with preoperative breast MRI? *Lancet*. Vol. 375, No. 9714, February 2010, pp. 528-530.

Mortellaro et al. (2009). Magnetic resonance imaging for axillary staging in patients with breast cancer. *J Magn Reson Imaging*. Vol. 30, No. 2, August 2009, pp. 309-312.

Murray et al. (2002) Dynamic contrast enhanced MRI of the axilla in women with breast cancer: comparison of pathology with excised nodes. *Br J Radiol* Vol. 75, No. 891, March 2002, pp. 220-228.

Nunes et al. (1997). Breast MR imaging: interpretation model. *Radiology*. Vol. 202, No. 3, March 1997, pp. 833-841.

Nunes et al. (2001). Update of breast MR imaging architectural interpretation model. *Radiology*. Vol. 219, No. 2, May 2001, pp. 484-494

Moy et al. (2009). Is breast MRI helpful in the evaluation of inconclusive mammography findings? *AJR Am J Roentgenol*. Vol. 193, No. 4, October 2009, pp. 986-993.

Orel et al. (1997). Breast carcinoma: MR imaging before re-excisional biopsy. *Radiology*. Vol. 205, No. 2, November 1997, pp. 429-436.

Orel et al. (1999). Breast MR imaging in patients with axillary lymph node metastases and unknown primary malignancy. *Radiology*. Vol. 212, No. 2, August 1999, pp. 543-549.

Peters et al. (2011). Preoperative MRI and surgical management in patients with non-palpable breast cancer: the MONET-randomised controlled trial. *Eur J Canc*. Vol. 47, No. 6, April 2011, pp. 879-886.

Pinker et al. (2009). A combined high temporal and high spatial resolution 3 Tesla imaging protocol for the assessment of breast lesions: initial experience. *Invest Radiol*. Vol. 44, No. 9, September 2009, pp. 553-558.

Raush et al. (2006). How to optimize clinical breast MR imaging practices and techniques on your 1.5-T system. *Radiographics*. Vol. 26, No. 5, September-October 2006, pp. 1469-1484.

Rinaldi et al. (2011). Extra-mammary findings in breast MRI. *Eur Radiol*. Epub ahead of print

Santamaria et al. (2010). Radiologic and pathologic findings in breast tumors with high signal intensity on T2-weighted MR images. *Radiographics*. Vol. 30, No. 2, March 2010, pp. 533-548.

Sardanelli et al. (2010). Magnetic resonance imaging of the breast: recommendations from the EUSOMA working group. *Eur J Canc*. Vol. 46, No. 8, May 2010, pp. 1296-1316.

Saslow et al. (2007). American Cancer Society guidelines for breast screening with MRI as an adjunct to mammography. *CA Cancer J Clin*. Vol. 57, No. 2, March-April 2007, pp. 75-89.

Schorn et al. (1999). MRI of the breast in patients with metastatic disease of unknown primary. *Eur Radiol*. Vol. 9, No. 3, pp. 470-473.

Schin et al. (2010). Comparison of mammography, sonography, MRI, and clinical examination in patients with locally advanced or inflammatory breast cancer who underwent neoadjuvant chemotherapy. *Br J Radiol*. Epub ahead of print

Siegmann et al. (2002). MR imaging-detected breast lesions: histopathologic correlation of lesions characteristics and signal intensity data. *AJR Am J Roentgenol*. Vol. 178, No. 6, June 2002, pp. 1403-1409.

Tse et al. (2007). Magnetic resonance imaging of breast lesions: a pathologic correlation. *Breast Cancer Res Treat*. Vol. 103, No. 1, May 2007, pp. 1-10.

Turnbull et al. (2010). Comparative effectiveness of MRI in breast cancer (COMICE) trial: a randomised controlled trial. *Lancet*. Vol. 375, No. 9714, pp. 563-571.

Uematsu et al. (2008). Comparison of magnetic resonance imaging, multidetector row computed tomography, ultrasonography, and mammography for tumour extension of breast cancer. *Breast Cancer Res Treat*. Vol. 112, No. 3, December 2008, pp. 461-474.

Weinstein et al. (2010). Breast MR imaging: current indications and advanced imaging techniques. *Radiol Clin N Am*. Vol. 48, No. 5, September 2010, pp. 1013-1042.

Yau et al. (2011). The utility of breast MRI as a problem-solving tool. *The Breast Journal*. Vol. 17, No. 3, March 2011, pp. 273-280.

Yeh et al. (2005). Prospective comparison of mammography, sonography, and MRI in patients undergoing neoadjuvant chemotherapy for palpable breast cancer. *AJR Am J Roentgenol*. Vol. 184, No. 3, March 2005, pp. 868-877.

Yeh. (2010). Breast magnetic resonance imaging: current clinical indications. *Magn Reson Imaging Clin N Am*. Vol. 18, No. 2, May 2010, pp. 155-169.

2

The Application of Breast MRI on Asian Women (Dense Breast Pattern)

Ting Kai Leung
Taipei Medical University & Hospital, Taipei, Taiwan

1. Introduction

1.1 Increase incidence of breast cancer in Taiwan and Asia

Although the incidence of breast cancer is lower in Asian countries, the cause-specific mortality in most Asian countries is much higher as compared to western countries (Agarwal et al., 2007; Shibuya et al., 2002). Although the overall picture of breast cancer is variable among different Asian countries and in different ethnic groups within individual countries, breast cancer has emerged as the largest cancer problem in Asian women. Breast cancer is also the largest cause of cancer-related deaths. It remains the second commonest malignancy in women in the rural areas of developing Asian countries (Agarwal et al., 2007). Breast cancer is gradually become one of the major public health problem and the most important issue to concern in order to decrease cancer mortality.

Base on the data from the Bureau of Health Promotion, Department of Health, Executive Yuan, Taiwan, indicate that the incidence of breast cancer in Taiwan increased from 27.9 to 49.2 per 100,000 women in the decade from 1995 to 2005, which is an annual increase of approximately 7%. As the decrease incidence of cervical cancer in the meanwhile, breast cancer is already the highest new number of malignancy diagnosis in Taiwan. Moreover, according to the data released from the World Health Organization, an incidence of Taiwanese breast cancer is reported as 52.8 per 100,000 women in 2008, which is the second place in Asia, only slightly lower than that seen in Singapore.

2. Characteristics and difficulty of early detection of breast tumor in Asian women

There are higher proportions of breast cancer patients in developing Asian countries are younger than patients in developed Asian and western countries (Agarwal et al., 2007; Amr et al., 1995). Given the huge population in the developing Asian nations, and the fact that up to 25% of all breast cancer patients in Asian countries are young, and also, young age by itself is a known indicator of poor prognosis in breast cancer patients (Agarwal et al., 2007; Amr et al., 1995). The first nation-wide mammographic screening program in Asia was started in Singapore during 2002 (Chuwa et al., 2009). By 2009, there is still no significant survival benefit could be demonstrated in the country, in the meanwhile, rapid increase of breast cancer incidence was reported. Singapore government choose for longer period of follow-up, expect for the benefit of mortality reduction in the population resulted from their mass mammography screening program (Chuwa et al., 2009). As we know, many therapeutic options for early detected breast cancer with small tumor size, the success rate of therapy for early stage cancer is higher than advanced stage disease.

In Taiwan, a national project of 2-year interval screening mammograms for 45- to 70-year-old women has detected significantly more early breast cancers (Chen et al., 2008). However, the major source of breast cancer detection is not arise from this screening program. The overall average detection size of breast cancer tumors in Taiwan is over 2 cm, which is larger than that detectable with the diagnostic capabilities in Europe and North America (Ng et al., 1998; Shen et al., 2005). The median age at diagnosis of breast cancer is 45–49 years in Taiwan, and this age group is more likely to present with a dense breast parenchyma pattern (DBPP). This median age is significantly lower than that of Caucasian women in Western countries, where breast cancer peaks between the ages of 70 and 74 years, and this older age group is more likely to present with a non-dense parenchyma pattern (NDBPP) (Huang et al., 2001; Shen et al., 2005). Breast cancer in this age group is reportedly more aggressive (Kwong et al., 2008). This pathological pattern is also commonly seen in our clinical practice in Taiwan (Leung et al., 2010b). Previous study have demonstrated that the prevalence of NDBPP (ACR types 1 and 2; ACR: American College of Radiology classification of breast parenchymal density in digital mammography) could be as high as 78%, compared with 22% for DBPP (ACR types 3 and 4), which is representative of most Western countries (Table 1) (Van Gils et al., 1999). The ratio of NDBPP to DBPP is reversed compared with their previous results. Although the case number is small, we believe that the results are representative of developed Asian countries such as Taiwan, Hong Kong, South Korea, Singapore, and Japan.

Breast pattern according to mammography	NDBPP	DBPP
Prevalence (%) in Taiwan (Leung et al in Taipei Medical university Hospital)	20.8	79.2
Prevalence (%) in Western countries	78	22

Table 1. Analysis of the prevalence of breast pattern in Taiwan and Western countries (Leung et al., 2010b; Van Gils et al., 1999).

Breast density is a major factor influencing the incidence of breast malignancy, and has been discussed extensively in the past two decades. In a normal woman, mammographic densities correspond to different amounts of fat and connective and epithelial tissue. Fat appears radiographically dark on film-screen mammograms, and radiographically opaque areas represent epithelial and connective tissues (Gram et al., 1997). Most cases of high mammographic density are not abnormalities, but varied distributions in healthy breast tissue. It was also found that high mammographic density may be related to a fourfold increased risk of developing breast cancer. It was found that the diagnostic sensitivity of mammography in women with a fatty breast pattern is 98% (Boyd et al., 1998; Kolb et al., 2002). Women with high mammographic breast densities are at higher risk of breast cancer; the incidence of breast cancer in NDBPP was 26.4% versus 73.4% in DBPP. It was discussed and investigated whether the women with DBPP should receive more frequent screening or screening with alternative techniques that increase the length of the preclinical detectable phase to reduce breast cancer mortality (Van Gils et al., 1999).

Data collected in Japan showed the successful result of a mass screening program using mammography on asymptomatic women over 50 years of age. The program had a 0.84 % cancer detection rate. The breast cancer cases screened from the program had not been detected by physical examination (Morimoto et al., 1994). The detection rates were higher in the sixth and seventh decades of life.

In a study of Japanese women, mammography missed 16 % of breast cancer occurrences (Uchida et al., 2008). Breast density was also confirmed as a significant determinant of breast cancer risk. They quantitatively measured the mammographic density, and found that a higher risk was associated with a larger breast size and with a higher proportion of glandular density, especially for extreme densities (Nagata et al., 2005). A study in Singapore showed an increased risk of breast cancer associated with a higher-density pattern with extensive nodular characteristics, and linear densities with a nodular size larger than normal lobules (Jakes et al., 2000).

Although breast cancer is the most common female cancer in South Korea, its early detection rate is low compared to developed Western countries (Ryu et al., 2008). The clinical characteristics of Korean breast cancer patients showed a pattern of a younger age (< 50 years old) and increasing early stage and asymptomatic cases. This finding reflects the need for more effective breast screening programs for young Korean women (Son et al., 2006).

Increased breast parenchyma density correlates with breast cancer risk and obscures the detection with the mammography of early stage, small-sized breast tumors. Asian women have smaller breasts and are affected by breast cancer at a younger age; both factors that are associated with DBPP (Leung et al., 2010b).

3. Limitation of conventional mammography in detecting early tumors in young Asian women with dense breast parenchyma pattern

In Western countries, mammography has been proven to detect breast cancer at an early stage and, when followed up with appropriate diagnosis and treatment, to reduce the mortality rate caused by breast cancer (Saslow et al., 2007).

Asian women have higher breast densities than Caucasian women, in addition, mammography is not a perfect screening tool for Asian women with DBPP. Mammography has lower sensitivity for invasive ductal carcinoma of breasts in patients with DBPP (Kolb et al., 2002).

The percentage of dense tissue to breast volume of both Chinese and Japanese women appeared to be higher than that in Caucasian women (Maskarineca et al., 2001). Despite the considerably smaller proportion of non-dense areas, the overall proportion of dense breast tissue in the breasts of Chinese and Japanese women is 20 % higher than in Caucasian women in the same age group (Huang et al., 2001; Maskarineca et al., 2001). Irrespective of race, women with lower mammographic densities have a lower risk of breast cancer.

Whether the presence of many dense areas in the breasts corresponds to a higher cancer risk is unclear (Boyd et al., 2005; Kolb et al., 2002; Maskarineca et al., 2001; Tseng et al., 2006). In fact, mammographic density usually reflects the opacity of epithelial and stromal tissue in the breast within the lucent background of non-dense fatty tissue. Ductal carcinoma *in situ* and infiltrative ductal carcinomas originate in epithelial cells, and therefore, areas of fibroglandular tissue with a greater number of cells are at a higher risk during increased epithelial proliferation (McCormack & Santos et al., 2006). The masking hypothesis proposed by Egan and Mosteller (1977) may also explain why radiographically dense patterns are associated with an increased risk of breast cancer. They found that breast cancer was easy to detect using mammography in breasts with non-dense glandular parenchyma, though it was unreliable for detecting cancer in dense glandular parenchyma. Cases of missed cancer detection during a first mammographic examination due to the masking effect of dense glandular tissue of the breast may be detected in subsequent mammographic examinations. The apparent excess of cancers detected in this specific group, with initial masking of the tumor in dense breasts, can cause the group to appear to be at a higher risk than those with non-dense breast tissue (Leung et al., 2010). Conventional mammography is also lower sensitivity to detect enlarged axillary and have no information on internal mammary chain. Probably due to some additional reasons, such as the screening program may cause call-back anxiety, psychological trauma by false positive results and radiation exposure (Leung et al., 2002), Hong Kong and most regions of mainland China currently have no mass screening programs for any age group.

Although some limitations of mammographic screening on DBPP women in Asia, we need give applause to health policy planners in the majority of developed Asian countries, such as Japan, Singapore, Taiwan, and South Korea, are believed helping us to bring early breast cancer awareness and provide cost-effective screening to prevent delay diagnosis of Asian breast cancer.

4. Application of breast MRI on Asian women and the dense breast parenchyma pattern

Digital mammography is reliable as a screening or diagnostic tool for Asian women with NDBPP. Mammography can reliably image microcalcifications and solid tumors with good contrast from the fatty background tissue of the breast. The aim of image production during mammography is to separate fatty tissue from glandular breast tissue of low contrast density based on different X-ray absorption characteristics. Mammographic density estimation is based on a single two-dimensional projection of the breast. In contrast, breast MRI distinguishes different tissue types based on their signal production after radiofrequency stimulation within a strong magnetic field. MRI evaluation of the breast is three-dimensional, and the image analysis is assisted by a post-enhanced kinetic curve, and subtraction techniques only allow contrast-enhanced lesions to be depicted (Figures 1&2).

Figure 1 presents a representative case in the NDBPP group showing that a large tumor and cluster of microcalcifications could be easily detected with both mammography and breast MRI. Figure 2, in contrast, shows a representative case from the DBPP group. The mammograms of the left breast under cranial-caudal and medial-oblique views show diffuse faint nodular shadows without major architectural distortion. The finding of malignancy could not be concluded due to a dense breast parenchyma background. However, breast MRI with a subtraction image demonstrated an enhanced tumor mass.

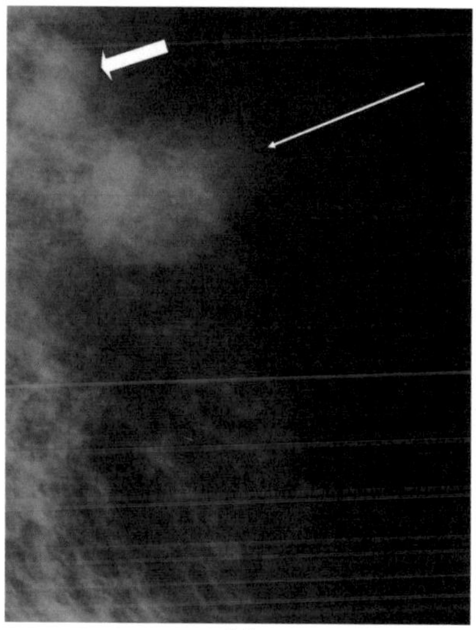

(a)

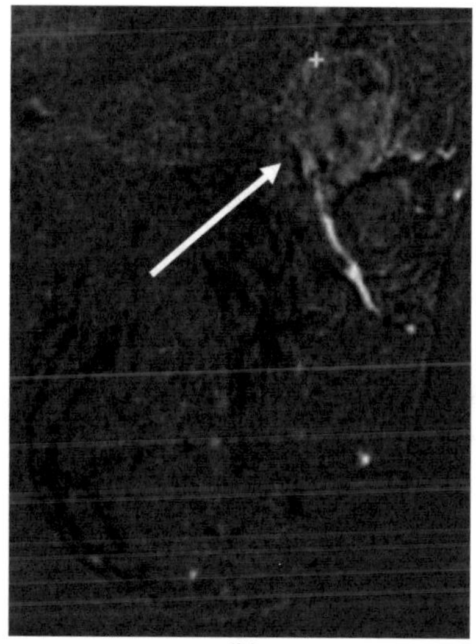

(b)

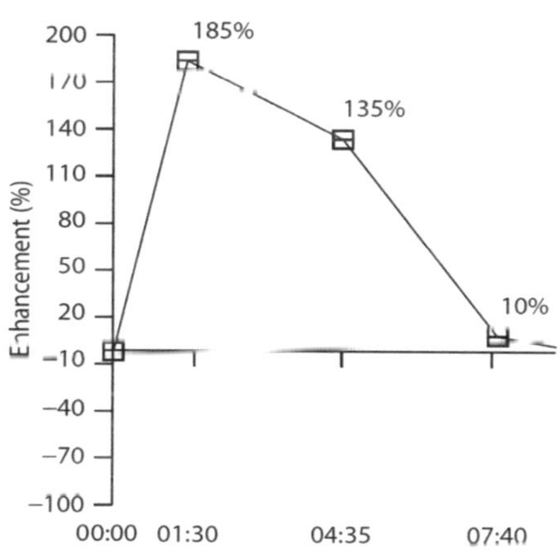

(c)

Fig. 1. (a) Mammogram of the non-dense parenchyma pattern group shows a large tumor and cluster of microcalcifications (thin white arrow) at the superior left breast with enlarged lymph nodes (thick white arrow), which was diagnosed as advanced infiltrative ductal carcinoma and lymph node metastasis. (b) The corresponding breast magnetic resonance imaging subtracted image of ESP (white arrow) matched the mammographic interpretation. (c) It shows a characteristic "wash-out" enhancing curve pattern, which is more likely to appear in malignancy.

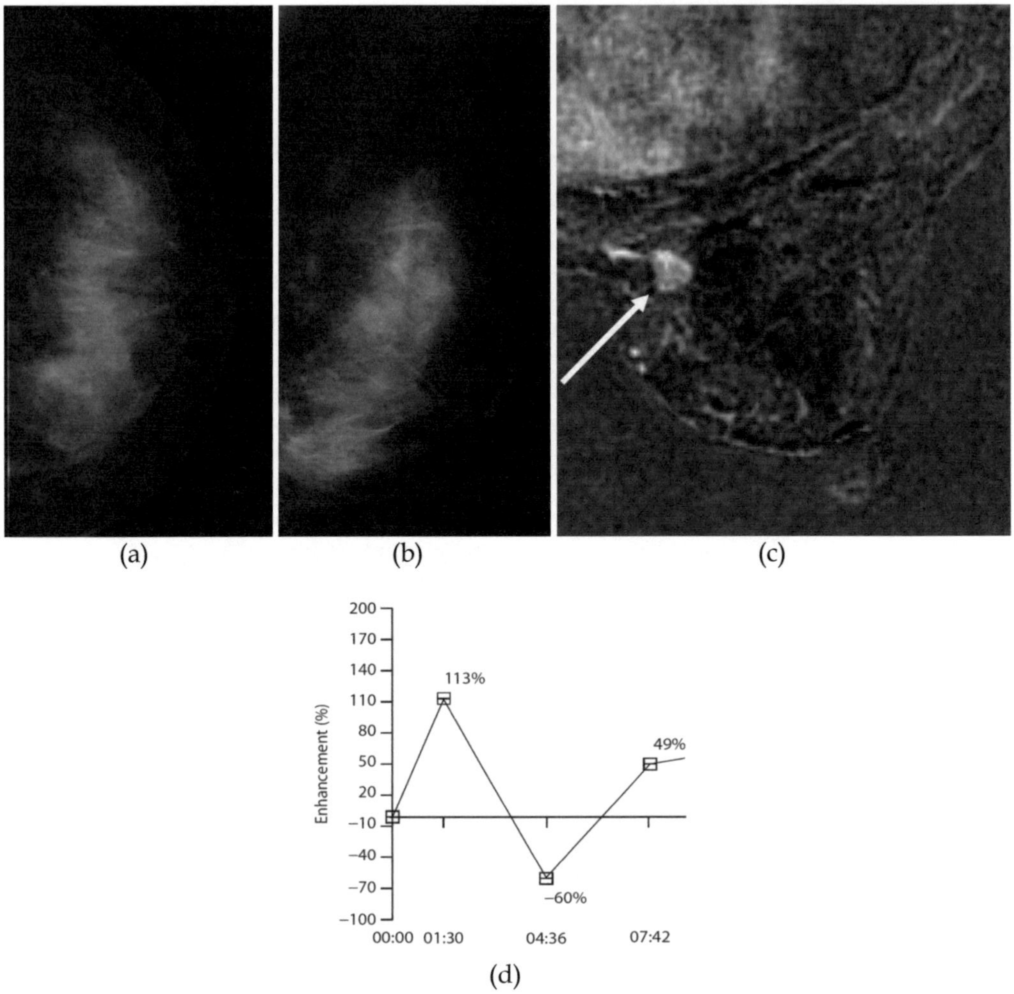

Fig. 2. Mammograms of the left breast under (a) cranial-caudal and (b) medial-oblique views of the dense parenchyma pattern group show diffuse faint nodular shadows without major architectural distortion. The finding of malignancy could not be concluded due to a dense breast parenchyma background. (c) However, follow-up breast magnetic resonance imaging with a subtraction image of ESP demonstrated an enhanced tumor mass (white arrow) at the medial aspect. (d) The corresponding enhanced curve analysis revealed a characteristic "wash-out" pattern.

Because the image is processed by subtraction of all the background tissue, a possible lesion can only be identified in the presence of extremely dense glandular tissue, different types of implantation, or fibrotic changes after chemotherapy with BRMRI (Thompson et al., 2009).

Previous study conducted by Kuhl et al (2010), have indicated that breast MRI is significantly more sensitive than mammography, sonography, and a combination of both. Breast MRI and mammography are more specific than sonography alone or in combination. In addition, the positive predictive value of breast MRI was 48%, higher than 39% of mammography and 36% of ultrasound.

5. MRI acts as a screening tool in a population of asymptomatic women

Mammography has well-recognized limitations for early breast cancer detection, especially for Asian women with DBPP. In the United States, MRI is provided as an adjunctive screening tool, mainly for women who may be at increased risk for the development of breast cancer. The Society of Breast Imaging and the Breast Imaging Commission of the ACR issue these recommendations to provide guidance to patients and clinicians on the use of imaging to screen for breast cancer. The recommendations are based on available evidence, or based on consensus opinions of professionals and experts from the executive committee of the Society of Breast Imaging and the members of the Breast Imaging Commission of the ACR. These recommendations are intended to suggest appropriate utilization of breast MRI for screening high-risk groups. They are not intended to replace sound clinical judgment and are not to be construed as representing the standard of care. Mammography should be remembered to be the only imaging modality that has been proven to decrease mortality from breast cancer. Before using breast MRI, the potential benefits, limitations, and harm from this additional screening modality should be reviewed (Lee et al., 2010; Saslow et al., 2007).

Similar to Western countries, a higher proportion of Asian women with breast cancer have at least one relative with breast cancer. This risk can be almost double that of the general population. However, the gene correlated with this is different from that found in Western countries. In addition, gene screening programs and services are poorly developed, even in the wealthiest Asian countries. To define the high-risk group in the population, the national screening mammography program in Taiwan provides services for women aged between 40-45 years with a family history of breast cancer. Considering the low sensitivity of mammography in young women, a more aggressive breast MRI screening at this age or lower is recommended. Adjuvant breast MRI screening should also be considered for women with lymphoma (Hodgkin's disease), women who received radiation treatment between the ages of 10 to 30 years, women with lobular carcinoma *in situ* (LCIS), atypical lobular hyperplasia (ALH), and atypical ductal hyperplasia (ADH), which may range from normal ductal hyperplasia to ductal carcinoma *in situ* (DCIS). Specifically, women with a personal history of breast cancer, including DCIS, should be included. As previously mentioned, DBPP has been shown to be an independent risk factor for breast cancer. Women with the highest breast density were found to have a 4- to 6-fold increased risk compared with women with the least dense breasts. In addition, malignant tumors of the breast are more likely to arise in the areas of greatest mammographic density than in fattier areas of the breast. Although the ACS recommendations for Breast MRI Screening as an adjunct to mammography are more detailed, the most suitable indications for Asian women are provided in the following table (**Table 2**; Lee et al., 2010; Saslow et al., 2007)

6. The value of breast MRI as an adjunct in the diagnosis of breast diseases

Breast MRI can be used as an adjunct in the diagnosis of breast diseases when inconclusive findings in conventional imaging exist, such as with mammography and sonography (BI-RADS 0). Therefore, MRI can be used as a problem-solving modality (Mann et al., 2008). Generally, breast MRI provides a relatively higher negative predictive value for excluding malignancy (Dorrius et al., 2009; Dorrius et al., 2010).

Breast MRI Screening as an adjunct to mammography is advised for women with a family history that may suggest a genetic predisposition to breast cancer (Lee et al., 2010; Saslow et al., 2007)
Breast MRI Screening recommendations for who received radiation therapy to the chest in their 2nd or 3rd decade (Saslow et al., 2007)
Breast MRI Screening recommendations for patients with lobular carcinoma *in situ* (LCIS) , atypical lobular hyperplasia (ALH), or atypical ductal hyperplasia (ADH) (Saslow et al., 2007)
Breast MRI Screening recommendations for heterogeneously or extremely dense breast tissue, disabling the mammograph from interpretation (Lee et al., 2010; Saslow et al., 2007)
Breast MRI Screening recommendations for personal history of breast cancer, including ductal carcinoma *in situ* (DCIS) (Lee et al., 2010; Saslow et al., 2007)

Table 2. MRI acts as a screening tool in a population of asymptomatic women with preselection is listed.

MRI is the most reliable imaging technique for measuring the tumor size, and it detects additional foci of the tumor in the ipsilateral breast in 10–30 % of patients (Mann et al., 2008). The sensitivity of breast MRI is, in the setting of preoperational evaluation, close to 100 %. MRI may be considered after breast-conserving therapy (BCT) as an evaluation tool for residual disease after positive tumor margins. Thus, breast MRI acts as a diagnostic tool for all patients who undergo BCT. Breast MRI is superior for evaluating suspected recurrence compared to clinical examination, mammography, or sonography (Kuhl et al., 2010). Postradiation changes usually occur up to 3 months after radiation therapy and do not reduce the accuracy of MRI for identifying residual or recurrent tumors. The presence of an implant does not seem to decrease the sensitivity of breast MRI. MRI is the most accurate modality in the evaluation of implant integrity. Its sensitivity for rupture is between 80 % and 90 %, and its specificity is approximately 90 %, whereas the sensitivity of mammography is approximately 25 %. MRI may aid explanation surgery as it documents the presence and extent of silicone leakage better than any other imaging modality. In patients with prosthesis and prior breast cancer, MRI may be used to evaluate suspected recurrent disease or as a postoperative screening modality (Mann et al., 2008). Although most MRI-detected lesions can be found (and biopsied) with a second sonography, many cannot. The specificity of MRI in a previous study was 88 %; a biopsy was recommended on the basis of a positive MRI in 13.9 % of the women, and 24.8 % of the biopsies resulted in a diagnosis of breast cancer (Lehman et al., 2007a). MRI resulted in 8.2 % of women undergoing biopsy compared with 2.3 % for mammography and 2.3 % for sonography (Lehman et al., 2007b). The Positve Predictive Values (PPVs) of biopsies obtained by using MRI (43 %) and mammography (50 %) were higher than those of the United States (25 %). Of the cancers identified by MRI alone, approximately 75 % were targeted under sonographic guidance. However, approximately 25 % were removed for biopsy under MRI guidance because only MRI demonstrated the accurate location (Lehman et al., 2007b). In addition, breast MRI identified high-grade DCIS and high-risk lesions that were missed by mammography (Hartman et al., 2004). The call-back and biopsy rates of MRI are higher than for mammography in high-risk populations, while the increased sensitivity of MRI leads to a higher call-back rate and a higher number of cancers detected (Saslow et al., 2007). Women at risk for familial breast cancer have shown an increased detection rate using this modality than with mammographic screening (Lee et al., 2010). Table 3 summarizes these values.

Backup for inconclusive findings and for more detail to evaluate the lesion characterization: Breast MRI may be indicated when other imaging examinations (sonography and mammography) and physical examinations are inconclusive for the presence of breast cancer **(Figure 14)**.
Occluded images: Certain conditions that may impair conventional breast imaging, such as silicone augmentation or radiographically dense breasts, may warrant breast MRI depending on clinical findings **(Figures 13,19)**.
Contralateral breast with breast malignancy: MRI can detect unsuspected disease in the contralateral breast (coincidence positive rate at 4-5% of breast cancer patients), which often provides false negative findings on mammography or sonography **(Figure 2)**.
To differentiate scars from real malignant mass: Breast MRI can help distinguish postoperative scarring or radiation scarring from recurrent cancer.
Suspect of breast cancer recurrence: Breast MRI may be indicated in women with a past history of breast cancer.
Metastatic adenopathy: MRI provides a full field of view in a single position and an image acquisition that covers major positions of the bilateral axillary lymph nodes and internal mammary chains, which may be missed by mammographic or physical findings **(Figure 4,5,12)**.
Determining true tumor extension: Breast MRI can locate the primary area of breast cancer and define the extent of the disease for definitive therapy. A negative breast MRI may exclude the breast as a potential primary site of cancer and avoid a mastectomy or help minimize the invasive procedure **(Figure 9,10,11)**.
For metastasis: Breast MRI helps evaluate the breasts in case of metastases of an unknown primary carcinoma.
For chemotherapy: Breast MRI helps evaluate therapy response in patients treated with neoadjuvant chemotherapy **(Figure 7-8)**.
Silicone and nonsilicone breast augmentation: Breast MRI is useful in the evaluation of patients with silicone implants and silicon injections, in which sonography and mammography are usually inconclusive in defining tumor mass, silicoma, granuloma, and intracapsular or extracapsular implant ruptures **(Figure 13,19)**.

Table 3. The value of breast MRI as an adjunct in the diagnosis of breast diseases (Mann et al., 2008).

7. Ability of MRI to describe multifocality and the extent of the disease

For women with newly diagnosed breast cancer, a single round of screening of the contralateral breast with MRI at the time of diagnosis might detect otherwise occult malignancy in approximately 3 % to 9 % of cases (Lee et al., 2010) (Figure 4).

MRI has been found to be more accurate in assessing tumor extent and multifocality in patients with dense breasts. MRI can improve the detection of cancer in the contralateral breast when added to a thorough clinical breast examination and mammographic evaluation at the time of the initial diagnosis of breast cancer. The increased rate of cancer detection comes with a false positive rate of 10.9 % and a relatively low risk of detecting benign disease on biopsy (9.4 %) (Lehman et al., 2007a).

8. Limitations of the breast MRI technique for screening in its current form

MRI is inappropriate for women at a low lifetime risk for breast cancer. Breast MRI is not meant to replace mammography (Lee et al., 2010). Under rare circumstances, such as DCIS with typical microcalcification clusters, mammography is superior to MRI for interpretation malignancy, which produces an image that is faint or equivocal (Lee et al., 2010).

The lesion-detecting specificity of MRI is highly influenced by reacted inflammation within a month after surgery. Thus, a time period should elapse post-surgery before an MRI (Mann et al., 2008). In addition, the dynamic breast MRI is highly influenced by hormonal fluctuations during the menstrual cycle, which may cause interpretative difficulties related to the uptake of gadolinium in normal breast tissue (Delille et al., 2005; Kriege et al., 2006). The call-back and biopsy rates of MRI are higher than for mammography in high-risk populations. This is because of the increased sensitivity of MRI. The net harm, benefits, and psychological impact of higher cancer detection rates should be considered (Saslow et al., 2007). Breast MRI screening is almost 10 times more expensive than mammographic screening, and generates higher diagnostic costs (Plevritis et al., 2006). Asian countries adopting unlimited breast MRI can face a heavy financial burden. Some concern exists regarding the clinical safety of the intravenous gadolinium-based contrast media used during breast MRI. In Hong Kong, the adverse reaction rate is reported at 0.48 %, and the incidence of severe anaphylactoid reaction is approximately 0.01 %. Although most of the symptoms are mild and transient, these adverse reactions must be documented and managed accurately (Li et al., 2006).

9. Advantages of a dedicated breast MRI (DBMRI) system with parameters of dynamic scan, 3D representation, and post processing techniques

The recent recommended standard for assessing MRIs to differentiate malignancies from benign lesions is the fourth edition of a breast MR lexicon (Morphological interpretation of BRMRI images using standards of the American College of Radiology's (ACR) BI-RADS-MRI lexicon for malignancy grading) (American College of Radiology, 2003; Erguvan-Dogan et al., 2006), which is a classification scheme used for the interpretation of breast cancer. Although universal standards for integrating different MRI systems and manufacturers are lacking, overall, characteristics based on BIRADS scoring of MRI descriptions depend on certain parameters. This is a report on my experience with a specific MRI system and pulse sequence.

The DBMRI system with a Spiral RODEO pulse sequence of a 1.5 T dedicated spiral breast MRI system (Aurora System; Aurora Imaging Technology Inc., North Andover, MA, USA, using the Spiral RODEO pulse sequence) is equipped with different post-processing techniques, including early subtracted phase (ESP), post-contrast kinetic curve, and MPR with ductal orientation, which can be independently applied in a DBMRI system (Leung et al., 2010a; Leung et al., 2010b; Leung et al., 2010c; Leung et al., in press). Axial and sagittal gradient echo T1 acquisitions were performed for both breasts with a bilateral breast coil. Sequences were performed before and after the infusion of 0.2 mmol/kg gadolinium, administrated as a bolus dose with a power injector followed by a 20 mL saline flush.

10. Lesion analysis using ESP image, kinetic curve patterns, color mapping, and morphology

In the DBMRI, for cases suspected of being malignant, an ESP image was obtained based on subtraction of the post-enhanced phase of images from 90 s non-enhanced images. Lesions that could be subtracted in the ESP (by subtraction of the post enhanced image at 90 s from the pre-contrast phase) were almost completely excluded from the possibility of being malignant (Figure 1b). Therefore, the lesions that could not be subtracted in the ESP required further analysis to assess the risk of malignancy.

Using the mean percentage calculation and comparing pre- and post-contrast kinetic data (calculated from 0 s, 90 s, and 4.5 min), the threshold point for lesion enhancement was displayed. According to the diagnostic observations of Dr. Christane Kuhl (1999), curved patterns of the plateau and washout with bound protein water and free water represent possible lesions. A stabilized enhancement without change in signal intensity between 90 s and 4.5 min was termed a "plateau" pattern. A "washout" pattern was indicated by a decline in signal intensity between 90 s and 4.5 min after the injection of contrast. Each lesion was characterized according to the strongest enhancement pattern visible over the entire lesion. Figures 1c show magnetic resonance imaging for differentiating lesions that are normal, benign, or display a washout pattern.

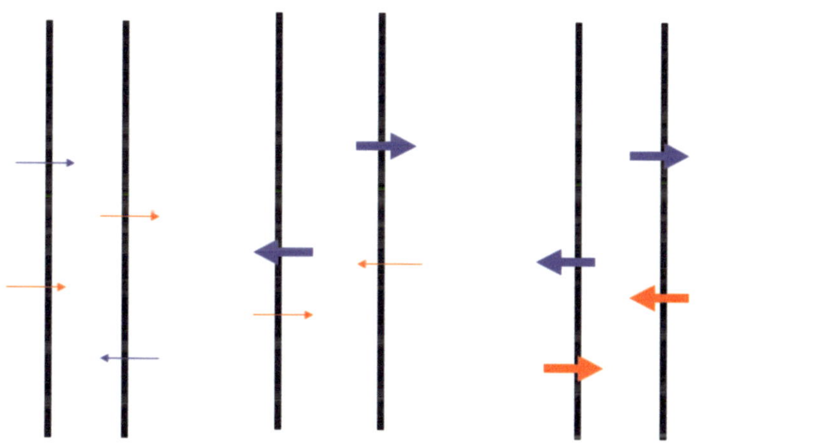

Fig. 3. In normal tissue, the contrast medium equally permeates in and out through the normal gaps in the vascular endothelial cells and interstitial space. In benign neoplasms, contrast does not permeate out of the microvessel to interstitial space, and the progressive accumulate increases the concentration which manifests itself in a progressively increased MRI signal.

The washout curve represents the initial increase in contrast concentration in the interstitial space and then a decrease, as it reverse permeates back through the abnormal gaps in the vascular endothelial cells. A final decreased contrast concentration in the tumor interstitial space can be detected.

A color mapping method was also adopted to assess the possibility of a malignancy. This reflects the overall curved patterns of the persistent-plateau (yellow color) and plateau-washout (red color), which is depends on the permeability of contrast medium through the capillary vessel of the neoplasm (Figure 3). This provided a tool for the subtle distinction of different grades of contrast-enhanced percentages so that the kinetic curve analysis of the region of interest (ROI) would be more convenient (Figure 1,2).

Morphological interpretation of BRMRI images uses standards of the American College of Radiology's (ACR) BI-RADS-MRI lexicon for malignancy grading (x). In this study, MRI studies were interpreted in conjunction with clinical history, family history of breast cancer, age, and menstrual status. Referring MRI-detected lesions for biopsy depended on characteristics of the ESP image, post-enhanced curve pattern, color mapping, and tumor morphology, such as spiculation, irregular margins, architectural distortion, and ductal or segmental enhancement (Figure 4). The lesion configuration was classified as focal mass enhancement or non-mass-like enhancement. The morphological parameters of focal mass enhancement were evaluated by its lesion shape and mass margin. Lesion shape was classified as round, oval, lobular, and irregular. Mass margins were classified as smooth, irregular, and spiculated. Non-mass-like enhancement included linear, ductal, regional, and segmental enhancement (Figure 4).

Morphological characteristics were considered the most important determining factor for benign or malignant masses. Any suspicious MR-enhanced lesions were described based on lesion shape, borders, distribution, kinetics, and internal architecture. The final MR assessment was classified on a six-point scale, which is summarized in the following table (Table 4).

Category	Interpretation and the suggestion
I	Negative for malignancy
II	Benign findings or benign lesions
IIIa	Probable benign lesion, suggest 6 months follow up with sonography focused on the MRI indicated position or in the other breast
IIIb	Probable benign lesion, suggest 3 months follow up with sonography focused on the MRI indicated position or in the other breast
IV	Could not rule out the possibility of malignancy, suggest biopsy
V	Malignancy is strongly suggested. Tumor staging and therapeutic planning suggested.
VI	Malignancy. Further treatment, including surgery, adjuvant chemical therapy, or radiation therapy is suggested.

Table 4. MRI is believed to be the most sensitive and accurate screening tool for breast cancer in Asian women. Thus, no Category 0 exists in the interpretation of breast MRI, which differs from mammography or sonography.

Examinations that provided an initial assessment of incomplete or 0 received a final MR assessment of Category I-V, based on the results of follow-up procedures. A lesion was identified as suspicious if a focal mass existed with irregular or speculated margins, if enhancement had a ductal distribution, if a solid lesion showed rim enhancement, or if there was intense regional enhancement in less than one quadrant. Benign lesions were identified as having smooth or lobulated margins (Lehman et al., 2007b).

A lesion of < 5 mm of enhancement, even with a washout curve or mixed washout/plateau kinetic curve and reddish color mapping, was not automatically referred for biopsy. This was because a tiny spot of enhancement of < 5 mm is known as a 'focus,' as described by the ACR Breast MRI Lexicon, and has a very low possibility of being a malignancy, and is, therefore, suitable for a short-interval follow-up (Liberman et al., 2006). MRI-guided biopsy, MRI-guided localization for an excisional biopsy, sono-guided biopsy, or surgical excision biopsy is employed in cases suggestive of or strongly suspected of being a malignancy.

The interpretation of breast MRI images using early phase subtraction, kinetic curve patterns, color mapping (based on the summing up of kinetic curve data from corresponding areas), and the morphology of the MR image, is helpful in differentiating malignancies from benign lesions. Dedicated breast MRI with ESP, kinetic curve, and morphology analysis was found to have an over 95% negative predictive value of ruling out malignancy and was helpful in identifying the characteristics of early-stage malignant lesions.

The usual applications, benefits and interpretations of breast MRI images are shown as Figure 4 -13.

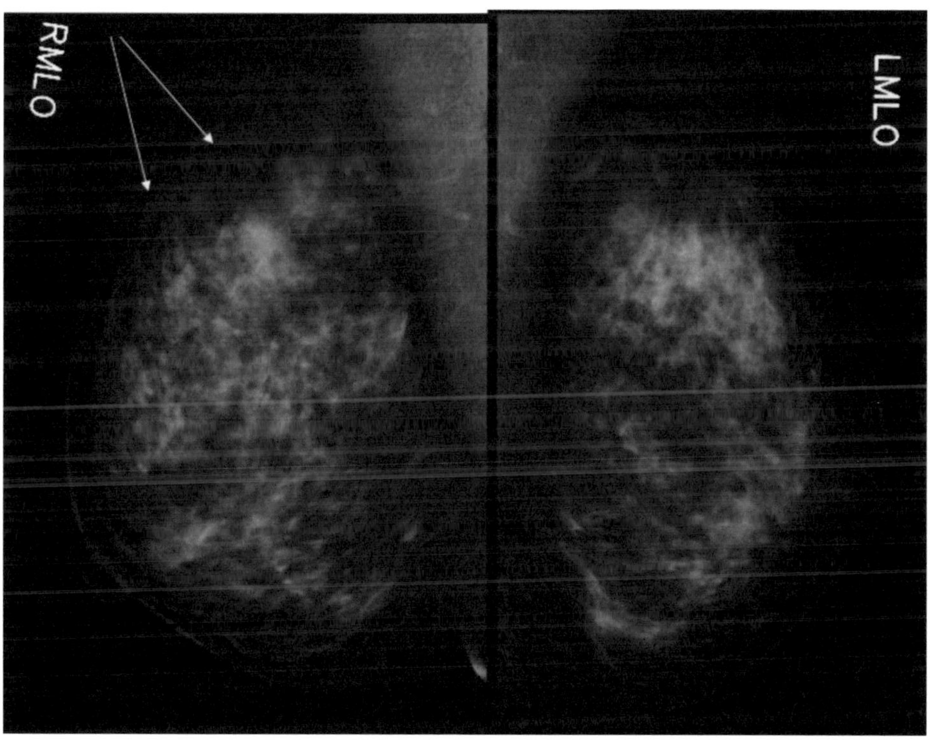

Fig. 4. (a)

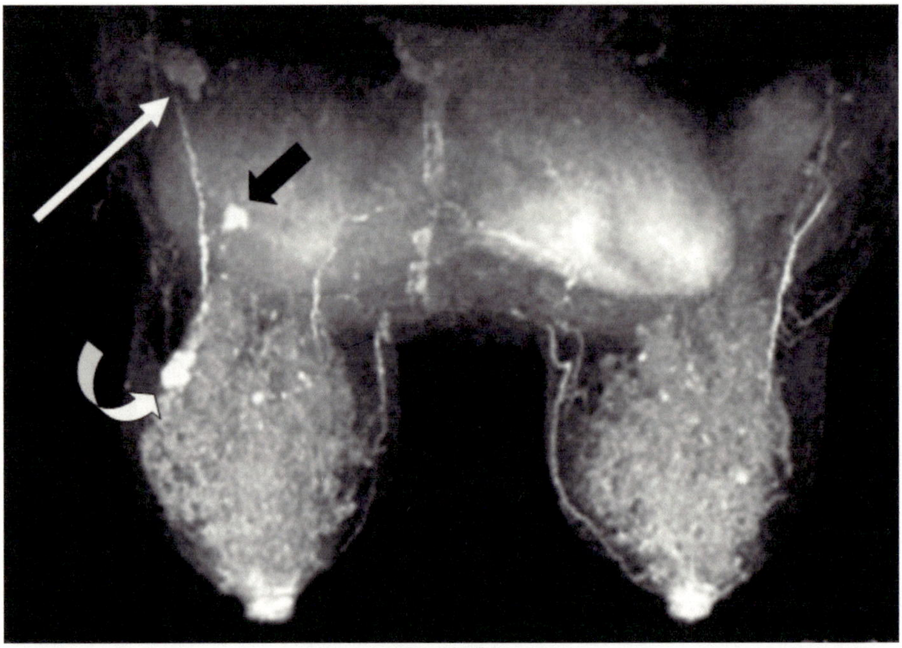

Fig. 4. (b)

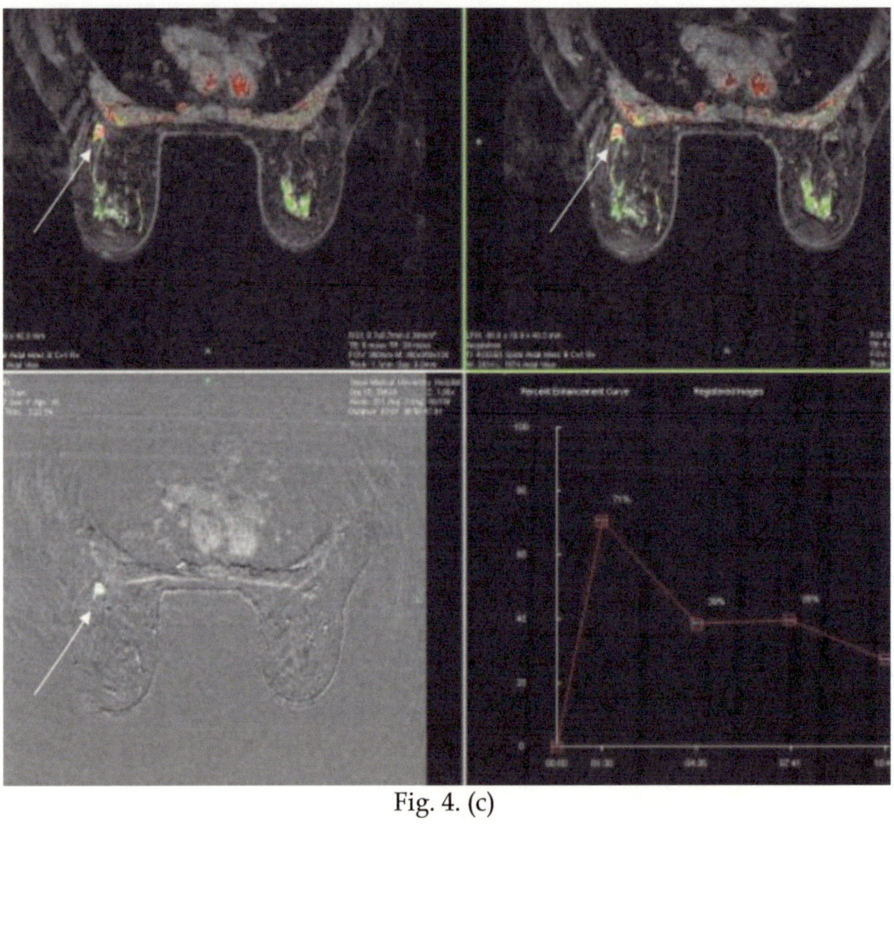

Fig. 4. (c)

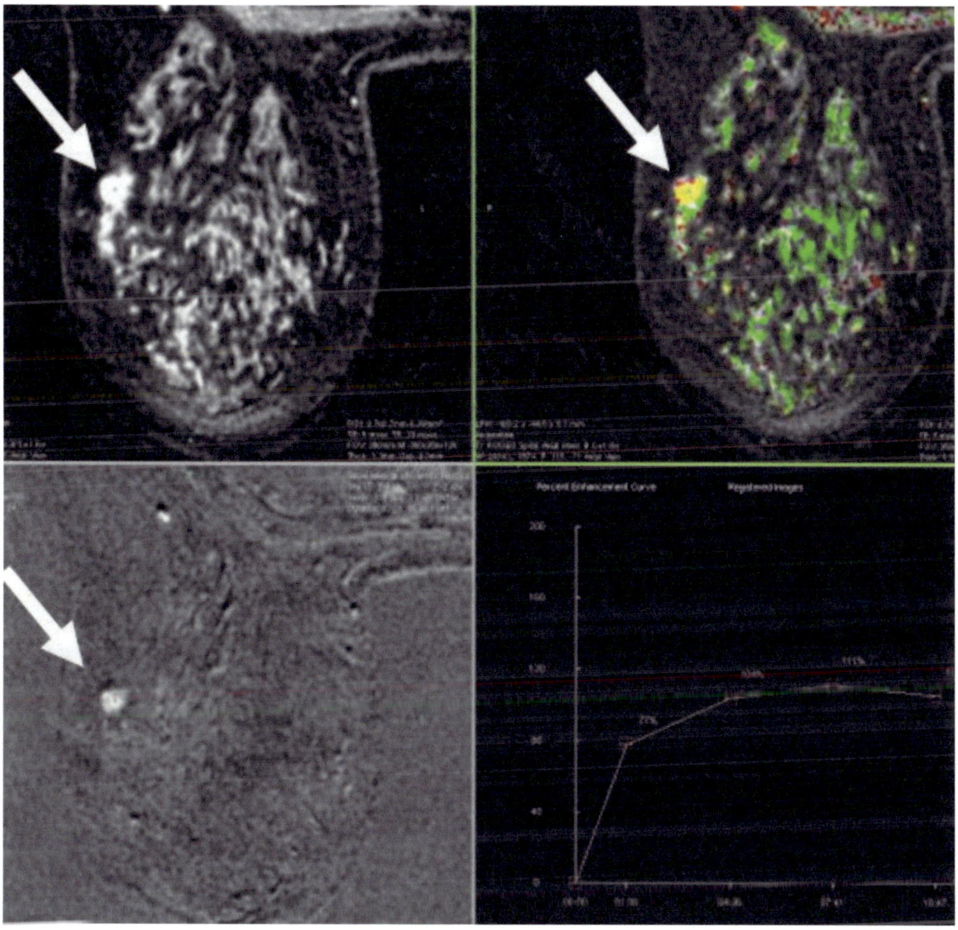

(d)

Fig. 4. (a) Digital mammography of an Asian women with DBPP showed two indistinct ill defined dense shadows noted at superior lateral of right breast. There is no enlarged axillary lymph node could be demonstrated. (b) Breast MRI simultaneously showed an enlarged right side axillary lymphadenopathy (long white arrow); first right superior mass (black arrow) and second right superior mass (white curve arrow). (c) Breast MRI with post processing software for analysis shows the first right superior mass remains high signal under ESP and exhibits 'washout' curve pattern. Pathological report indicate a small invasive ductal carcinoma. (d) It shows the second right superior mass remains high signal under ESP but exhibits a 'persistent' curve pattern. Pathological report as benign fibroadenoma.

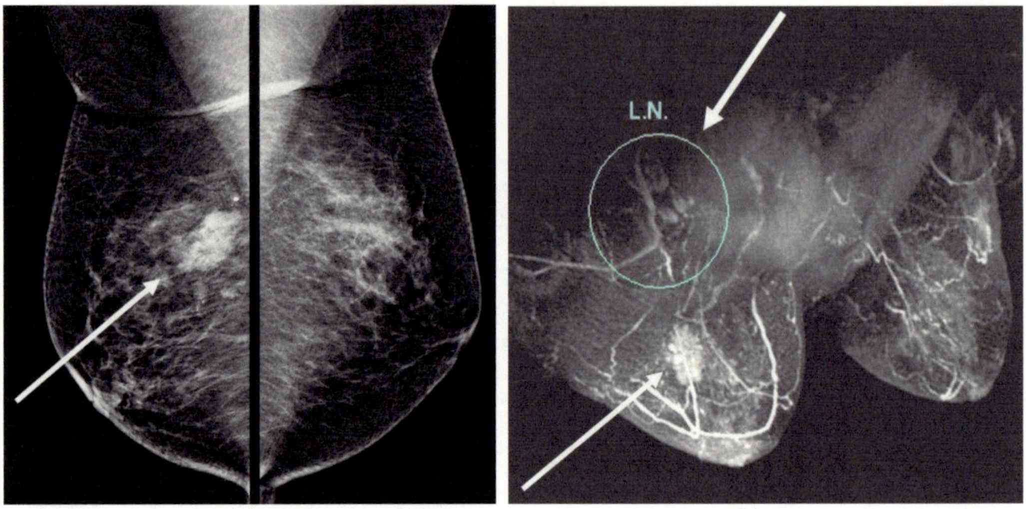

(a) (b)

Fig. 5. (a) Digital mammography showed an ill defined hyperdense mass (thin arrow) locate at superior right breast, but it could not demonstrate ipsilateral axillary lymph node. (b) Breast MRI with 3D MIP (maximum intensity projection) shows the first right superior mass remains high signal under ESP and exhibits 'washout' curve pattern. Pathological report indicates a small invasive ductal carcinoma.

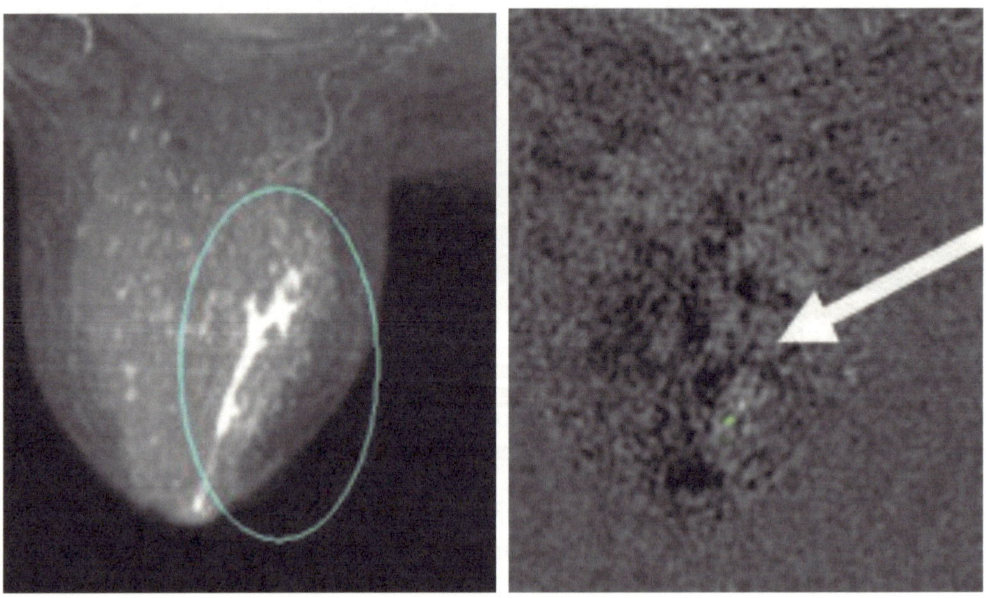

Fig. 6. Breast MRI image of an Asian woman with bloody discharge with clinical diagnosis as malignancy, it shows high signal intensity content within intraductal appearance under 3D MIP (a: with circle); but the signal being almost subtracted under ESP (b: arrow). Pathological report indicates benign papilloma.

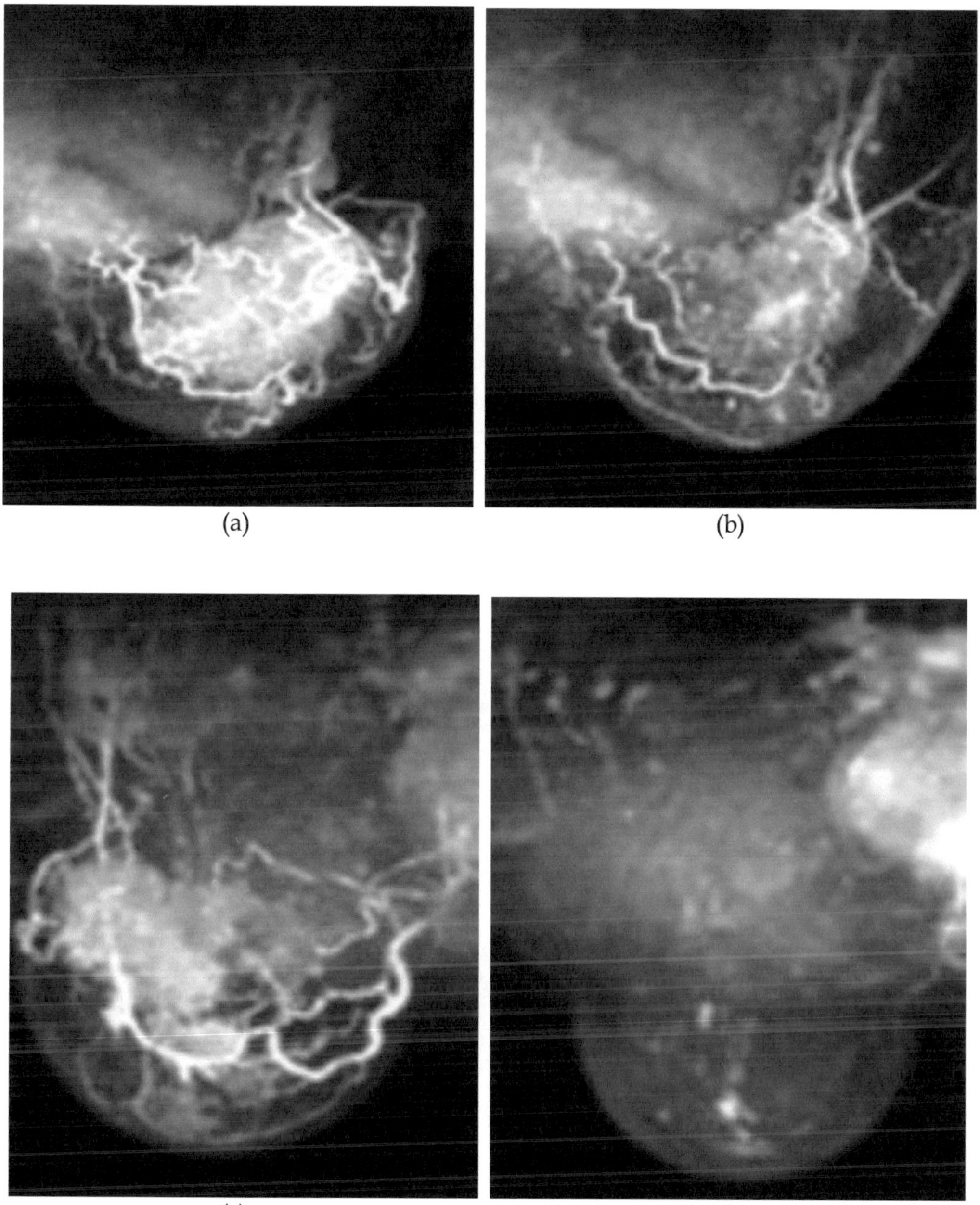

(a) (b)

(c) (d)

Fig. 7. Breast MRI has the merit on the clinical response assessment for chemotherapy. (a)(b) A patient with a huge size tumor of IDC at the left breast; after five cycles of chemotherapy, the tumor was shrinkage. (c)(d) In another patient, a similar huge size IDC mass in right breast, is finally almost completely regress after adjuvant and targeting chemotherapy.

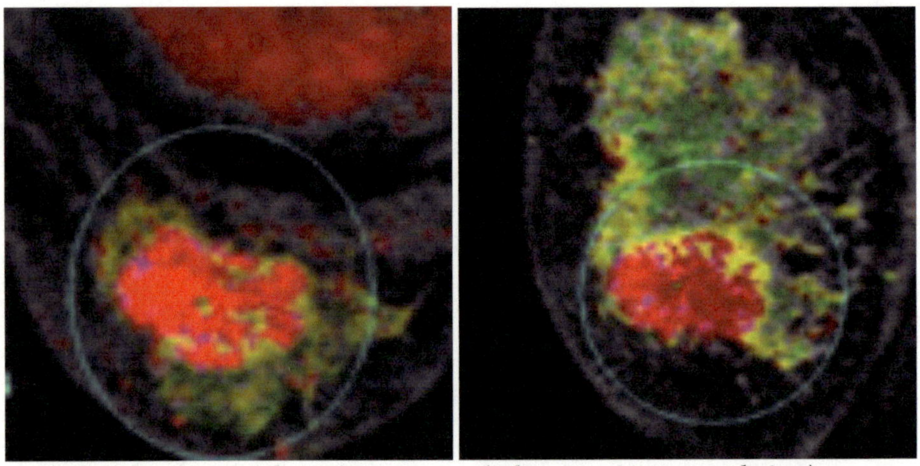

(color mapping, axial view) (color mapping, coronal view)

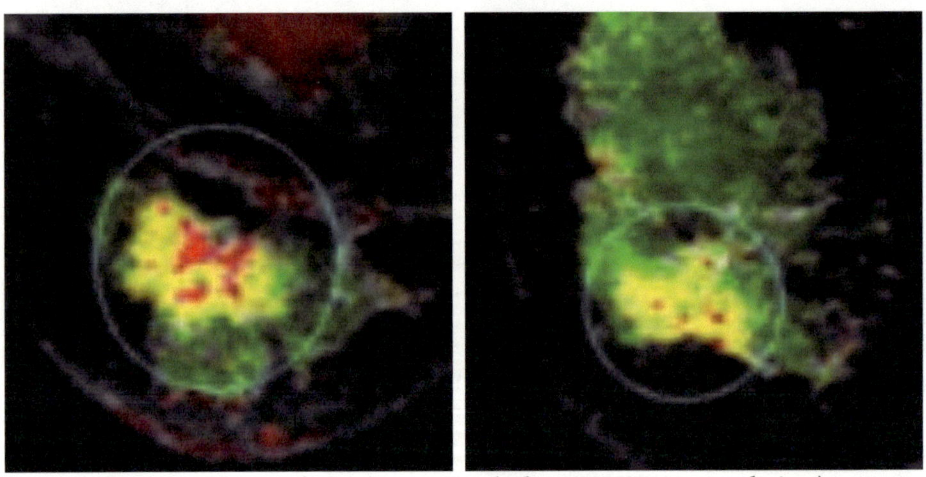

(color mapping, axial view) (color mapping, coronal view)

Fig. 8. By using color mapping of post processing breast MRI technique, more lively to demonstrate initial result of chemotherapy, even though the tumor size is not remarkable shrinkage. (a)(b) Red color area (represent active viable malignant cell with 'washout' contrast enhanced kinetic curve pattern) occupy the major part of the IDC tumor, in the right breast. (c)(d) After two cycles of chemotherapy, the red color shrinkage to less than 20% area of the tumor. This result encouraged both clinician and patient to continue this effective protocol of chemotherapy.

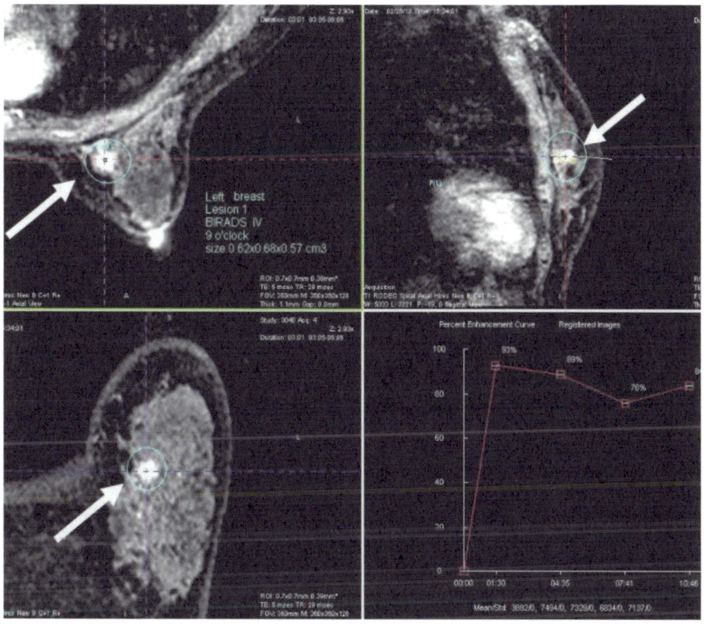

(a)

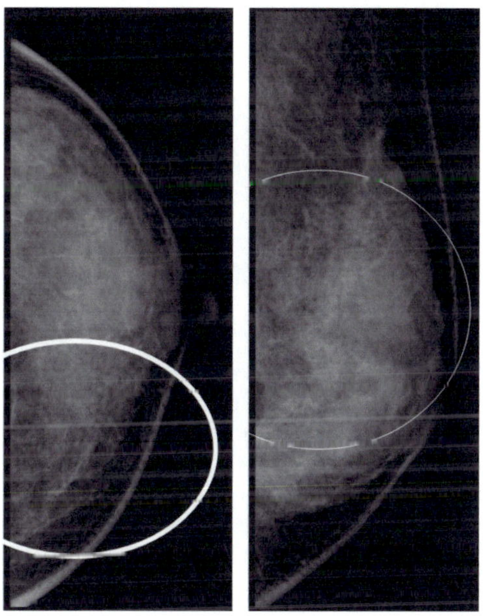

(b)

Fig. 9. Breast MRI adjunct the conventional breast modality with no limitation of breast size and breast dense pattern. (a) In this Breast MRI image of Asian woman, a 1.5 cm IDC tumor showed on left breast by all axial, sagittal and coronal views and associate 'washout' kinetic curve pattern. (b) As we retrospectively to review the digital mammography of this patient (both CC & MLO views), the mentioned mass is not capable to demonstrate due to the deep location and dense parenchyma occult effect of the breast.

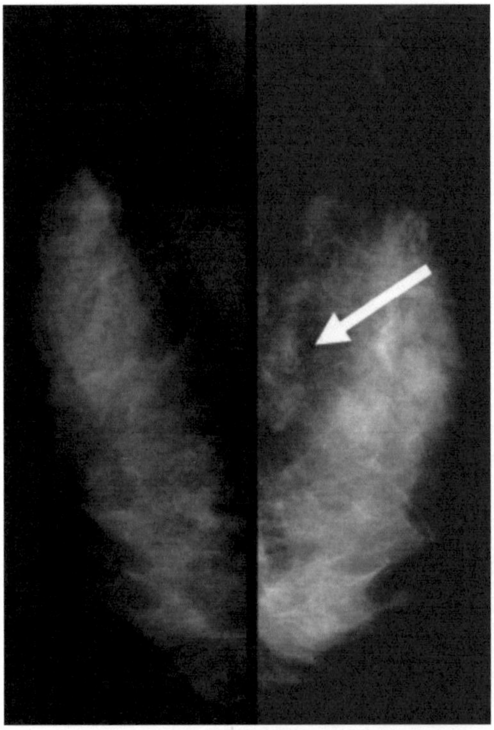

(a)

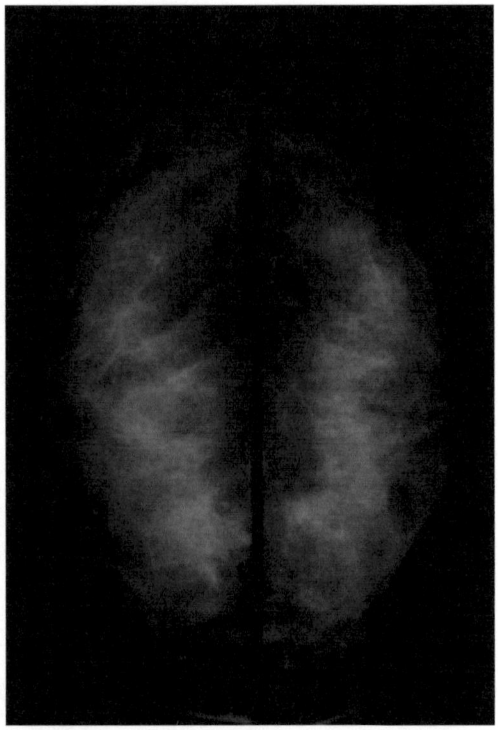

(b)

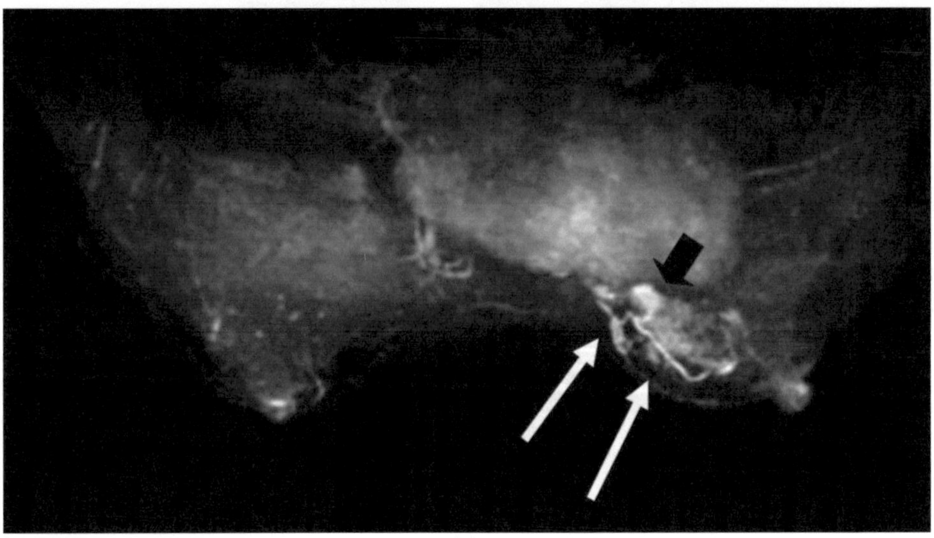

(c)

Fig. 10. (a)(b) An Asian woman with DBPP who received digital mammography, it shows suspicious mass locate at deep superior of left breast under MLO view (white arrow), but the CC view could not demonstrate the tumor location. (c) Breast MRI (oblique view of 3D MIP) is more clearly to demonstrate multiple foci of malignant masses by different tumor location and tumor sizes . Pathological proved as IDC and DCIS.

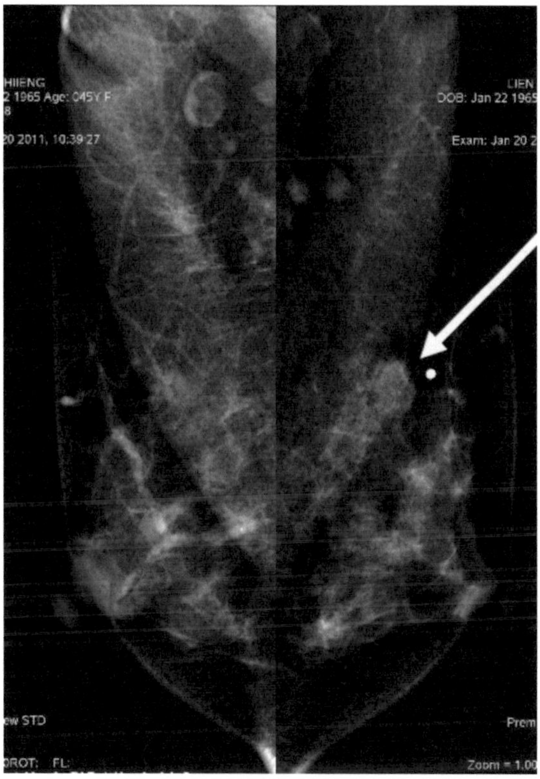

(a)

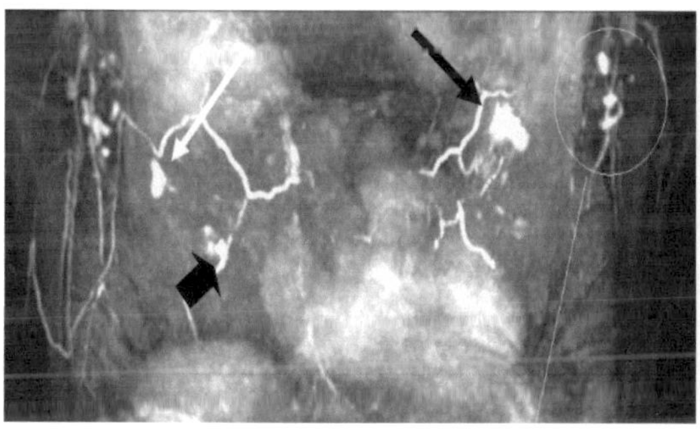

(b)

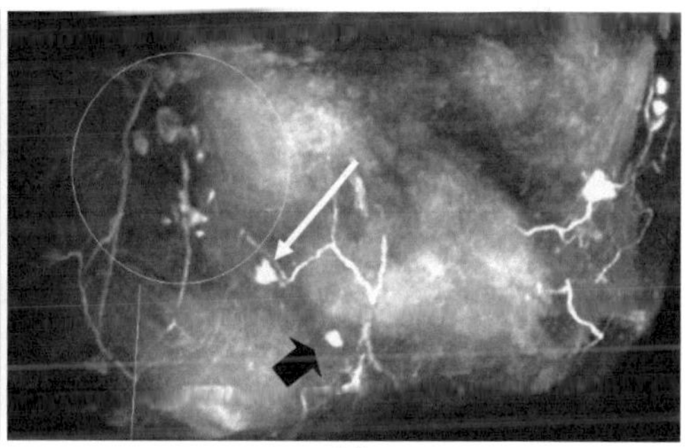

(c)

Fig. 11. (a) Breast MRI have the merit on the describing multifocality and the detection of asymptomatic cancer on the contralateral breast. In this Asian patient, digital mammography shows a single isodense palpable mass at superior of left breast (white arrow with metal beam). (b)(c)The follow up breast MRI shows another two enhanced tumor masses, with ill defined margin at superior lateral of right breast (long white arrow), which was proved as IDC. There is also a well defined enhanced mass with smooth margin, locate at paramedial aspect of left breast (black thick arrow), which was proved as fibroadenoma. Besides, the stronger enhancement of left axillary lymph nodes (circle on 11b) indicate the metastasis, compared with the weaker enhancement of right axillary lymph nodes (circle on 11c).

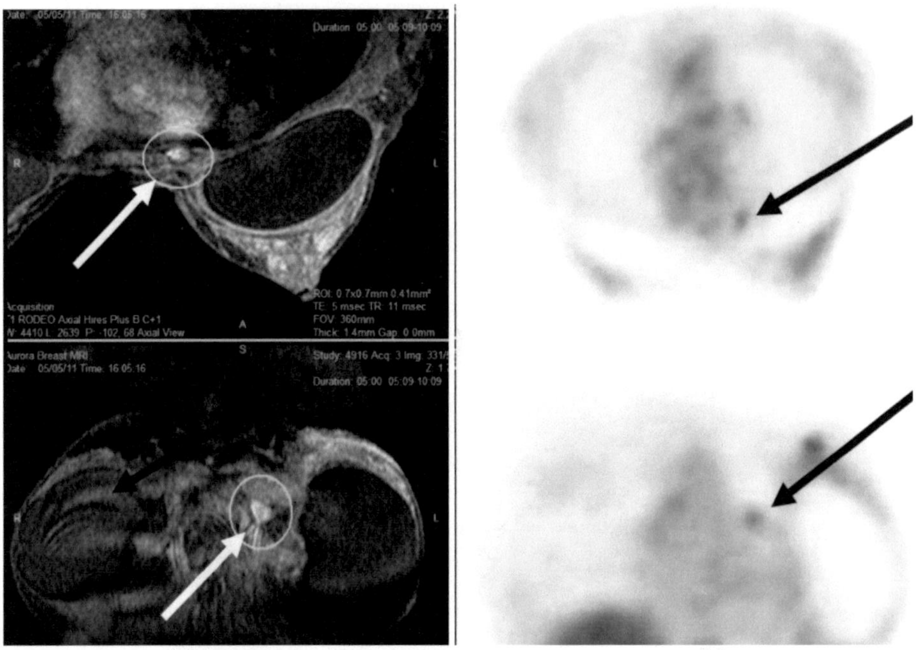

(a) (b)

Fig. 12. (a) Breast MRI shows suspect enlarged lymph node at left side internal mammary chain (white arrows), (b) which proven by PET scan (black arrows).

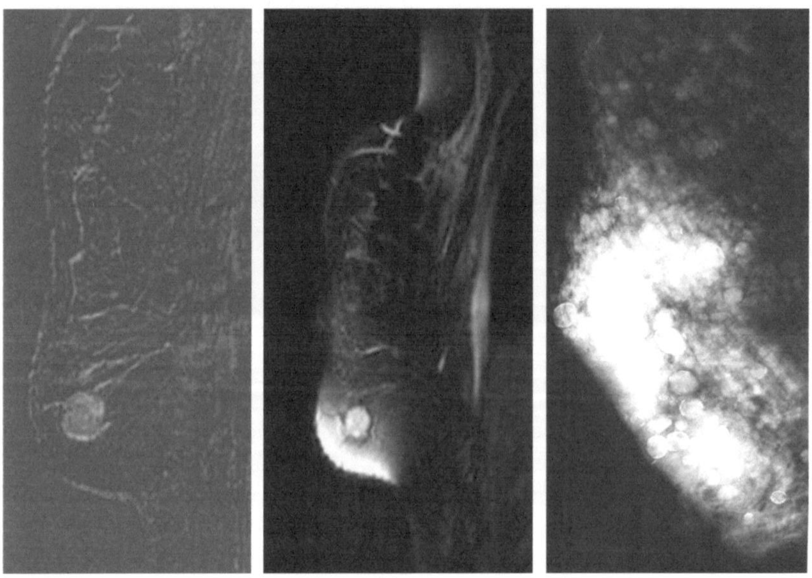

(a) (b) (c)

Fig. 13. Free silicon injection with silicoma and calcified granuloma formations usually occult the possible tumor growth on mammography (a); MRI with sagittal T2 plus fat saturation (b) and post enhanced subtracted image (c) provide a satisfactory detective rate on cancer on this group of patient.

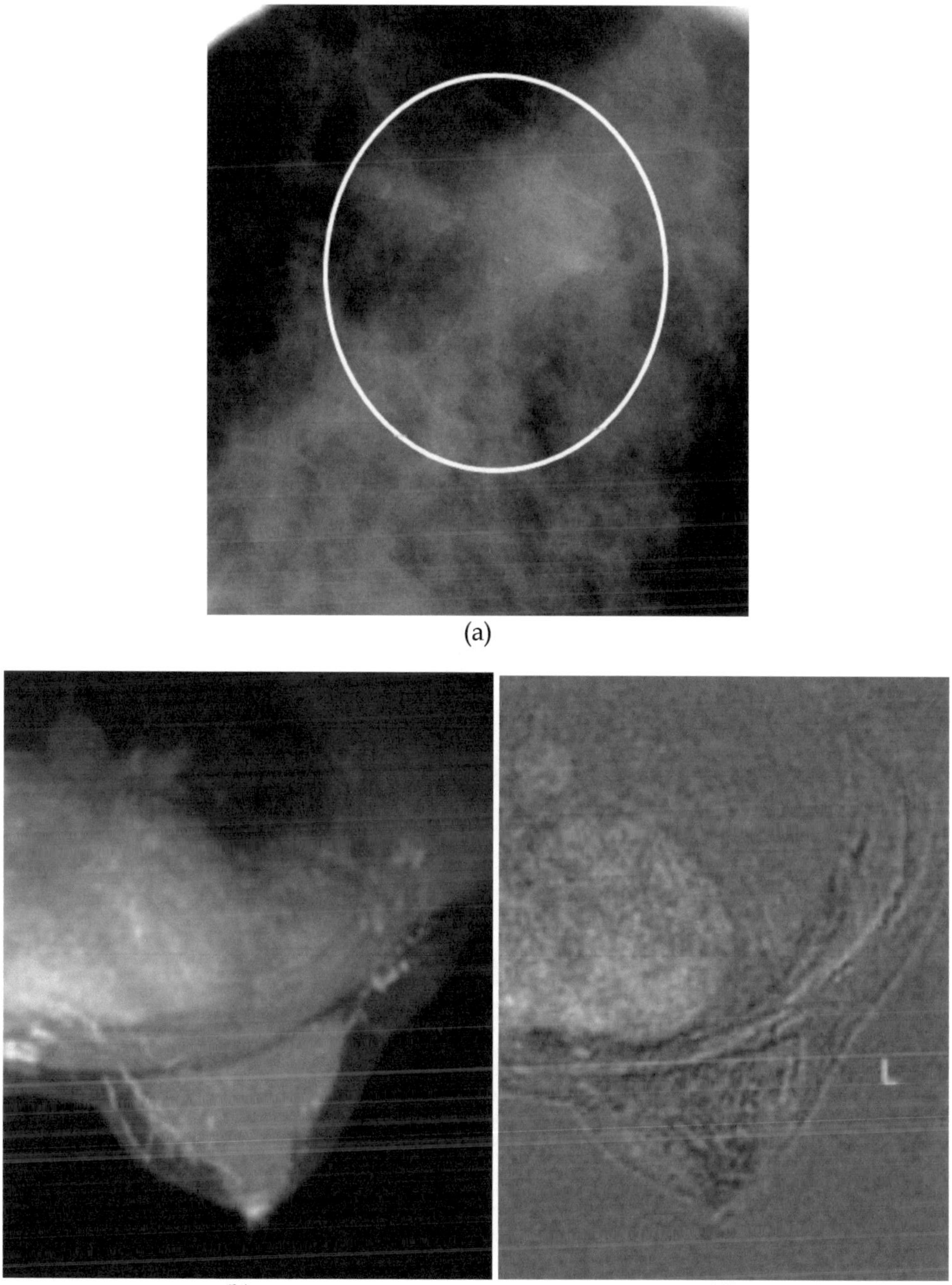

(a)

(b) (c)

Fig. 14. Breast MRI may decrease unnecessary biopsy base on interpretation of screening mammography. In this Asian patient, digital mammography with spot compression view on left breast (a) demonstrate some cluster of faint microcalcifications. However, the follow up breast MRI shows no enhanced lesion in both 3D MIP (b) and subtracted image (c), thus, the schedule of call-back mammographic guide biopsy was cancelled.

11. Using a dedicated breast MRI system with the application of postprocessing techniques for multiplanar reformation (MPR) on mammary ductal orientation, for three-dimensional (3D) anatomical demonstration

Surgeons are required to localize accurately malignant tumors of the breast. Preoperative evaluation using DCIS or IDC is helpful for determining the surgical method and the necessity of lymphadectomy or preoperative chemotherapy. Compared to mammography and sonography, magnetic resonance imaging (MRI) is the most sensitive tool for breast cancer detection. Its ability for 3D anatomical representation has also become more important for pre-surgical evaluation.

Although the incidence of DCIS of the breast seems to be gradually increasing in Taiwan and other Asian countries, the proportion of small tumors detected is lower than in Western countries (Leung et al., 2010c; Huang et al., 2001; Shen et al., 2005).

The early stage of ductal carcinoma in situ (DCIS) appears as a spread-out distribution pattern, extending toward the nipple and is occasionally seen in the breast tissue peripheral to the infiltrating carcinoma. Only 3D imagery demonstrates the correlation of image and pathology. Sonography and mammography are incapable of showing the anatomical and spatial relationship between the lesion and the ductal structures within the breast (Figure 15) (Leung et al., 2010c).

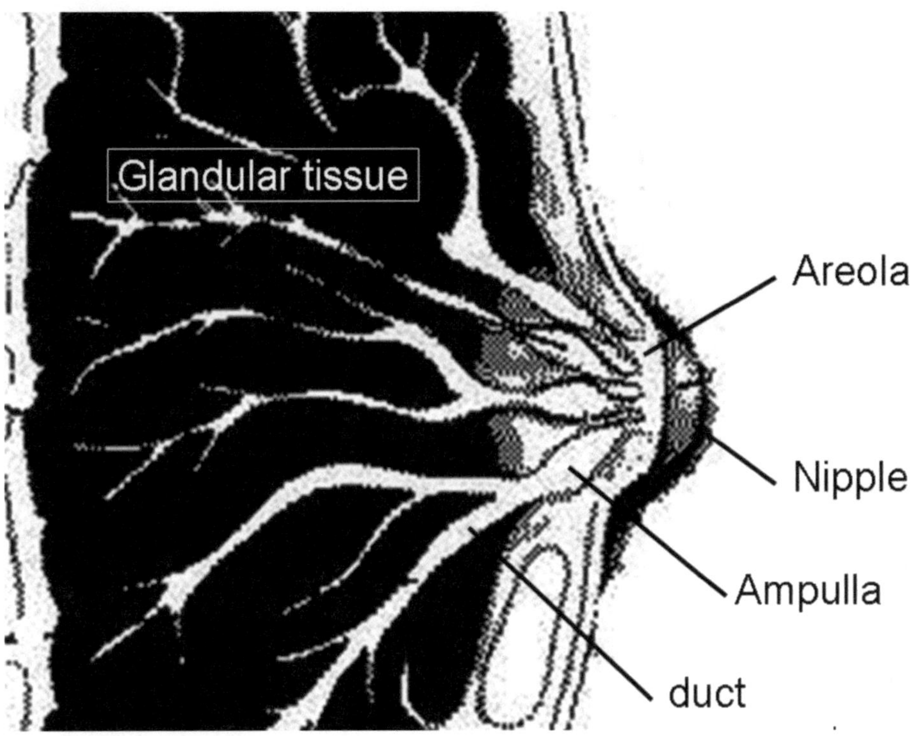

Fig. 15. shows the relationship between the mammary duct, the glandular tissue, and the nipple (Leung et al., 2010c).

The following figures demonstrate the application of DBMRI with the MPR technique, based on the AurorCad 4.0's oblique display protocol (Aurora System; Aurora Imaging Technology Inc., North Andover, MA, USA). The 3D maximum intensity projection (MIP) image outputs the selected plane of orientation as an oblique MPR on side-by-side display windows. The user controls the rotation of the 3D MIP from any angle, and the MPR pane is updated to match the slice, while having the same orientation as the MIP (Figures 16a & 16b).

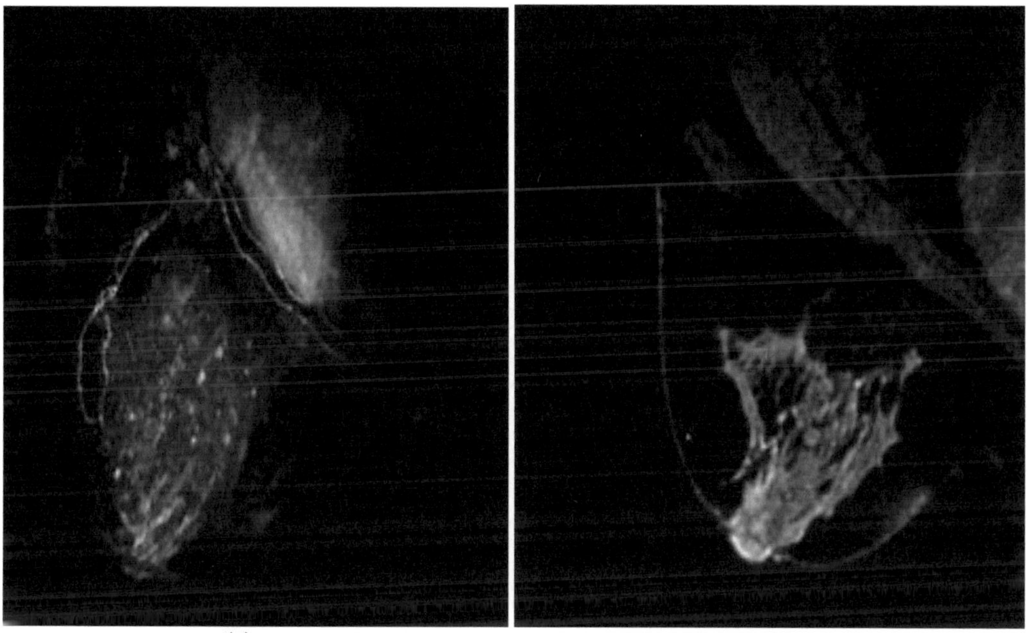

(a) (b)

Fig. 16. While controlling the rotation of the 3D MIP (Maximum Intensity Projection) (a) from any angle of rotation, the MPR (multi-planar reformation) pane updates to match the slice in the same orientation as the new orientation of the MIP (b).

Ductal carcinoma *in situ* (DCIS) is a preinvasive condition that appears as tumor lesions of the ducts with severe atypical proliferation of epithelial cells. DCIS shows different grades of malignant potential, and certain subtypes of DCIS are more likely to recur. Approximately 60 % of women with DCIS will progress to invasive ductal carcinoma (IDC) over an 8–10-year period, and poor prognostic outcomes are likely when IDC develops. Thus, the early detection of DCIS through imaging studies that permit accurate assessment of size and distribution is important.

Breast MRI is a useful tool for staging invasive cancers like IDC. However, traditional breast MRI systems have limitations in the analysis of early DCIS using the sagittal and coronal planes. Although MRI provides a 3D representation of the enhanced tissues, the borders between DCIS and its surrounding benign processes are often indistinguishable, especially when DCIS is sparsely scattered. The actual size is also difficult to measure accurately during pathological examinations. This is because of the anatomy of the breast ducts are distributed in three dimensions and histological sections show only two. Measuring scattered and widely distributed DCIS is difficult, which is one possible explanation for the frequent mismatch between MRI and pathological findings.

Screening for cases with ductogram appearance were performed to find if a significant correlation between DCIS and ductograms exists. The term 'ductogram' was used for image phenomenon that occurred when peri-ductal infiltration in the tissues immediately adjacent to the mammary duct was observed. The ductogram image shows non-contrast ductal structures differing from the enhanced periductal tumor infiltration if the ductal orientation is in phase using multiplanar reformation (MPR) (Leung et al., 2010c) (Figure 17).

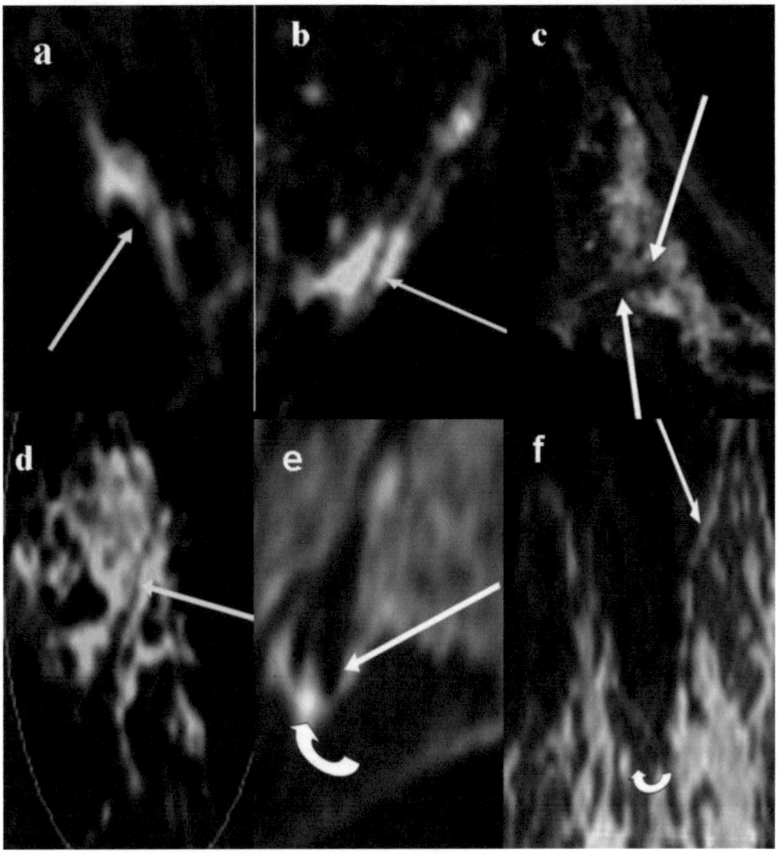

Fig. 17. (a) A characteristic ductogram appearance (long arrow) is visualized in case 1. (b) A characteristic ductogram appearance (long arrow) is visualized in case 2. (c) Case 3 shows characteristics of a ductogram pattern along the lactiferous sinus and duct to the areola, within a background of stripping and non-mass signal intensity. (d) Case 4 shows that pure DCIS is an intermediate grade of malignancy with delayed surgical treatment, in which the ductogram appearance is preserved. The MPR for ductal orientation is visualized by a non-mass with strip appearance, and lesion cross-over glandular tissue. (e) Case 5 shows pure DCIS visualized by its non-mass like intensity (curved arrow) and ductogram appearance. (f) Case 6 shows pure DCIS appearing with non-mass of intensity (arrow is the true DICIS area). The MRI overestimates tumor size over pathological size by over 200% (the curved arrow shows the false area).

Non-DCIS early ductal lesions, including intraductal papilloma, ductal hyperplasia, and early focal IDC, can be visualized using MPR with ductal orientation. Although certain characteristics of the lesion morphology (Figure 18) are similar to the pictures in terms of tumor size and the spreading along glandular tissue, not all lesions exhibit a ductogram appearance. However, additional analysis using early subtracted image and a post-contrast kinetic curve may further confirm the image diagnosis.

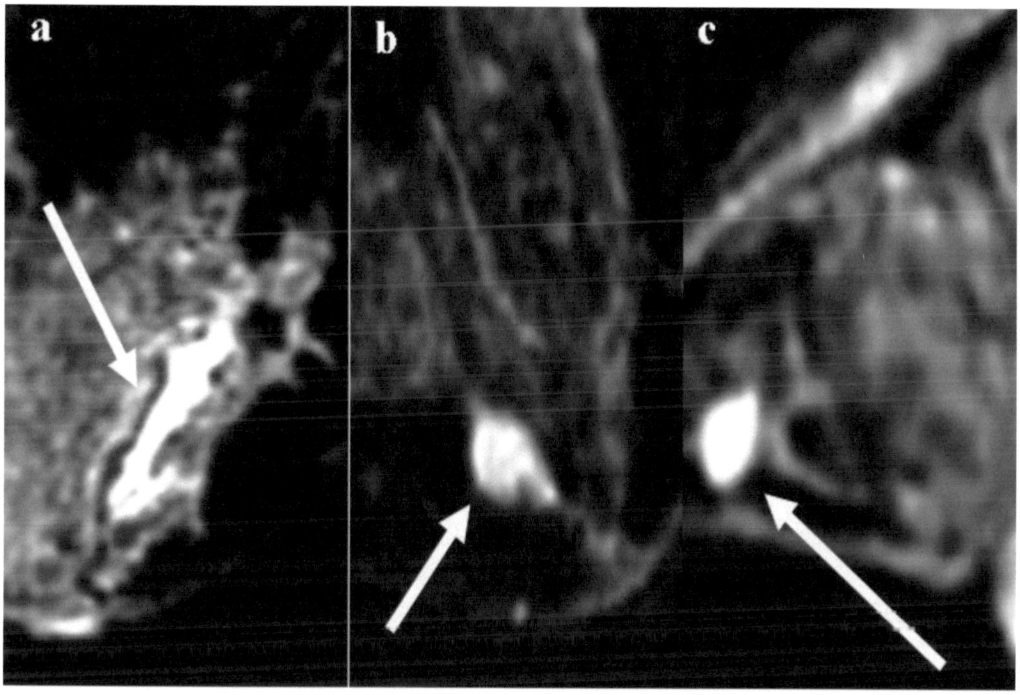

Fig. 18. Three types of non-DCIS lesions, both benign and malignant, under MPR with ductal orientation. (a) MPR shows enhanced thick strip-like intensity with an irregular contour, which spreads along the intraductal structure (arrow) and within the network (intraductal papilloma). (b) MPR shows an enhanced and well-defined smooth nodular lesion with a tadpole morphology, which occupies the intraductal area of the non-dilated side (ductal hyperplasia; arrow). (c) MPR shows a focal lesion with enhancement (arrow), which crosses over the ducts of the surrounding glandular structures and is not continuous with the ductal structures (early focal intraductal carcinoma).

A traditional MRI system can provide coronal, sagittal, and coronal images of the whole breast and is capable of visualizing lesions (Menellet et al., 2005). However, the borders between DCIS and its surrounding benign processes are often indistinguishable, especially when DCIS is sparsely scattered. The actual size, based on the pathologic examination, is also difficult to accurately measure. This is because the anatomy of the breast ducts is distributed in three dimensions, while histological sections are in two dimensions. Measuring scattered and widely distributed DCIS is difficult, which is one possible explanation for the frequent mismatch between MRI and pathologically determined tumor size. In addition, heterogeneous DCIS lesions more often exist alongside benign active tissue or lesions, such as adenosis, sclerosing adenosis, inflammation, and proliferative fibrocystic changes. Therefore, the image size acquired in DBMRI is usually overestimated and larger than the actual pathological size of the lesion. MPR with a ductal orientation for anatomical localization and 3D demonstration was found to be a useful technique for increasing the detection rate for early stage DCIS. Detection is performed using characteristic findings that include a strip morphology, the spreading along glandular tissue, and a ductogram appearance. Moreover, MPR is excellent for visualizing the anatomical pattern of spreading early intraductal carcinoma which extends towards the nipple. In addition, MPR can show the spatial relationship between the carcinoma and the surrounding breast tissue. These findings should be considered for surgical strategy in segmental resections or partial mastectomy. Breast MRI with MPR for ductal orientation improves the early detection rate and exhibits higher specificity because of improved anatomical interpretation of mammary ducts. However, the existence of adenosis, fibroadenomas, and some specific benign proliferative processes may still interfere with the characteristic pattern of the MRI findings. This can lead to an overestimation of the true size and scope of the distribution (Viehweg et al., 2000). For cases of IDC with a DCIS component, distinguishing the DCIS from the IDC region is difficult. Some pitfalls exist when matching the three-dimensional DCIS distribution with the routine two-dimensional histology sectioning. Using a DBMRI system with Spiral Rodeo pulse sequence, those lesions that could be subtracted in the ESP were almost completely excluded from the possibility of being a malignancy (Figure 6b).

To improve the correlation between image diagnosis of tumor size and pathological size, the pathologist should be notified of the MRI findings, the estimated lesion size, and the mammary ductal orientation before planning sectioning of a specimen that is scheduled for microscopic study. In the future, better integration of radiologists, surgeons, and pathologists to propose working guidelines would create an environment for better correlation of imaging studies and pathology. The accumulation of experience will provide a more accurate estimation of the DCIS volume and improve preoperative image assessment (Mariano et al., 2005; Neubauer et al., 2003).

12. Probably benign interpretations of Breast MRI and False positive biopsy results base on MRI interpretation

Breast MRI is a very sensitive modality for breast lesion, but the specificity for real malignancy is the issue that long been concerned. People may think breast MRI can pick up a lot of things, but these things are not necessarily abnormal. Besides malignant lesions, Breast MRI may also highlight fibrocysts, fibroadenomas, and other benign conditions. Breast MRI reported to have false positive rate, range from 13% to 83% (Hoogerbrugge et al., 2008), which means that it may misdiagnosis for lesions that not cancer. Breast MRI reading radiologists have the responsibility, through restlessly of receiving new MRI knowledge and collecting clinical experience, to achieve higher specificity of tumor differentiation and image diagnosis. By our self assessment in Taipei Medical University hospital, benign lesions reported by pathology accounted for 15.2%, which were initially suspected of being malignancy based on the MRI. In our experience, the pathological results of those false positive MRI interpretations are included atypical ductal hyperplasia, adenosis/apocrine metaplasia, radial scar, sclerosing adenosis, phylloides tumor, infectious mastitis and fat necrosis with hemorrhage.

In both North America and in Asia, the frequency of benign proliferative breast lesions, particularly among women under 40 years of age, is progressively increasing (Schnitt et al.,

1993). Breast neoplasm is a developing disease, and initially the possible risk cannot be precisely determined by a single biopsy result. A study conducted by Liberman el al. demonstrated that 24% of all breast MRI cases studied were interpreted as 'probably benign' in the initial readings. Within seven months, however, nearly 10% of them were subsequently proven to be malignancies (Buadu et al., 1996). One study based on over 120,000 individual cases collected in ten years that received breast biopsies, had been diagnosed as benign disease. However, 50% of the lesions were associated proliferative changes, of which nearly 10% had atypical ductal hyperplasia. Within this latter group, 15% eventually developed invasive carcinoma (London et al., 1992). Atypical hyperplasia and other benign results at the first time of biopsied, is significantly increased risk of breast cancer (London et al., 1992). In another study, about 2% of cases interpreted as probably benign were subsequently identified as malignancies (Liberman et al., 2003).

Accordingly, we cannot negate the possibility to those probably benign lesions or suspected malignant lesions that based on MRI's interpretation that initially proven to be benign(as false positive lesions) may further malignant development, although it is not yet to have a precise predictive percentage value. Thus, of the proven benign cases, it is essential to have long-term imaging follow-up. To our limited knowledge, not able to explain the possible reasons of false positive interpretation of MRI, there is still lack of study on direct biomolecular correlation with MRI images. In the future, we believe that further understanding of tumor transformation will improve our interpretation of dynamically enhanced breast MRI, according to the kinetic curve analysis. This will help in evaluating lesions as well as identifying angiogenesis, microvessel density, and microvascular endothelial permeabilities. The investigation should also include image-pathology correlations of tumor behavior, biological activity, nuclear pleomorphism, mitotic count, and histological grading (Bone et al., 1998; Mussurakis et al., 1997; Narisada et al., 2006; Szabo et al., 2003).

13. Screening by DBMRI with breast augmentations

DBMRI can differentiate breast glandular tissue and pathological lesions from silicone/saline bag implants. It can also better visualize intracapsular rupture of breast implantation. Breast augmentation has become popular among different age groups in Asia, especially in the developed countries. In our breast image center, over 30% of breast MRI candidates have received at least one or two different types of breast implant surgery. Silicon can cause major complications. Silicone compounds primarily consist of fluids, gels, rubbers, sponges, foams, and resins (Ojo-Amaize et al., 1994). Although silicone is relatively inert and biocompatible with biological tissue, it is polymeric, has hydrophobic characteristics, and possesses electrostatic charges. The organic side groups have potentially immunogenic factors, especially over the long-term. Silicone induces inflammatory responses in women with breast implants who have several types of autoantibodies against different self-antigens (Van Gilset al., 1999). The symptoms and signs of preoperative diagnosis for breast implant rupturing based on physical examination are usually vague, especially when the fibrous capsule encloses the rupture. This situation may become complicated when active inflammation and malignancy are suspected. Image studies are, then, necessary for localization and preoperative differentiation (Scaranelo et al., 2004).

Intense images followed up with sonography may find minor changes in implanted breast pathology. However, in most situations, breast sonography provided no definite way to differentiate benign from malignant conditions. When mammography is arranged, well-trained radiological technicians may help provide good quality pictures as the implantation is being compressed and differentiate the implant from normal breast glandular tissue, in order to detect possible lesions. Poor technique for patients with breast implants are increase the risk of iatrogenic ruptures. In this situation, sonographic guided or mammographic guided biopsy may be indicated. If DBMRI is available, further analysis with noninvasive techniques is preferred before a biopsy is suggested.

In our center, a breast MRI with a dedicated breast acquisition system was arranged using the Aurora Spiral Rodeo pulse sequence (Figure 19). The Silicone and water Rodeo image mode was adopted to subtract implanted silicone and water bag material as low signal intensity background before and after contrast injection. Post processing of the images could be performed using silicon and water material subtraction techniques followed by the AurorCad 4.0's color mapping display protocol. The same procedure may also apply to other breast augmentation material, such as hyaluronic acid (HA) and an individual's own breast tissue.

Although it is difficult to identify the malignancies when the rupture of implants was coexisted, MRI is considered the most accurate modality for detecting breast cancer in the presence of silicone (Azavedo & Bone, 1999). The MR images of ruptured implants usually showed low-signal-intensity bands, linguine appearance, and a mass within the gel of the implants, while of malignancies were irregular margin and showed reddish of color mapping. However, free silicone may be hypothesized to induce a foreign body reaction with dense fibrosis and granulomatous formations. In this situation, distinction of inflammation areas and malignancies remains problematic.

In case of rupture, silicone from an implant can leak out into the space around the implant. An intracapsular rupture (silicone contained within the fibrous capsule) can progress to the outside of the, becoming an extracapasular rupture (silicone present outside the fibrous capsule) (Everson et al., 1994). These conditions indicate the need for removal of the implant. Previous study results establish a rupture rate of 8.0 percent at 11 years for silicone breast implants (Hedén et al., 1994). If clinical examination by a skillful surgeon is the only diagnostic tool for identifying implant rupture, it is not reliable, and neither the sensitivity nor the specificity is acceptable (Holmich et al., 2005). Physical examination is inadequate to evaluate a suspected rupture, as experienced plastic surgeons accurately detect only 30% of ruptures in asymptomatic patients, compared to 86% detected by MRI (Hedén et al., 1994). Mammography is a highly sensitive and specific modality for diagnosing extracapasular silicone rupture, and it can detect silicone gel migration through the glandular parenchyma. On the other hand, the diagnosis of intracapsular rupture is difficult to detect via mammography (Gorczyca et al., 1994; Scaranelo et al., 1994). A change in implant shape is the most important mammographic pattern (Gorczyca et al., 1994). Breast sonography has been used in breast implant integrity evaluation for several years. A great variety of sonography signs detect anywhere from 10% to 17% of ruptured implants (Scaranelo et al., 1994). Breast sonography can be the first test in the assessment of breast implants in asymptomatic patients, followed by mammography. This is because breast sonography has greater ability to detect intracapsular rupture than mammography does (Chung et al., 1996;

Harris et al., 1993; Venta et al., 1996). There is limitation for sonogram to rule out extracapsular rupture, but accurate diagnosis requires magnetic resonance imaging (Chung et al., 1996; Harris et al., 1993; Venta et al., 1996). As a result, the FDA has recommended that MRIs be considered for use in screening for silent ruptures starting at three years after implantation, and every two years thereafter (Allergan, 2006; FDA, 2004). The following figures show a special case with initially neither breast sonography nor mammography was able to detect the intracapsular rupture of the implant. Although mammography reveals microcalcifications that might be malignancy, but the final suggestion for surgery is based on MRI images. In our opinion, MRI should be a first-line diagnostic tool for implant rupture when coexisting malignancy is suspected (Paetau et al., 2010) (Figure 19).

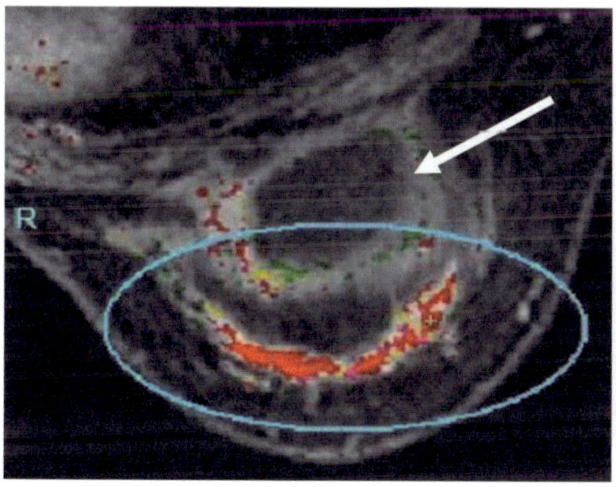

(a)

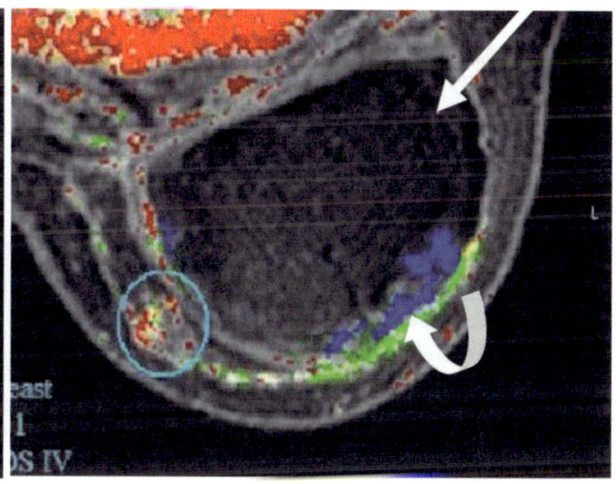

(b)

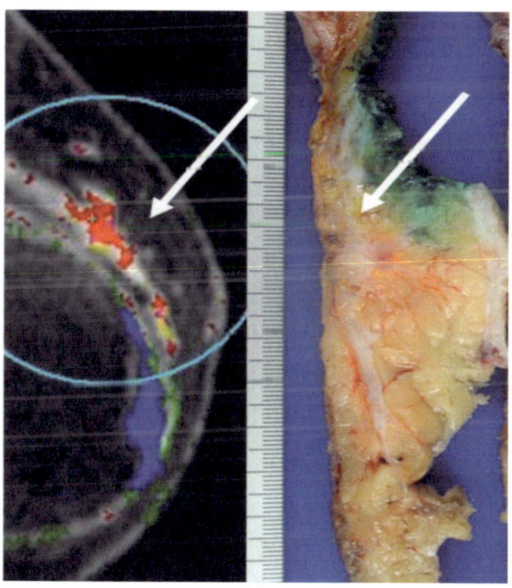

(c)

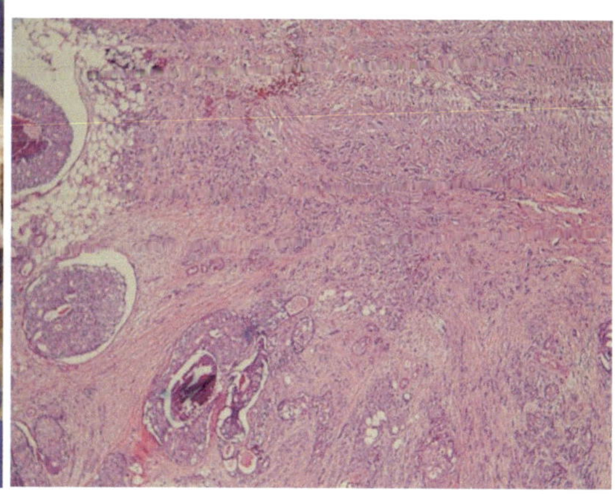

(d)

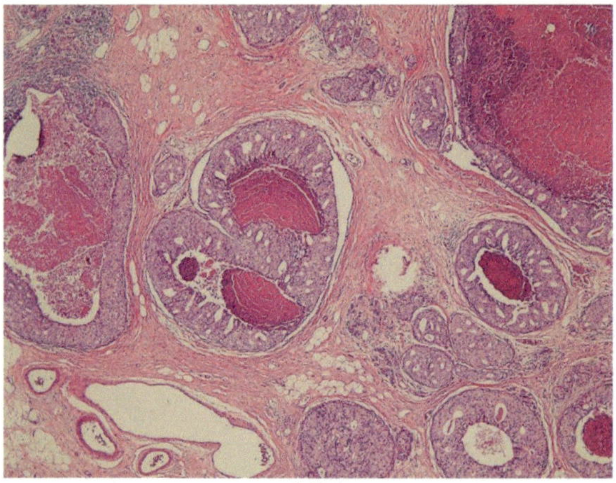

(e)

Fig. 19. (a) The breast MRI showed an ill-defined, non-mass enhanced area with red under color mapping, located in the deep superior anterior portion of the left breast (region1); the silicon implantation is showed by white arrow. (b) The breast MRI showed an enhanced focus with heterogenous red and yellow color mapping (marked by blue circle) at about 9 o'clock from the nipple of the left breast (region2); Blue area (by curved arrow) respresents intracapsular rupture within the implanted silicon bag (white arrow). (c) The mass (region1) of irregular red and yellow by color mapping (by white arrow) showed by DBMRI is corresponding to the excised specimen and is palpable as firm mass by surgeon (by white arrow). (d) Pathological results revealed a mass of invasive ductal carcinoma (IDC) on the region 1. (e) Pathological results also showed extensive high-grade ductal carcinoma in situ (DCIS) on region 2.

14. Reference

Agarwal, G., Pradeep, P.V., Aggarwal, V., Yip, C.H. & Cheung, P.S. (2007). Spectrum of Breast Cancer in Asian Women. *World Journal of Surgery,* Vol. 31, No. 5, pp. 1031-1040, ISSN 0364-2313.

Allergan. (2006). *Important Information for Women about Breast Augmentation with INAMED Silicone-Filled Breast Implants.*

American College of Radiology. (2003). *Breast imaging reporting and data system (BIRADS),* (fourth ed.), Reston, VA.

Amr, S.S., Sa'di, A.R., Ilahi, F. & Sheikh, S.S. (1995). The Spectrum of Breast Diseases in Saudi Arab Females: A 26 Year Pathological Survey at Dhahran. *Annals of Saudi Medicine,* Vol. 15, No. 2, pp. 125-132 , ISSN 0256-4947.

Azavedo, E. & Bone, B. (1999). Imaging Breasts with Silicone Implants. *European Radiology,* Vol. 9, No. 2, pp. 349-355.

Bone, B., Aspelin, P., Bronge, L. & Veress, B. (1998). Contrast-enhanced MR imaging as a prognostic indicator of breast cancer. *Acta Radiologica,* Vol. 39, No. 3, pp. 279-284, ISSN 0284-1851.

Boyd, N.F., Lockwood, G.A., Byng, J.W., Tritchler, D.L. & Yaffe, M.J. (1998). Mammographic Densities and Breast Cancer Risk. *Cancer Epidemiology, Biomarkers & Prevention,* Vol. 7, pp. 1133-1144.

Boyd, N.F., Rommens, J.M., Vogt, K., Lee, V., Hopper, J.L., Yaffe, M.J. and Peterson, A.D. (2005). Mammographic Breast Density as an Intermediate Phenotype for Breast Cancer. *Lancet Oncology*, Vol. 6, pp. 798-808, ISSN 1470-2045.

Buadu, L.D., Murakami, J., Murayama, S., Hashiguchi, N., Sakai, S., Masuda, K., Toyoshima, S., Kuroki, S. & Ohno, S. (1996). Breast Lesions: Correlation of Dynamic Contrast Enhancement Patterns on MR Images with Tumor Angiogenesis. *Radiology*, Vol. 200, No.3, pp. 639-649.

Chen, C.Y., Tzeng, W.S., Tsai, C.C., Mak, C.W., Chen, C.H. & Chou, M.C. (2008). Adjusting Mammography-Audit Recommendations in a Lower-Incidence Taiwanese Population. *Journal of the American College of Radiology*, Vol. 5, pp. 978-985.

Chung, K.C., Wilkins, E.G., Beil, R.J., Helvie, M.A., Ikeda, D.M., Oneal, R.M., Forrest, M.E. & Smith, D.J. (1996). Diagnosis of Silicone Gel Breast Implant Rupture by Ultrasonography. *Plastic and Reconstructive Surgery*, Vol. 97, No. 1, pp. 104-109.

Chuwa, E.W., Yeo, A.W., Koong, H.N., Wong, C.Y., Yong, W.S., Tan, P.H., Ho, J.T., Wong, J.S. & Ho, G.H. (2009). Early Detection of Breast Cancer through Population-Based Mammographic Screening in Asian Women: A Comparison Study between Screen-Detected and Symptomatic Breast Cancers. *The Breast Journal*, Vol. 15, No. 2, pp. 133-139.

Delille, J.P., Slanetz, P.J., Yeh, E.D., Kopans, D.B. & Garrido, L. (2005). Physiologic Changes in Breast Magnetic Resonance Imaging during the Menstrual Cycle: Perfusion Imaging, Signal Enhancement, and Influence of the T1 Relaxation Time of Breast Tissue. *The Breast Journal*, Vol. 11, No. 4, pp. 236-241.

Dorrius, M.D., Pijnappel, R.M. & Oudkerk, M. (2009). Breast Magnetic Resonance Imaging as a Problem-Solving Modality? *Imaging Decisions MRI*, Vol. 13, No. 3-4, pp. 126-129.

Dorrius, M.D., Pijnappel, R.M., Sijens, P.E., van der Weide, M.C. & Oudkerk, M. (2011). The negative predictive value of breast Magnetic Resonance Imaging in noncalcified BIRADS 3 lesions. *European Journal of Radiology*, in press.

Egan, R.L. & Mosteller, R.C. (1977). Breast Cancer Mammography Patterns. *Cancer*, Vol. 40, pp. 2087-2090.

Erguvan-Dogan, B., Whitman, G.J., Kushwaha, A.C., Phelps, M.J. & Dempsey, P.J. (2006). BI-RADS-MRI: A Primer. *American Journal of Roentgenology*, Vol. 187, No. 2, pp. W152-W160, ISSN 0361-803X.

Everson, L.I., Parantainen, H., Detlie, T., Stillman, A.E., Olson, P.N., Landis, G., Foshager, M.C., Cunningham, B. & Griffiths, H.J. (1994). Diagnosis of Breast Implant Rupture: Imaging Findings and Relative Efficacies of Imaging Techniques. *American Journal of Roentgenology*, Vol. 163, No. 1, pp. 57-60, ISSN 0361-803X.

FDA. (2004). *FDA Breast Implant Consumer Handbook.*

Gorczyca, D.P., DeBruhl, N.D., Ahn, C.Y., Hoyt, A., Sayre, J.W., Nudell, P., McCombs, M., Shaw, W.W. & Bassett, L.W. (1994). Silicone Breast Implant Ruptures in An animal Model: Comparison of Mammography, MR Imaging, US, And CT. *Radiology*, Vol. 190, No. 1, pp. 227-232.

Gram, I.T., Funkhouser, E. & Tabar, L. (1997). The Tabar Classification of Mammographic Parenchymal Patterns. *European Journal of Radiology*, Vol. 24, No. 2, pp.131-136.

Harris, K.M., Ganott, M.A., Shestak, K.C., Losken, H.W. & Tobon, H. (1993). Silicone Implant Rupture: Detection with US. *Radiology*, Vol. 187, No. 3, pp. 761-768.

Hartman, A.R., Daniel, B.L., Kurian, A.W., Mills, M.A., Nowels, K.W., Dirbas, F.M., Kingham, K.E., Chun, N.M., Herfkens, R.J., Ford, J.M. & Plevritis, S.K. (2004). Breast Magnetic Resonance Image Screening and Ductal Lavage in Women at High Genetic Risk for Breast Carcinoma. *Cancer,* Vol. 100, No. 3, pp. 479-489.

Hedén, P., Nava, M.B., van Tetering, J.P., Magalon, G., Fourie le, R., Brenner, R.J., Lindsey, L.E., Murphy, D.K. & Walker, P.S. (2006). Prevalence of Rupture in Inamed Silicone Breast Implants. *Plastic and Reconstructive Surgery,* Vol. 118, No. 2, pp. 303-308.

Holmich, L.R., Fryzek, J.P., Kjoller, K., Breiting, V.B., Jorgensen, A., Krag, C. & McLaughlin, J.K. (2005). The Diagnosis of Silicone Breast-Implant Rupture: Clinical Findings Compared with Findings at Magnetic Resonance Imaging. *Annals of Plastic Surgery,* Vol. 54, No. 6, pp. 583-589.

Hong Kong Cancer Registry. (2004). *Cancer Registry Annual Report,* Hong Kong SAR: Hong Kong Hospital Authority, Hong Kong.

Hoogerbrugge, N., Kamm, Y.J., Bult, P., Landsbergen, K.M., Bongers, E.M., Brunner, H.G., Bonenkamp, H.J., de Hullu, J.A., Ligtenberg, M.J. & Boetes, C. (2008). The Impact of a False-Positive MRI on the Choice for Mastectomy in BRCA Mutation Carriers is Limited. *Annals of Oncology,* Vol. 19, No. 4, pp. 655-659.

Huang, C.S., Chang, K.J. & Shen, C.Y. (2001). Breast Cancer Screening in Taiwan and China. *Breast Disease,* Vol. 13, pp. 41-48.

Jakes, R.W., Duffy, S.W., Ng, F.C., Gao, F. & Ng, E.N. (2000). Mammographic Parenchymal Patterns and Risk of Breast Cancer at and After a Prevalence Screen in Singaporean Women. *International Journal of Epidemiology,* Vol. 29, No. 1, pp. 11-19, ISSN 0300-5771.

Kolb, T.M., Lichy, J. & Newhouse, J.H. (2002). Comparison of the Performance of Screening Mammography, Physical Examination, and Breast US and Evaluation of Factors that Influence Them: An Analysis of 27,825 Patient Evaluations. *Radiology,* Vol. 225, No. 1, pp. 165-175.

Kriege, M., Brekelmans, C., Obdeijn, I., Boetes, C., Zonderland, H., Muller, S., Kok, T., Manoliu, R., Besnard, A., Tilanus-Linthorst, M., Seynaeve, C., Bartels, C., Kaas, R., Meijer, S., Oosterwijk, J., Hoogerbrugge, N., Tollenaar, R., Rutgers, E., Koning, H. & Klijn, J. (2006). Factors Affecting Sensitivity and Specificity of Screening Mammography and MRI in Women with an Inherited Risk for Breast Cancer. *Breast Cancer Research and Treatment,* Vol. 100, No. 1, pp. 109-119.

Kuhl, C., Weigel, S., Schrading, S., Arand, B., Bieling, H., König, R., Tombach, B., Leutner, C., Rieber-Brambs, A., Nordhoff, D., Heindel, W., Reiser, M. & Schild, H.H. (2010). Prospective multicenter cohort study to refine management recommendations for women at elevated familial risk of breast cancer: the EVA trial. *Journal of Clinical Oncology,* Vol. 28, No. 9, pp. 1450-1457.

Kuhl, C.K., Mielcareck, P., Klaschik, S., Leutner, C., Wardelmann, E., Gieseke, J. & Schild, H.H. (1999). Dynamic Breast MR Imaging: Are Signal Intensity Time Course Data Useful for Differential Diagnosis of Enhancing Lesions? *Radiology,* Vol. 211, No. 1, pp. 101-110.

Kwong, A., Cheung, P., Chan, S. & Lau, S. (2008). Breast Cancer in Chinese Women Younger than Age 40: Are They Different from Their Older Counterparts? *World Journal of Surgery,* Vol. 32, No. 12, pp. 2554-2561, ISSN 0364-2313.

Lee, C.H., Dershaw, D.D., Kopans, D., Evans, P., Monsees, B., Monticciolo, D., Brenner, R.J., Bassett, L., Berg, W., Feig, S., Hendrick, E., Mendelson, E., D'Orsi, C., Sickles, E. & Burhenne, L.W. (2010). Breast Cancer Screening with Imaging: Recommendations from the Society of Breast Imaging and the ACR on the Use of Mammography, Breast MRI, Breast Sonography, and Other Technologies for the Detection of Clinically Occult Breast Cancer. *Journal of the American College of Radiology,* Vol. 7, No. 1, pp. 18-27.

Lehman, C.D., Gatsonis, C., Kuhl, C.K., Hendrick, R.E., Pisano, E.D., Hanna, L., Peacock, S., Smazal, S.F., Maki, D.D., Julian, T.B., DePeri, E.R., Bluemke, D.A. & Schnall, M.D. (2007). MRI Evaluation of the Contralateral Breast in Women with Recently Diagnosed Breast Cancer. *The New England Journal of Medicine,* Vol. 356, No. 13, pp. 1295-1303.

Lehman, C.D., Isaacs, C., Schnall, M.D., Pisano, E.D., Ascher, S.M., Weatherall, P.T., Bluemke, D.A., Bowen, D.J., Marcom, P.K., Armstrong, D.K., Domchek, S.M., Tomlinson, G., Skates, S.J. & Gatsonis, C. (2007). Cancer Yield of Mammography, MR, and US in High-Risk Women: Prospective Multi-Institution Breast Cancer Screening Study. *Radiology,* Vol. 244, No. 2, pp. 381-388.

Leung, G.M., Lam, T.H., Thach, T.Q. & Hedley, A.J. (2002). Will Screening Mammography in the East Do More Harm Than Good? *American Journal of Public Health,* Vol. 92, No. 11, pp. 1841-1846.

Leung, T.K., Chu, J.S., Huang, P.J., Lee, C.M., Lin, Y.H., Chen, C.S., Tai, C.J. & Wu, C.H. (2010). Breast MRI for Monitoring Images of an 'Adenomyoepithelioma with Malignant Features', Before, During, and After Chemotherapy. *The Breast Journal,* Vol. 16, No. 6, pp. 652-653.

Leung, T.K., Huang, P.J., Chen, C.S., Lin, Y.H., Wu, C.H. & Lee, C.M. (2010). Is Breast MRI Screening More Effective Than Digital Mammography in Asian Women? *Journal of Experimental & Clinical Medicine,* Vol. 2, No. 5, pp. 245-250.

Leung, T.K., Huang, P.J., Lee, C.M. & Chen, C.S. Silicone Breast Implant with Intracapsular Rupture Coexisting with Locally Advanced Carcinoma. *The Breast Journal,* in press.

Leung, T.K., Huang, P.J., Lee, C.M., Chen, C.S., Wu, C.H. & Chao, J.S. (2010). Can Breast Magnetic Resonance Imaging Demonstrate Characteristic Findings of Preoperative Ductal Carcinoma In Situ in Taiwanese Women? *Asian Journal of Surgery,* Vol. 33, No. 3, pp 143-149.

Li, A., Wong, C.S., Wong, M.K., Lee, C.M. & Yeung, M.C. (2006). Acute Adverse Reactions to Magnetic Resonance Contrast Media--Gadolinium Chelates. *British Journal of Radiology,* Vol. 79, No. 941, pp. 368-371.

Liberman, L., Mason, G., Morris, E.A. & Dershaw, D.D. (2006). Does Size Matter? Positive Predictive Value of MRI-Detected Breast Lesions as a Function of Lesion Size. *American Journal of Roentgenology,* Vol. 186, No. 2, pp. 426-30.

Liberman, L., Morris, E.A., Benton, C.L., Abramson, A.F. & Dershaw, D.D. (2003). Probably Benign Lesions at Breast Magnetic Resonance Imaging Preliminary Experience in High-Risk Women. *Cancer,* Vol. 98, No. 2, pp. 377-388.

London, S.J., Connolly, J.L., Schnitt, S.J. & Colditz GA. (1992). A Prospective Study of Benign Breast Disease and the Risk of Breast Cancer. *Journal of the American Medical Association,* Vol. 267, No. 7, pp. 941-944.

Mann, R.M., Kuhl, C.K., Kinkel, K. & Boetes, C. (2008). Breast MRI: Guidelines from the European Society of Breast Imaging. *European Radiology,* Vol. 18, No. 7, pp. 1307-18.

Mariano, M.N., van den Bosch, M.A., Daniel, B.L., Nowels, K.W., Birdwell, R.L., Fong, K.J., Desmond, P.S., Plevritis, S., Stables, L.A., Zakhour, M., Herfkens, R.J. & Ikeda, D.M. (2005). Contrastenhanced MRI of Ductal Carcinoma *In Situ*: Characteristics of a New Intensity-Modulated Parametric Mapping Technique Correlated with Histopathologic Findings. *Journal of Magnetic Resonance Imaging,* Vol. 22, No. 4, pp. 520-526.

Maskarineca, G., Menga, L. & Ursinb, G. (2001). Ethnic differences in mammographic densities. *International Journal of Epidemiology,* Vol. 30, pp. 959-965, ISSN 0300-5771.

McCormack, V.A. & dos Santos, S. (2006). Breast Density and Parenchymal Patterns as Markers of Breast Cancer Risk: A Meta-Analysis. *Cancer Epidemiology, Biomarkers & Prevention,* Vol. 15, No. 6, pp. 1159-1169.

Menell, J.H., Morris, E.A., Dershaw, D.D., Abramson, A.F., Brogi, E. & Liberman, L. (2005). Determination of the Presence and Extent of Pure Ductal Carcinoma in Situ by Mammography and Magnetic Resonance Imaging. *The Breast Journal,* Vol. 11, No. 6, pp. 382-390.

Morimoto, T., Sasa, M., Yamaguchi, T., Harada, K. & Sagara, Y. (1994). High Detection Rate of Breast Cancer by Mass Screening Using Mammography in Japan. *Japanese Journal of Cancer Research,* Vol. 85, No. 12, pp. 1193-1195.

Mussurakis, S., Buckley, D.L. & Horsman, A. (1997). Dynamic MR Imaging of Invasive Breast Cancer: Correlation with Tumor Grade and Other Histologic Factors. *British Journal of Radiology,* Vol 70, No. 833, pp. 446-451, ISSN 0007-1285.

Nagata, C., Matsubara, T., Fujita, H., Nagao, Y., Shibuya, C., Kashiki, Y. & Shimizu, H. (2005). Mammographic Density and the Risk of Breast Cancer in Japanese Women. *British Journal of Cancer,* Vol. 92, No. 12, pp. 2102-2106.

Narisada, H., Aoki, T., Sasaguri, T., Hashimoto, H., Konishi, T., Morita, M. & Korogi, Y. (2006). Correlation between Numeric Gadolinium-Enhanced Dynamic MRI Ratios and Prognostic Factors and Histologic Type of Breast Carcinoma. *American Journal of Roentgenology,* Vol. 187, No. 2, pp. 297-306, ISSN 0361-803X.

Neubauer, H., Li, M., Kuehne-Heid, R., Schneider, A. & Kaiser, W.A. (2003). High Grade and Non-High Grade Ductal Carcinoma *in Situ* on Dynamic MR Mammography: Characteristic Findings for Signal Increase and Morphological Pattern of Enhancement. *British Journal of Radiology,* Vol. 76, No. 901, pp. 3-12.

Ng, E.H., Ng, F.C., Tan, P.H., Low, S.C., Chiang, G., Tan, K.P., Seow, A., Emmanuel, S., Tan, C.H., Ho, G.H., Ng, L.T. & Wilde, C.C. (1998). Results of Intermediate Measures from A Population-Based, Randomized Trial of Mammographic Screening Prevalence and Detection of Breast Carcinoma Among Asian Women: The Singapore Breast Screening Project. *Cancer,* Vol. 82, No. 8, pp. 1521-1528.

Ojo-Amaize, E.A., Conte, V., Lin, H.C., Brucker, R.F., Agopian, M.S. & Peter, J.B. (1994). Silicone-Specific Blood Lymphocyte Response in Women with Silicone Breast Implants. *Clinical and Diagnostic Laboratory Immunology,* Vol. 1, No. 6, pp. 689-695.

Paetau, A.A., McLaughlin, S.A., McNeil, R.B., Sternberg, E., TerKonda, S.P., Waldorf, J.C. & Perdikis, G. (2010). Capsular Contracture and Possible Implant Rupture: Is Magnetic Resonance Imaging Useful? *Plastic and Reconstructive Surgery,* Vol. 125, No, 3, pp. 830-835, ISSN 0032-1052.

Plevritis, S.K., Kurian, A.W., Sigal, B.M., Daniel, B.L., Ikeda, D.M., Stockdale, F.E. & Garber, A.M. (2006). Cost-Effectiveness of Screening BRCA1/2 Mutation Carriers with Breast Magnetic Resonance Imaging. *Journal of the American Medical Association,* Vol. 295, No. 20, pp. 2374-2384.

Ryu, E., Ahn, O., Baek, S.S., Jeon, M.S., Han, S.E., Park, Y.R. & Ham, M.Y. (2008). Predictors of Mammography Uptake in Korean Women Aged 40 Years and Over. *Journal of Advanced Nursing,* Vol. 64, No. 2, pp. 168-175, ISSN 0309-2402.

Saslow, D., Boetes, C., Burke, W., Harms, S., Leach, M.O., Lehman, C.D., Morris, E., Pisano, E., Schnall, M., Sener, S., Smith, R.A., Warner, E., Yaffe, M., Andrews, K.S. & Russell, C.A. (2007). American Cancer Society guidelines for breast screening with MRI as an adjunct to mammography. American Cancer Society Breast Cancer Advisory Group. *A Cancer Journal for Clinicians*, Vol. 57, No. 2, pp. 75-89.

Scaranelo, A.M., Marques, A.F., Smialowski, E.B. & Lederman, H.M. (2004). Evaluation of the Rupture of Silicone Breast Implants by Mammography, Ultrasonography and Magnetic Resonance Imaging in Asymptomatic Patients: Correlation with Surgical Findings. *Sao Paulo Medical Journal,* Vol. 122, No. 2, pp. 41-47.

Scaranelo, A.M., Marques, A.F., Smialowski, E.B. & Lederman, H.M. (2004). Evaluation of the rupture of silicone breast implants by mammography, ultrasonography and magnetic resonance imaging in asymptomatic patients: correlation with surgical findings. *Sao Paulo Medical Journal,* Vol. 122, No. 2, 41-47.

Schnitt, S.J., Jimi, A. & Kojiro, M. (1993). The Increasing Prevalence of Benign Proliferative Breast Lesions in Japanese Women. *Cancer,* Vol. 71, No. 8, pp. 2528-2531.

Shen, Y.C., Chang, C.J., Hsu, C., Cheng, C.C., Chiu, C.F. & Cheng, A.L. (2005). Significant Difference in the Trends of Female Breast Cancer Incidence between Taiwanese and Caucasian Americans: Implications from Age-Period-Cohort Analysis. *Cancer Epidemiology, Biomarkers & Prevention,* Vol. 14, No. 8, pp. 1986-1990.

Shibuya, K., Mathers, C.D., Boschi-Pinto, C., Lopez, A.D. & Murray, C.J. (2002). Global and Regional Estimates of Cancer Mortality and Incidence by Site: II. Results for the Global Burden of Disease 2000. *BMC Cancer*, Vol. 2, No. 37, ISSN 1471-2407.

Son, B.H., Kwak, B.S., Kim, J.K., Kim, H.J., Hong, S.J., Lee, J.S., Hwang, U.K., Yoon, H.S. & Ahn, S.H. (2006). Changing Patterns in the Clinical Characteristics of Korean Patients with Breast Cancer during the Last 15 Years. *Archives of Surgery,* Vol. 141, No. 2, pp. 155-160.

Szabo, B.K., Aspelin, P., Kristoffersen, W.M., Tot, T. & Boné, B. (2003). Invasive breast cancer: correlation of dynamic MR features with prognostic factors. European Radiology, Vol. 13, No. 11, pp. 2425-2435.

Thompson, J., Leach, M.O., Kwan-Lim, G., Gayther, S.A., Ramus, S.J.,Warsi, I., Lennard, F., Khazen, M., Bryant, E., Reed, S., Boggis, C.R., Evans, D.G., Eeles, R.A., Easton, D.F. & Warren, R.M. (2009). Assessing the Usefulness of a Novel Mribased Breast Density Estimation Algorithm in a Cohort of Women at High Genetic Risk of Breast Cancer: The UK MARIBS Study. *Breast Cancer Research,* Vol. 11, No. 6, pp. R80.

Tseng, M., Byrne, C., Evers, K.A., London, W.T., Daly, M.B. (2006). Acculturation and Breast Density in Foreign-Born, U.S. Chinese Women. *Cancer Epidemiology, Biomarkers & Prevention,* Vol. 15, No. 7, pp. 1301-1305.

Uchida, K., Yamashita, A., Kawase, K. & Kamiya, K. (2008). Screening Ultrasonography Revealed 15% of Mammographically Occult Breast Cancers. *Breast Cancer*, Vol. 15, No. 2, pp. 165-168.

Van Gils, C.H., Otten, J.D., Hendriks, J.H., Holland, R., Straatman, H. & Verbeek, A.L.M. (1999). High Mammographic Breast Density and Its Implications for the Early Detection of Breast Cancer. *Journal of Medical Screening*, Vol. 6, pp. 200-204, ISSN 0969-1413.

Venta, L.A., Salomon, C.G., Flisak, M.E., Venta, E.R., Izquierdo, R. & Angelats, J. (1996). Sonographic Signs of Breast Implant Rupture. *American Journal of Roentgenology*, Vol. 166, No. 6, pp. 1413-1419, ISSN 0361-803X.

Viehweg, P., Lampe, D., Buchmann, J. & Heywang-Köbrunner, S.H. (2000). In Situ and Minimally Invasive Breast Cancer: Morphologic and Kinetic Features on Contrast-Enhanced MR Imaging. *Magnetic Resonance Materials in Physics, Biology and Medicine*, Vol. 11, No. 3, pp. 129-137.

Scintimammography - Molecular Imaging: Value and New Perspectives with ^{99m}Tc(V)-DMSA

Vassilios Papantoniou, Pipitsa Valsamaki and Spyridon Tsiouris
University General Hospital "Alexandra", Athens
Greece

1. Introduction

Breast cancer is the most common non-skin cancer and the second leading cause of cancer death in women. Despite advances in the adjuvant treatment of early stage disease, many women will have breast cancer relapse that often is not amenable to complete surgical excision [Eubank et al., 2005]. There are 40,000 women per year dying of breast cancer in the United States, and most breast cancer victims die of progressive metastatic disease.

Currently, the detection and staging of breast cancer involves physical examination, fine needle aspiration (FNA) biopsy and imaging methods, namely mammography, ultrasonography, breast magnetic resonance imaging (MRI) and scintimammography. Screening mammography is widely available and evaluates patients with low cost, yet it bears a sensitivity ranging from 45% to 90% and low specificity, especially in cases of dense breasts, fibrocystic change and scars. Ultrasonography differentiates cystic from solid masses. Scintimammography by the use of various common radiotracers such as technetium-99m hexakis 2-methoxyisobutyl isonitrile (^{99m}Tc-sestamibi), ^{99m}Tc-6,9-bis (2-ethoxyethyl)-3, 12-dioxo-6, 9-diphosphatetradecane (^{99m}Tc-tetrofosmin), thallium-201 chloride (^{201}TlCl), ^{99m}Tc-methylene diphosphonate (^{99m}Tc-MDP) and pentavalent ^{99m}Tc-dimercaptosuccinic acid [^{99m}Tc(V)-DMSA], constitutes not only a complementary modality, but a significant method of choice in particular clinical settings, as summarized in Table 1.

Nuclear medicine methods enormously contribute to breast cancer clinical management due to the following reasons; (a) the recent technological advance in the detection and processing systems. Single photon emission computed tomography (SPECT) is progressively used more often in parallel with traditional planar scintigraphy with considerable improvement of the resolution and sensitivity of the scintigraphic image, mainly pertaining to lymph node involvement. The detection limit regarding malignant lesions approaches the corresponding one obtained by traditional radiological methods. Another important innovative improvement is positron emission tomography (PET), a technique which is based on the use of precursor metabolites (amino acids, hormones, monosaccharites), which are labelled with isotopes with very short half life that emit positrons. The pioneer characteristics of this technique enable the study of tumor biology accurately and non-invasively, providing interesting perspectives for research and clinical applications. PET is gradually used more extensively in oncology and seems to have particular value in breast cancer; (b) the introduction of new radiotracers has allowed the acquisition of images reflecting on biological and functional parameters that can characterize specific tumor features, like perfusion, mitotic and metabolic activity and receptor status. The significance of these parameters lies upon the fact that apart from defining the extent of the disease, they could also be regarded as prognostic indices of response to treatment and tumor behavior, and thus have major impact on designing and monitoring local and systemic therapy. Among the developed radiopharmaceuticals, the tracers described in Table 2 may play significant role in investigating breast cancer, with particular detection accuracy.

Traditional established indications
High-risk patients with difficult mammographic evaluation (dense breasts, breast structural abnormalities, implants)
Patients with multiple suspicious lesions or calcifications
Lobular carcinoma
Scars from previous biopsy visible on mammography
Palpable breast mass, not detectable by mammography or ultrasound staging
Evaluation of response to pre-operative chemotherapy
Detection of residual disease following mastectomy
Patients with palpable axillary lymph nodes with unknown primary focus
Novel clinical applications for ^{99m}Tc(V)-DMSA [Papantoniou et al., 2006-2011]
Patients with potentially premalignant mammary conditions (pre- and post-chemopreventive treatment)
Patients with increased serum CGRP
Selection of patients with metastatic breast cancer for treatment with ^{188}Re(V)-DMSA

Table 1. Indications for scintimammography

Nuclear medicine modality	**Radiopharmaceuticals**
Scintimammography: tumor-seeking tracers with specific metabolic features	^{99m}Tc-sestamibi, ^{99m}Tc-tetrofosmin, ^{201}TlCl
Scintimammography: tumor-seeking tracer with proliferation-seeking properties	^{99m}Tc(V)-DMSA [Papantoniou et al., Denoyer et al., Al Scheidauer et al.]
Hydroxyapatite crystals/amorphous calcium phosphate-seeking scintigraphy	^{99m}Tc-MDP
Lymphoscintigraphy	^{99m}Tc-labelled nanocolloids
Radioimmunoscintigraphy	Labelled monoclonal antibodies
Receptor scintigraphy	Labelled peptides with affinity for specific receptors
PET	^{18}F-FDG*

*^{18}F-FDG: fluorine-18 fluorodeoxyglucose

Table 2. Synopsis of nuclear medicine exams and tracers applied in breast cancer

Furthermore, during the past few years the scintigraphic recognition of mammary lesions retaining a considerable potential to progress to breast cancer has been introduced in association with risk factors involved in the carcinogenic process such as breast density (BD) and calcitonin gene-related peptide (CGRP) [Papantoniou et al. 2010b, 2011].

Specifically, ^{99m}Tc(V)-DMSA scintimammography in combination with mammography may substantially contribute toward the visualization of these lesions [Papantoniou et al. 2005-2007, 2010, 2011].

Considering that besides cytotoxic chemotherapy, various systemic options including hormonal and other biologically targeted therapies are now available, the detection potential of the imaging modalities currently employed at such early premalignant stages, is limited. Therefore, this review focuses on current and future applications of traditional scintimammography (planar and SPECT) and PET to breast cancer, highlighting the significant advantages, the clinically crucial role and the perspectives of molecular imaging by ^{99m}Tc(V)-DMSA scintimammography.

2. Scintimammography - molecular imaging

2.1 Scintimammography with γ-emitting tumor-avid agents

^{99m}Tc-sestamibi and *^{99m}Tc-tetrofosmin* are lipophilic cations which accumulate in the cell and in mitochondria due to the negative transmembrane potential. This happens mainly in cells with high-energy metabolism (and hence rich in mitochondria), including neoplastic cells. ^{99m}Tc-sestamibi imaging of breast cancer was first reported in a patient under investigation due to myocardial infarction [Chiti A et al., 1994]. As opposed to ^{99m}Tc-sestamibi, ^{99m}Tc-tetrofosmin mostly localizes within the cytosol, with only a fraction passing into the mitochondria. Nevertheless, considering that both tracers pass through an intact cell membrane, their cellular uptake and retention mainly reflects on the viability of lesion cells, their perfusion and their metabolic status, including cellular proliferative activity as a major driving force. Moreover, scintimammography using ^{99m}Tc-sestamibi/tetrofosmin is not influenced by mammographic limitations, like dense breast and scars. The method demonstrates 85-95% sensitivity and specificity regarding primary tumor imaging, although somewhat lower values are expected for non-palpable lesions and axillary lymph node invasion. In general, these two tracers present greater sensitivity than ^{201}TlCl. The method can help the surgeon localize the tumor during planning biopsy or surgery. In addition, sestamibi is associated with prognostic significance due to the correlation between radiopharmaceutical uptake and tumor angiogenesis or, most importantly, between tumor uptake and tissue P-glycoprotein expression, which is encoded by the multi-drug resistance (MDR) gene. P-glycoprotein is a membrane protein that acts as an ATP-dependent drug efflux pump, excreting anticancer pharmaceuticals and radiopharmaceutical imaging agents outside the tumor cell. Thus, prediction of P-glycoprotein-mediated response to anticancer agents is identified *in vivo* by sestamibi retention or efflux.

According to the scintimammographic protocol, the patient is asked to accommodate at prone position, in order for anterior, lateral and 30° posterior oblique images to be obtained. The latter projection is helpful for distinguishing lesions localized at the posterior breast segment from the ones at the thoracic wall and for axillary lesions. The planar images (10min/image) are acquired at 5-10 min and 60 min after intravenous (IV) injection of 740 MBq of radiotracer activity.

^{201}TlCl exhibits kinetic behavior as a potassium-analogue tracer and shows intense uptake in all proliferating cases with increased cell number. Planar scintigraphy, including anterior and lateral images, takes place 3 h post IV injection of 111 MBq of the tracer. This

radioligand is indicated in women bearing benign or malignant breast lesions, since it demonstrates a sensitivity of 80-96%. Its specificity varies from relatively poor, with a false-positive rate of 23% due to adenomas, to high (96%) in benign fibrocystic disease, which shows no ^{201}TlCl uptake. Unfortunately, the tracer appears weak in detecting axillary metastases with a reported sensitivity of only 57%. The study seems more suitable in the differential diagnosis of palpable lesions, providing useful indications for the selection of patients for biopsy, rather than pre-operative staging [Waxmann AD et al., 1989, Lee VW et al., 1993]. Of note are the unfavorable radiation characteristics of this tracer when compared to ^{99m}Tc-labelled compounds, with increased radiation burden to the patient and inferior image quality.

^{99m}Tc-methylene diphosphonate (MDP) is another radioligand applied in breast lesions and was first proposed by Piccolo S et al. (1995) reporting that a) in a portion of breast lesions MDP uptake with optimal tumor-to-background (T/Bg) ratio occurs a little after the radiopharmaceutical administration. This phenomenon could be attributed to the particularly increased tumor perfusion due to neo-angiogenesis and c) this it could be useful in the differential diagnosis of mammographically equivocal lesions, or in the diagnosis of lesions in dense breasts, in which mammography shows limited value. Protocol guidelines include image acquisition at anterior and posterior positions at 4 min, 10–20 min and 2 h post IV injection of 740 MBq of the tracer. Ninety-two percent of breast cancer lesions appear as a focus of ^{99m}Tc-MDP uptake in the 10–20 min-image, with mean T/Bg ratio: ~4.3, as opposed to the 2 h-image which is positive in 38% of cases. In addition, the method provides prognostic information by the traditional whole-body study identifying skeletal metastases.

2.1.1 ^{99m}Tc(V)-DMSA scintimammography

^{99m}Tc(V)-DMSA is a well-known tumor-seeking radiotracer with affinity for neuroendocrine and soft tissue tumors, such as medullary thyroid carcinoma and lung, breast, brain, and metastatic bone lesions [Ohta et al., 1984, Babbar et al., 1991, Kashyap et al., 1992, Hirano et al., 1995, Atasever et al., 1997, Lam et al., 1997, Kiratli et al., 1998, Papantoniou et al., 2002, 2004-2007, 2010, 2011, Denoyer et al., 2004, 2005, Tsiouris et al., 2007, Al-Saeedi, 2007]. These tumor-seeking properties have lead to the use of ^{99m}Tc(V)-DMSA in scintimammographic studies. In our studies the radiotracer is prepared using a domestically available kit (DMS(V)/Demoscan, National Center of Physical Sciences, Institute of Radioisotopes and Radiodiagnostics "Demokritos", Athens, Greece) labelled with ^{99m}Tc within our Department. Scintimammography is performed on a single-head gamma camera (Sophycamera DS7, Sopha Medical Vision International, Buc Cedex, France) equipped with a high-resolution, parallel-hole collimator and connected to a dedicated computer (Sophy NxT, Sopha Medical Vision International). The matrix is set at 256 x 256 pixels, and the photopeak centered at 140 keV, with a symmetric 10% window. Lateral and anterior prone early and late planar images (at approximately 10–20 and 60–70 minutes, respectively) are acquired after IV administration of 925 to 1,100 MBq tracer activity. Acquisitions are obtained using a special positioning pad (PBI-2 Scintimammography Pad Set, Pinestar Technology Inc., Greenville, PA). Breast radiotracer uptake in early and late images is first evaluated visually. Any focally increased accumulation is regarded as associated with invasive pathology, whereas any other pattern of a more widespread diffuse uptake has been found to correspond to pre-invasive lesions (ductal carcinoma *in situ* (DCIS), epithelial

hyperplasia) [Papantoniou et al., 2005a, 2006a]. Semiquantitative analysis is also performed. Radiotracer uptake area is calculated at the late (60-minute) images by drawing regions of interest (ROI) encompassing the total breast and the area of focally and/or diffusely increased tracer uptake in the lateral view; then the number of pixels within these two regions is divided. The aforementioned procedure is repeated in the anterior scintigraphic image, and the average tracer uptake area of these two views is considered the tracer uptake area of the breast under investigation.

Our research over the last two decades has been increasingly focused on the behavior, kinetics and properties of ^{99m}Tc(V)-DMSA in a variety of breast lesions, based on the postulation that breast cancer is the end-result of a continuum, i.e. a pathway leading to malignant transformation upon which intervention possibilities may emerge and early avoid disease development and progression. Therefore this research was initially limited on evaluating invasive ductal carcinoma (IDC) and was continued backwards through the pathway of malignant transformation, i.e. to include DCIS and to reach even some cases of the early stages of epithelial hyperplasia, occasionally representing a state of a so-called "activated" normal epithelium, which could eventually progress to a premalignant state and eventulally to malignant transformation, though lacking such evidence or suspicion on any available imaging modality or even biopsy. Based on *in vivo* scintigraphic studies, we advocated that its cellular uptake mechanism is closely related to cellular proliferation, as expressed by the Ki-67 immunohistologic index [Papantoniou et al., 2004-2006] and at the same time is independent from estrogen receptor (ER) status [Babbar et al., 1991, Kashyap et al., 1992]. It has been further demonstrated that the uptake of ^{99m}Tc(V)-DMSA is related to cell proliferation, focal adhesion kinase (FAK) activation, neo-angiogenesis and overexpression of several growth factors, including CGRP and platelet-derived growth factor (PDGF) [Papantoniou et al., 2005-2007, 2010, 2011]. Denoyer and colleagues elucidated the exact mechanisms; notably, the tracer reflects phosphate ion (Pi) transport and metabolism, entering cancer cells specifically via the type III Na/Pi co-transporter, this uptake being driven by the cellular levels of phosphorylated (i.e. activated) FAK, a keystone of accelerated proliferation [Denoyer et al., 2004, 2005].

With reference to the scintimammographic diagnostic yield, we have demonstrated that in cases of clinical and/or mammographic suspicion, both ^{99m}Tc-sestamibi and ^{99m}Tc(V)-DMSA exhibit high sensitivity (88.4%), specificity (93.3%), positive predictive value (PPV) (95%), negative predictive value (NPV) (82% & 80%), and accuracy for the primary lesion (90 & 89%, respectively). Notably, in lesions of less than 1 cm in diameter, the planar imaging sensitivity drops to ~75%, a percentage which is considerably improved by SPECT. Regarding lymph node involvement, the tracers have been reported to show 78.9% sensitivity and 86.3% specificity. Pre-invasive lesions, like DCIS and lobular carcinoma *in situ* (LCIS) are detected with high sensitivity by ^{99m}Tc(V)-DMSA, whereas with high specificity by ^{99m}Tc-sestamibi [Papantoniou et al., 2001, 2002].

Moreover, in breast cancer we have determined tumor size and Ki-67 as independent parameters of ^{99m}Tc-sestamibi and ^{99m}Tc(V)-DMSA uptake, respectively; hence tumors which accumulate ^{99m}Tc(V)-DMSA sustain increased cell proliferation and are in fact more aggressive [Papantoniou et al. 2002].

Relatively recent *in vivo* and *in vitro* studies have demonstrated that ^{99m}Tc(V)-DMSA possesses the potential to depict increased cellular proliferation, compatible with increased

Ki-67 expression, not only in IDC (Figure 1) but also in some cases of epithelial hyperplasia of the usual type and in pre-invasive mammary lesions like DCIS, independently of the presence of estrogen or progesterone receptors [Boyd et al., 1998, Papantoniou et al., 2004-2007, Denoyer et al., 2004, 2005, Tamimi et al., 2007]. Characteristic diffuse and intense ^{99m}Tc(V)-DMSA uptake is depicted in a case of usual ductal breast hyperplasia in Figure 2 (a) & (b), though no corresponding findings are observed by ^{99m}Tc-sestamibi (Figure 2 (c) & (d)).

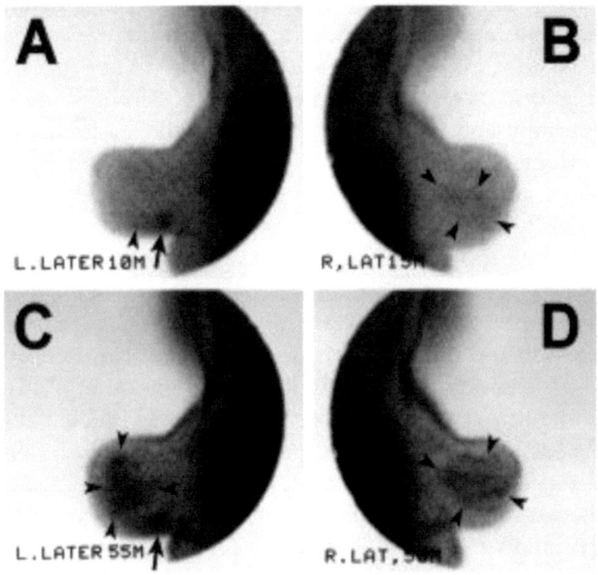

Fig. 1. ^{99m}Tc(V)-DMSA scintimammography (lateral projections) in a 58-year-old woman bearing a 2.5-cm, grade III, left-sided IDC with a coexistent 5-cm DCIS, both diagnosed histologically. **A**. The round-shaped focal tracer accumulation (arrow) corresponds to the invasive lesion and is noticeable since the early (10-minute) acquisition. Anterior to it lies a restricted, hardly visible region of diffuse tracer uptake (arrowhead). **B**. On the contralateral breast, there is also a rather faint extended area of diffuse uptake (arrowheads). **C**. In the late (55-minute) image, the focal ^{99m}Tc(V)-DMSA accumulation intensifies and its margins expand and become less sharply demarcated from the surrounding breast (arrow). The diffuse tracer uptake, corresponding to the *in situ* component, substantially increases and extends above and anterior to the invasive lesion, occupying an area of the gland seemingly normal on early imaging. **D**. Likewise, the inhomogeneous diffuse uptake area on the normal right breast becomes clearer and expands over time. No biopsy for histologic confirmation was performed on this breast; nonetheless, based on our experience from similar histologically-verified scintimammographic patterns, the finding is suspicious of representing a widespread pre-invasive lesion (DCIS and/or epithelial hyperplasia) [Papantoniou et al., 2007].

At the same time, our continuing research shed light to the intensified CGRP expression and neoangiogenesis in IDC with a coexistent *in situ* and/or hyperplastic component, in association with the tendency of the proliferation depicter ^{99m}Tc(V)-DMSA to image pre-invasive breast pathologies. The CGRP/^{99m}Tc(V)-DMSA correlation could be indicative of

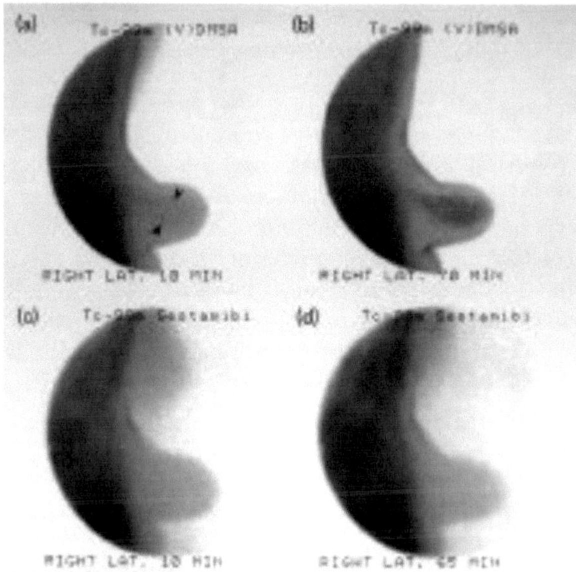

Fig. 2. Dual-tracer study in usual breast hyperplasia. Usual ductal hyperplasia of the right breast in a 68-year-old woman. Scintimammography, right lateral projection; ^{99m}Tc(V)-DMSA at (**a**) 10 min and (**b**) 70 min. Diffusely increased tracer uptake in the area corresponding to the lesion is observed, barely visible during early acquisition (arrowheads), but clearly perceptible at 70 min (lesion-to-background ratios: L/B_{early} =1.32 and L/B_{late}=1.83). ^{99m}Tc-sestamibi at (**c**) 10 min and (**d**) 65 min. No increased tracer activity is identified in the corresponding area throughout the study (L/B_{early}=1.12 and L/B_{late} =1.14). [Papantoniou et al., 2006b]. As a cell proliferation tracer, ^{99m}Tc(V)DMSA evaluates the invasive potential in a case of usual ductal breast hyperplasia, i.e. identifies mammary tissue with increased cellular proliferation, a state of so-called "activated" epithelium, which is related to Ki-67 expression and thus could provide some indication of its probability to progress towards atypical ductal hyperplasia, DCIS and IDC, i.e. the malignant transformation pathway upon which intervention possibilities may aid in early avoidance of disease development and progression.

an additional proliferative role for CGRP, possibly exerted through the PDGF/PDGF-receptor system. In this study, the preferential CGRP expression in low- rather than in high-grade IDC added support to the hypothesis of its precocious role primarily during the early stages of mammary malignant transformation [Papantoniou et al., 2007].

Furthermore, in a recent retrospective study we aimed at identifying a possible relationship between mammographic BD and scintimammographic ^{99m}Tc(V)-DMSA uptake in various breast histologies. We also investigated whether women with dense breasts, possibly expressing a proliferative potential, could be discriminated visually or on the basis of semiquantitative analysis of ^{99m}Tc(V)-DMSA uptake intensity and benefit from biopsy and possible proper chemoprophylactic treatment. Our findings support that increased BD correlates with the presence of florid epithelial hyperplasia and mixed DCIS+IDC but not with pure IDC or mild epithelial hyperplasia. Its close relationship to the proliferation-seeking ^{99m}Tc(V)-DMSA, which also showed an affinity to florid epithelial hyperplasia, indicates that stromal microenvironment may constitute a specific substrate leading to progression to different subtypes of cancerous lesions (i.e. DCIS+IDC) that are totally different from pure IDC originating from particular pathways.

In another prospective study of ours enrolling women with breast epithelial hyperplastic lesions, a relatively short (4-week) scheme of daily oral intake of the non-steroidal anti-inflammatory drug (NSAID) ibuprofen (400 mg) resulted in the reduction of diffuse ^{99m}Tc(V)-DMSA uptake (Figure 3) [Papantoniou et al., 2010]. Other recent studies have shown that cyclo-oxygenase-2 (COX-2) inhibitors may reduce the risk of breast cancer [Harris et al., 2006]. The biokinetic characteristics of ^{99m}Tc(V)-DMSA support our suggestion that the observed reduction in its uptake could be attributable to ibuprofen-induced COX inhibition and may indicate a "switch off" mechanism on activated FAK, rather than a slowing down of the proliferation rate *per se*. ^{99m}Tc(V)-DMSA cellular uptake is linked to FAK activation and cell proliferation, which is a precocious stage of malignant transformation [Papantoniou et al. 2004, Le Jeune et al. 2005, Al-Saeedi, 2007]. Compared to invasive lesions, the exact mechanism of ^{99m}Tc-(V)DMSA accumulation in benign proliferating diseases and in some non-proliferating diseases with higher lesion-to-background tracer uptake ratios is not yet clear [Papantoniou et al. 2004, 2006b]. Nevertheless, based on the imaging properties and biokinetic characteristics of ^{99m}Tc(V)-DMSA in relation to mammographic density and its ability to visualize potentially pre-invasive lesions, the clinical impact of various chemopreventive agents may be evaluated by quantifying their effect on ^{99m}Tc(V)-DMSA breast uptake.

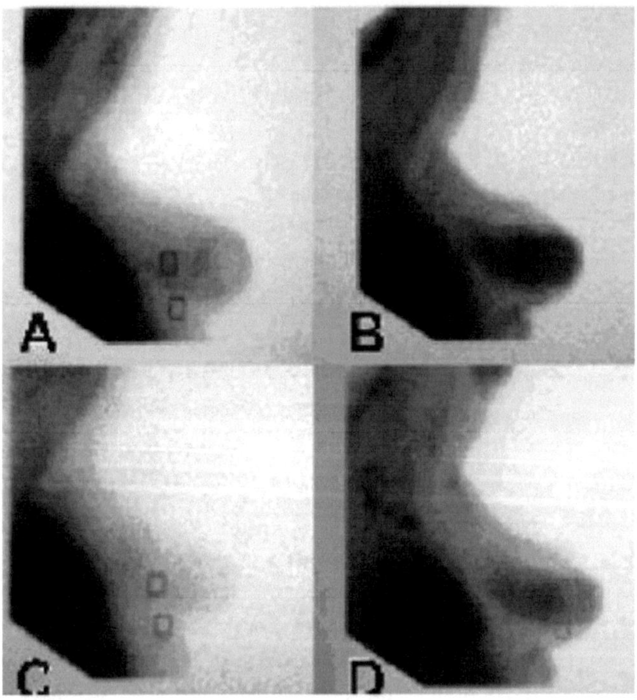

Fig. 3. Early (**A**) and late (**B**) images of ^{99m}Tc(V)-DMSA breast distribution at baseline and corresponding acquisitions after a monthly oral course of ibuprofen (**C** and **D**, respectively). After the NSAID treatment the diffuse tracer uptake is notably diminished on both early and late imaging [Papantoniou et al., 2010]

We also studied prospectively the variation of the serum neo-angiogenic neuropeptide CGRP levels in women bearing histologically confirmed benign and malignant breast lesions and evaluated its possible correlation with mammographic BD. Among the various lesions, including mild, florid and atypical epithelial hyperplasia as well as DCIS and pure IDC, women suffering from mixed DCIS+IDC demonstrated significantly higher serum CGRP levels, which also correlated with BD. These findings further support that DCIS+IDC represents a discrete pathological entity which is evoked by an interdependent mechanism between BD and serum CGRP expression. In addition, in the near future serum CGRP levels could constitute a useful pre-operative index regarding the nature and type of a mammographically suspicious lesion, in order for the proper therapeutic scheme to be planned, and potentially for the challenging innovative perspective of introducing adjunctive therapeutic administration of anti-CGRP peptides.

Finally, in advanced breast cancer stages, ^{99m}Tc(V)-DMSA uptake in metastatic lesions may guide therapeutic ^{188}Re(V)-DMSA administration, as propounded by Papantoniou and colleagues. Currently this protocol has just started being processed in collaboration with Djokic and colleagues (Vince Institute of Nuclear Sciences, Belgrade, Serbia).

2.2 Lymphoscintigraphy and lymphoimmunoscintigraphy

The development of distant metastases and breast cancer patient survival appear to be related to lymphoscintigraphic positivity [Casara et al., 1992, Uren et al., 1995]. Based on the used radiotracers, the following techniques have been applied:

i. Lymphoscintigraphy using labelled colloids. The used radiolabelled particles are 10-30 nm in size, pass through the extracellular space into the lymph capillaries and are then transferred by the lymph to the regional lymph nodes, to be recruited by macrophages. The colloids used are labelled with ^{99m}Tc and include antimony/sulphur/colloids, b) rhenium/sulphur/microcolloids and c) albumin nanocolloids.

   Protocol guidelines indicate injection of ~37 MBq radioactivity in the extracellular space (intradermal, subcutaneous or submucosal) and the injection site depends on the lymph node region under investigation. In breast cancer, the tracer is usually injected in the interdigital spaces of the hand when examining axillary lymph nodes, at the periareolar zone when intramammary lymph nodes are studied, parasternally by the xiphoid process in order for the internal mammary chain to be investigated, or intercostally or close to the tumor.

   For over the past decade the strategic importance of the pre-operative determination of lymph node invasion at the mammary region has encouraged the application of lymphoscintigraphy using colloids for lymphatic mapping and detection of the sentinel lymph node (SLN) (100% PPV and 96% NPV). Lymphoscintigraphy can be successfully applied in breast cancer management, if conducted intra-operatively by the use of γ-probe and in combination with blue dye; this technique can identify axillary lymph node invasion and through SLN detection may allow planning strategy and extent of the surgical operation [Krag et al., 1993, De Cicco et al., 1997]. Unfortunately, the method lacks adequate specificity. Therefore, particular attention has been paid to alternative methods:

ii. Lymphoscintigraphy using tumor-seeking tracers that can localize neoplastic tissue, like ^{99m}Tc-sestamibi, which localizes invaded lymph nodes with 80% PPV and NPV; and
iii. Lymphoimmunoscintigraphy using monoclonal antibodies (MAbs) administered IV, subcutaneously or directly into lymphatics [Khalkhali et al., 2001]. The first lymphoimmunoscintigraphic studies were performed in 1984 and since then various $^{123/131}$I, ^{111}In or ^{99m}Tc-labelled MAbs have been applied, including anti-breast MAb (^{131}I-RCC-1), MAbs raised against human milk fat globulins (^{131}I-anti-HMFG$_1$, anti-HMFG$_2$) and anti-carcinoembryonic antigen MAbs (^{99m}Tc- or ^{131}I-labelled anti-CEA, ^{99m}Tc-BW 431/26) [Thompson et al., 1984, Athanassiou et al., 1988, Kairemo., 1990]. MAbs approved by the United States Food and Drug Administration (FDA) include the anti-CEA and B72.3, prepared against the tumor-associated glycoprotein- TAG-72. In most cases, breast cancer cell lines produce CEA, although only a slight increase of serum CEA levels above normal may appear [Lind et al., 1991]. Regarding the detection of lymph node breast cancer metastases by arcitumomab, the commercially applied kit of anti-CEA MAb (CEA-Scan, Immunomedics, Morris Plains, NJ, USA), it has achieved 75% sensitivity, 83% specificity, 80% accuracy, 75% PPV and 83% NPV [Nabi, 1997, Goldenberg et al., 1999]. The method has not gained access into routine clinical practice though, because false-positive results are frequent due to tracer uptake by inflammatory lymph nodes, the technique is relatively complex owing to the slow tracer kinetics and biodistribution and the radiolabelled MAbs can hardly be obtained. Nevertheless the inherent biologic property of MAbs to accumulate selectively in the tumor as well as in metastases could be useful in both imaging and treatment of breast cancer. Specifically, "cold" or "hot" monoclonal antibodies may be applied therapeutically, with or without chemotherapeutic agents, thereby propounding significant changes in overall breast cancer management and survival [Stipsanelli et al., 2005]. Hence, further research may assist in most effectively applying lymphoimmunoscintigraphy to aid decision upon conservative or surgical approach, monitoring response to treatment and evaluating treatment regimes.

2.3 Radioimmunoscintigraphy

Radioimmunoscintigraphy may play a major role in the diagnosis of multifocal breast cancer by revealing residual or recurrent tumors, and also occult metastases. Several labelled MAbs, already mentioned above, have been hitherto used in breast cancer and new immuno-substrates continue to be proposed. The c-*erb*B-2 (also known as HER$_2$) oncogene receptor is overexpressed in 25%-30% of breast cancer cell lines and is associated with poor prognosis. The expression of the products of HER$_2$ oncogene in malignant mammary tissue and lymph node metastases has been studied *in vivo* by radioimmunoscintigraphy using anti-c-*erb*B-2 oncoprotein MAb labelled with ^{99m}Tc and has been targeted by "cold" or "hot" synthetic therapeutic immuno-agents. Specifically, the recombinant humanized "cold" anti-HER$_2$ MAb (or trastuzumab) has been widely used in the United States to treat breast cancer, either alone or combined with chemotherapy. Moreover, radioimmunotherapy comprises systemically administered MAbs, linked to high-energy, beta-emitting radionuclides, such as yttrium-90 (^{90}Y-BrE-3, ^{90}Y-m170) and ^{131}I- or ^{90}Y-labelled L6 antibody, yielding partial or rarely complete responses. Adjuvant peripheral blood stem cells transfusion prevents myelotoxicity.

Scintigraphic protocol guidelines suggest planar or SPECT imaging following tracer administration in the extracellular space or more often IV and rarely via an alternative route (e.g. intraperitoneally).

The higher PPV and NPV for anti-CEA-MAb SPECT as compared to mammography (100% vs 91% and 78%-80% vs 25%, respectively) allows for prompt biopsy or lumpectomy in MAb-positive lesions. High scintigraphic yield has also been reported for ^{99m}Tc- or ^{111}In-labelled m170 with 90% sensitivity, 93% specificity and 92% accuracy concerning the detection of both primary and metastatic breast cancer lesions measuring less than 1 cm in diameter [McEwan et al., 1994]. Similar results for breast cancer detection have been shown by the use of satumomab (OncoScint, Cytogen Corp, Princeton, NJ USA), which consists of 2 mg of B72.3 MAb labelled with ^{111}In [Nabi., 1997, Khalkhali I et al., 2001].

Overall, suggested applications of the technique do not mainly aim at diagnosing the primary tumor, but at identifying regional lymph node spread and distant metastases (bone and soft tissue), which are not otherwise visualized during pre-operative staging and at post-treatment follow-up.

2.4 Receptor imaging

Another radiopharmaceutical category of potential interest for imaging breast lesions comprises substances with high affinity for receptors. Receptor imaging may be applied in the diagnosis, staging, restaging, response to therapy and prognosis of breast cancer patients. Radiolabelled estradiol has been under investigation *in vivo* by traditional scintiscan (with 16-a,17-b-iodo-estradiol- ^{123}IE2) and by PET. In patients with suspected breast cancer, it has shown ≥66% sensitivity. Nevertheless, differential diagnosis of a lesion's benign or malignant nature is difficult to be based solely on this technique, mainly because fibrocystic breast disease is also characterized by ER expression [Scheidauer et al., 1991, Rijks et al., 1996].

An interesting alternative approach utilizes radiolabelled somatostatin analogues, e.g. ^{111}In-pentetreotide. Upon investigating 52 breast cancer patients, somatostatin receptor expression has been reported to reach 85% in ductal and 56% in lobular histologies; a total of 75% detection rate regarding the primary lesion, but only 30% sensitivity for axillary lymph node status. Overall, despite the *in vivo* breast cancer somatostatin receptor depiction, the method is inferior to the use of traditional ^{99m}Tc-labelled scintimammographic agents, owing to comparatively unfavorable dosimetry and cost-effectiveness [Van Eijck et al., 1994].

2.5 Other molecular metabolic imaging modalities: positron emission tomography (PET)

Initial PET studies on breast cancer were performed by Beany and colleagues in 1984. They demonstrated that breast tumors sustain higher perfusion than normal tissues and that despite the increased total oxygen consumption by the neoplastic tissue, oxygen extraction within the tumor is significantly decreased compared to normal tissues. Later on Mintun and colleagues described the visualization of primary tumors and a great percentage of lymh node invasion by the IV injection of steroid hormones labelled with positron-emitting nuclides, specifically ^{18}F-16-a fluoroestradiol (FES). Hormone receptor imaging constitutes a major functional approach of PET on breast cancer research. A subsequent study revealed 93% sensitivity for ^{18}F-a-FES in the detection of the primary tumor, metastases or relapse. At the same time, clearly decreased radiotracer lesion accumulation was observed in patients receiving anti-estrogen treatment. Thus, the ability to estimate and evaluate ^{18}F-a-FES uptake highlights the important role of PET on assessing breast cancer patients' response to endocrine treatment [Flanagan et al., 1996]. On the contrary, frustrating were the first attempts to depict progestin receptors (PgR) using fluoro-16a-ethyl-19-norprogesterone (FENP) labelled with ^{18}F. According to Dehdashti and colleagues (1991), the inherent radiotracer disadvantage is its non-specific uptake resulting in background uptake to the skeleton, normal mammary tissue and blood circulation. Other interesting PET radiotracers that may eventually allow for *in vivo* breast tumor characterization, comprise carbon-11 methionine (^{11}C-MET) as a tumor protein metabolism indicator; ^{11}C-thymidine or the most promising ^{18}F-fluoro-L-thymidine (FLT) as markers for cellular proliferation; ^{64}Cu-labelled peptide agonists of alphavbeta3 integrin as possible markers for angiogenesis; and ^{18}F-fluoromisonidazole as a marker for tumor hypoxia [Khalkhali et al., 2001, Chen et al., 2004]. PET studies retain the major advantage of true quantification of the radiotracer distribution.

The most widely used radiopharmaceutical in clinical PET is ^{18}F-FDG, a tracer focusing on the study of tumor glucose metabolism. Protocol guidelines indicate the IV administration of 370 MBq of the tracer to a fasting patient (blood Glu< 200mg/dL) with concurrent hydration and imaging after 60-180 min.

^{18}F-FDG-PET applications in breast cancer patients have attempted detection, staging, and monitoring treatment response. According to a large series, the sensitivity for detecting tumors less than 1 cm is reported to be 57%, compared to 91% for tumors larger than 1 cm [Avril N et al., 2000]. The sensitivity for detecting carcinoma *in situ* appears even lower at 25%. A significantly higher false-negative rate has been observed in infiltrating lobular carcinoma (ILC) compared to IDC (65% vs 24%, respectively), possibly due to a higher metabolic activity associated with poor prognosis. The specificity of FDG-PET in differentiating benign from malignant lesions approaches 90% in most of the studies, with the false positive results mostly attributable to inflammatory conditions. Overall sensitivity in the detection of the primary tumor has been reported to reach 80%-100% and specificity 75%-100%. The verified prognostic significance of FDG uptake in the primary tumor has yet to be clarified with reference to the driving biochemical mechanisms evoking enhanced glucose metabolism. Yet, based on various research reports, its proven accuracy in detecting the primary tumor and axillary staging, does not surpass its most important current clinical application, i.e. the detection and definition of the extent of recurrent or metastatic breast cancer and monitoring response to treatment. FDG-PET is complementary to conventional staging methods in terms of higher sensitivity in identifying metastatic nodal and lytic (or mixed) bone lesions (95% sensitivity and specificity vs. 93% sensitivity and 79% specificity by conventional imaging). Regarding distant metastases, PET appears to be more accurate compared to conventional staging modalities, with the exception of brain and osteoblastic bone metastases. Nevertheless, its sensitivity and specificity ranging from 57% to 100% and 66% to 100%, respectively in various series, PET cannot be a substitute for traditional staging by computed tomography (CT) and bone scintigraphy [Eubank WB et al., 2005]. The evaluation and follow-up of the response of metastases and locally advanced disease to treatment consists the mainstay of clinical PET in breast cancer. Precocious metabolic response, as compared to the delayed tumor size reduction, is demonstrated by FDG-PET, thus permitting earlier assessment of response to neo-adjuvant chemotherapy administered in locally advanced disease (after 1 or 2 cycles instead of 3 to 4 required by conventional morphological imaging modalities). This early metabolic amendment potentially indicates cancer cell resistance to apoptosis [Eubank et al., 2005].

2.6 Developing horizons

Small tumor size is perhaps the most significant limiting factor of conventional planar scintimammography. The development of small field-of-view, dedicated breast γ-cameras with high-resolution CdZnTe (CZT) detectors seems to contribute greatly to increasing the diagnostic accuracy of the modality even for lesions below the 1-cm range [Spanu et al., 2008, 2009].

Limitations of FDG uptake including small tumor size, increased breast density, more well-differentiated histologic subtypes (tubular carcinoma and CIS) and lobular carcinomas, have urged for technological improvements. The spatial resolution has been further enhanced with the introduction of the hybrid PET/CT scanner, which shows higher sensitivity and specificity than either PET or CT used separately.

Dynamic contrast-enhanced CT (DCECT) can measure the regional blood flow and volume along with mean transit time of blood through the capillaries and thus tumor perfusion. Combined FDG-PET/DCECT can assess not only tumor glucose metabolism, but also tumor vascularity.

These two parameters can be used in the differential diagnosis between benign and malignant lesions, assessment of tumor aggressiveness and prognosis, localisation of residual disease, treatment selection and follow-up, assessment of response to treatment and radiotherapy planning.

Furthermore, since PET using $H_2{}^{15}O$ for tumor perfusion evaluation is not readily available, the method has not entered clinical practice. Contrast-enhanced dynamic MRI and FDG-PET may obtain similar results, which seem advantageous over DCECT due to the lack of ionizing radiation and possible reactions to the IV contrast media.

In general, the coordination of multiple methods for breast imaging is expected to improve detection, diagnosis and clinical management of breast cancer patients. Detection and diagnosis of breast cancer may be based initially on mammography. Suspicious lesions should be elucidated by SPECT or PET and MRI, in order to avoid unnecessary biopsies. While PET differentiates malignant lesions by their most enhanced metabolic activity and thus intense imaging, MRI provides the exact morphologic information about lesion site, which is required for planning biopsy or radiotherapy [Baum, 2008]. In addition, maximal benefit from PET and MRI may be obtained by spatial alignment and fusion in a single image. Difficulties resulting from the soft and easily deformed tissue may be overcome by using identical patient positioning and fiducial skin markers visible in both PET and MRI, which should be taped to predetermined locations on the skin of the breast prior to image acquisition. By this technique, it is posssible to estimate marker and nodule motions based on surface and oncometric coefficients using specific software heat transfer module.

Another approach towards a better PET/MRI image utilizes PET/CT scanner. Synchronized CT and PET acquisition may permit further accuracy in corresponding breast sites in conjunction with MRI skin markers. Positron emission mammography (PEM) is conducted by concurrent acquisition using two planar detectors and a traditional mammographic system and its role in screening or diagnosis still constitutes a field under investigation, although it does sustain the potential capability of detecting smaller and less FDG-avid tumors than the conventional whole-body PET.

Finally, other SPECT or PET assessments using proper tracers may determine selection of treatment for breast cancer patients through: a) quantification of the therapeutic target by receptor imaging, radioimmunoscintigraphy and ^{99m}Tc(V)-DMSA-depicted cell proliferation in a CGRP-related neo-angiogenic background, introducing e.g. the ER (tamoxifen and letrozole), HER2 (trastuzumab [Herceptin]), EGFR (gefitinib [Iressa]) and angiogenesis factors (bevacizumab [Avastin]), considering that tumor expression may also be examined *in vitro* on biopsy specimens, b) identification of resistance factors, i.e. anti-HER_2 MAb-depicted HER_2 expression which evokes resistance to hormone therapy, ^{99m}Tc-sestamibi-depicted P-glycoprotein expression which denotes resistance to chemotherapy (doxorubicin, taxanes) and c) measurement of early response to treatment, as indicated by reduction of cell proliferation shown by ^{99m}Tc(V)-DMSA or ^{18}F-FLT.

3. Conclusion

In the era of rapidly developing technology, improvements in mammographic and molecular diagnostics appear promising, keeping up with the progress and corresponding demands raised by therapeutic oncology. The combination of multiple imaging methods (PET/CT, PET/MRI etc.) may concurrently evaluate both morphological and functional parameters and may directly influence the clinical management of patients bearing breast lesions, especially in recurrent or metastatic disease.

Scintimammography on its own is a simple, safe, non-invasive and widely available conventional nuclear medicine technique, which provides valuable multilevel information in the clinical management of breast lesions. The method visualizes the lesion site and also reflects specific biological and functional lesion features, including perfusion, proliferative potential, metabolic activity and receptor status. Thus, scintimammography represents not only a complementary method, but also a study of choice by applying the proper radioligand in the corresponding clinical background. It is noteworthy that the whole-body absorbed radiation dose for scintimammography is equivalent with that of mammography.

Current innovative scintimammographic findings using ^{99m}Tc(V)-DMSA and ^{99m}Tc-sestamibi add to our understanding of the process of malignant transformation, tumor biology and further propound individualized treatment strategy by improving our ability to depict and possibly quantify the therapeutic target, identify drug remission and resistance factors, measure and predict early response and possibly apply novel therapeutics such as ^{188}Re(V)-DMSA or anti-CGRP peptides.

Hence, the clinical impact of the recent scintimammographic findings could be of great value in terms of preoperative evaluation –on a molecular basis– of the extent and the nature of a suspected breast lesion, i.e. extent of the DCIS component in a mixed DCIS+IDC, lesion multicentricity or lymph node involvement. Furthermore, possible chemoprophylactic treatment with tamoxifen, aromatase inhibitors or anti-CGRP peptides in pre-cancerous lesions, or even prophylactic administration of NSAIDs in florid hyperplastic lesions could be considered in patients with diffuse breast uptake patterns on ^{99m}Tc(V)-DMSA. Finally, treatment with ^{188}Re(V)-DMSA in cases of advanced disease with osseous and soft tissue metastatic spread could be considered if these lesions are depicted by breast and whole-body ^{99m}Tc(V)-DMSA scintigraphy.

4. References

Al-Saeedi FJ. (2007). Role of ^{99m}Tc(V)-DMSA in detecting tumor cell proliferation. *Anal Chem Insights,* Vol.2, (2007), pp.81-83, ISSN 1177-3901

Atasever, T; Gundogdu, C; Vural, G; et al. (1997). Evaluation of pentavalent Tc-99m DMSA scintigraphy in small cell and nonsmall cell lung cancers. *Nuklearmedizin,* Vol.36, No.7, (October 1997), pp.223-227, ISSN 0029-5566

Athanassiou, A; Pectasides, B; Pateniotis, K; et al. (1988). Immunoscintigraphy with ^{131}I-labelled HMFG2 and HMFG1 F(ab')$_2$ in the pre-operative detection of clinical and subclinical lymph node metastases in breast cancer patients. *Int J Cancer,* Vol.41. Suppl.S3, (1988), pp.89-95, ISSN 0020-7136

Avril, N; Rose, CA; Schelling, M; et al. (2000). Breast imaging with positron emission tomography and fluorine-18]-fluorodeoxyglucose: use and limitations. *J Clin Oncol,* Vol.18, No.20, (October 2000), pp.3495-3502, ISSN 0732-183X

Babbar, A; Kashyap, R; Chauhan, UP. (1991). A convenient method for the preparation of 99mTc-labelled pentavalent DMSA and its evaluation as a tumour imaging agent. *J Nucl Biol Med,* Vol.35, No.2, (April-June 1991), pp.100-104, ISSN 0392-0208

Baum, KG. (2008). Multimodal Breast Imaging: Registration, Visualization, and Image Synthesis. *PhD Dissertation,* Rochester Institute of Technology, Chester F. Carlson Center for Imaging Science, 2008.

Beaney, RP; Lammertsma, AA; Jones, T; McKenzie, CG; Halnan, KE. (1984). Positron emission tomography for in vivo measurement of regional blood flow, oxygen utilisation, and blood volume in patients with breast carcinoma. *Lancet,* Vol.1, No.8369, (January 1984), pp.131-134, ISSN 0140-6736

Boyd, NF; Lockwood, GA; Byng, JW; et al. (1998). Mammographic densities and breast cancer risks. *Cancer Epidem Biomark Prev,* Vol.7, (December 1998), pp.1133-1144, ISSN 1055-9965

Casara, D; Rubello, D; Saladini, G; Masarotto, G; Calzavara, F. (1992). Significance of internal mammary lymphoscintigraphy (IML) in clinical staging and prognosis of breast cancer. *Eur J Lymphology,* Vol.3, (1992), pp.103-109, ISSN 0778-5569

Chen, X; Liu, S; Hou, Y; et al. (2004). MicroPET imaging of breast alphav-integrin expression with 64Cu-labelled dimeric RGD peptides. *Mol Imaging Biol,* Vol.6, No.5, (September-October 2004), pp.350-359, ISSN 1536-1632

Chiti, A; Maffioli, L; Castellani, M; Gasparini, M; Capri, G; Bombardieri, E. (1994). Case report: technetium-99m-hexakis-2-methoxy-isobutyl-isonitrile imaging of breast cancer and myocardial infarction in the same patient. *Tumori,* Vol.80, (1994), pp.480–481, ISSN 0300-8916

Dehdashti, F; McGuire, AH; Van Broclin, HF; Siegel, BA; Andriole, D; Griffeth, LK; Pomper, MG; Katzenellenbogen, JA; Welch, MJ. (1991). Assessment of 21-[18F]fluoro-16aethyl-19-norprogesterone as a positron-emitting radiopharmaceutical for the detection of progestin receptors in human breast carcinomas. *J Nucl Med,* Vol.32, No.8, (August 1991), pp.1532-1537, ISSN 0161-5505

Denoyer, D; Perek, N; Le Jeune, N; et al. (2004). Evidence that ^{99m}Tc-(V)-DMSA uptake is mediated by NaPi cotransporter type III in tumour cell lines. *Eur J Nucl Med Mol Imaging,* Vol.31, No.1, (January 2004), pp.77-84, ISSN 1619-7070

Denoyer, D; Perek, N; Le Jeune, N; et al. (2005). Correlation between ^{99m}Tc-(V)-DMSA uptake and constitutive level of phosphorylated focal adhesion kinase in an in vitro model of cancer cell lines. *Eur J Nucl Med Mol Imaging,* Vol.32, No.7, (July 2005), pp.820-827, ISSN 1619-7070

De Cicco, C; Cremonesi, M; Chinol, M; Bartolomei, M; Pizzamiglio, M; Leonardi, L; Fiorenza, M; Paganelli, G. (1997). Optimization of axillary lymphoscintigraphy to detect the sentinel node in breast cancer. *Tumori,* Vol.83, No.2, (March-April 1997), pp.539-541, ISSN 0300-8916

Eubank, WB; Mankoff DA. (2005). Evolving Role of Positron Emission Tomography in Breast Cancer Imaging. *Semin Nucl Med,* Vol.35, No.2, (April 2005), pp.84-99, ISSN 0001-2998

Flanagan, FL; Dehdashti, F; Mortimer, JE;, Siegel, BA; Jonson, S; Welch, MJ. (1996). PET assessment of response to tamoxifen therapy in patients with metastatic breast cancer. *J Nucl Med,* Vol.37, (1996), pp.99P, ISSN 0161-5505

Goldenberg, DM; Nabi HA. (1999). Breast cancer imaging with radiolabelled antibodies. *Semin Nucl Med,* Vol.29, No.1, (January 1999), pp.41-48, ISSN 0001-2998

Harris, RE; Beebe-Donk, J; Alshafie, GA. (2006). Reduction in the risk of human breast cancer by selective cyclooxygenase-2 (COX-2) inhibitors. *BMC Cancer,* Vol.6, (January 2006), pp.27, ISSN 1471-2407

Hirano, T; Otake, H; Yoshida, I; Endo, K. (1995). Primary lung cancer SPECT imaging with pentavalent technetium-99m-DMSA. *J Nucl Med,* Vol.36, No.2, (February 1995), pp.202-207, ISSN 0161-5505

Hirano, T; Otake, H; Kazama, K; et al. (1997). Technetium-99m(V)-DMSA and thallium-201 in brain tumor imaging: correlation with histology and malignant grade. *J Nucl Med,* Vol.38, No.11, (November 1997), pp.1741-1749, ISSN 0161-5505

Le Jeune, N.; Perek, N.; Denoyer, D. & Dubois, F. (2005). Study of monoglutathionyl conjugates TC-99M-sestamibi and TC-99M-tetrofosmin transport mediated by the multidrug resistance-associated protein isoform 1 in glioma cells. *Cancer Biother Radiopharm,* Vol.20, No.3, (June 2005), pp.249-259, ISSN 1084-9785

Kairemo, KJ. (1990). Immunolymphoscintigraphy with Tc-99m-labelled monoclonal antibody (BW 431/26) reacting with carcinoembryonic antigen in breast cancer. *Cancer Research,* Vol.50, Suppl.3 (1990), pp.949s-954s, ISSN 0008-5472

Kashyap, R; Babbar, A; Sahai, I; et al. (1992). Tc-99m(V) DMSA imaging. A new approach to studying metastases from breast carcinoma. *Clin Nucl Med,* Vol.17, No.2, (February 1992), pp.119-122, ISSN 0363-9762

Khalkhali, I; Maublant, JC; Goldsmith, SJ. (2001). *Nuclear oncology. Diagnosis and therapy.* 1st edn. Philadelphia: Lippincott Williams and Wilkins; (2001).

Kiratli, H; Kiratli, PO; Ercan, MT. (1998). Scintigraphic evaluation of tumors metastatic to the choroid using technetium-99m(V)-dimercaptosuccinic acid. *Jpn J Ophthalmol,* Vol.42, (1998), pp.60-65, ISSN 0021-5155

Krag, DN; Weaver, DL; Alex, JC; Fairbank, JT. (1993). Surgical resection and radiolocalization of the sentinel lymph node in breast cancer using a gamma probe. *Surg Oncol,* Vol.2, No.6, (December 1993), pp.335-339, ISSN 0960-7404

Lam, AS; Kettle, AG; O'Doherty, MJ; et al. (1997). Pentavalent 99mTc-DMSA imaging in patients with bone metastases. *Nucl Med Commun,* Vol.18, No.10, (March 1997), pp.907-914, ISSN 0143-3636

Lee, VW; Sax, EJ; McAneny, DB; Pollack, S; Blanchard, RA; Beazley, RM; Kavanah, MT; Ward, RJ. (1993). A complementary role for thallium 201 scintigraphy with mammography in the diagnosis of breast cancer. *J Nucl Med,* Vol.34, No.12 (December 1993), pp.2095–2100, ISSN 0161-5505

Lind, P; Smola, MG; Lechner, P; et al. (1991). The immunoscintigraphic use of Tc-99m-labelled monoclonal anti-CEA antibodies (BW 431/26) in patients with suspected primary, recurrent and metastatic breast cancer. *Int J Cancer,* Vol.47, No.6, (April 1991), pp.865-869, ISSN 0020-7136

McEwan, AJB; MacLean, GD; Goldberg, L; et al. (1994). Evaluating radioimmunoscintigraphy in patients with breast cancer (abstr.). *Eur J Nucl Med,* Vol.21, (1994), P748, ISSN 1619-7070

Nabi, HA. (1997). Antibody imaging in breast cancer. *Semin Nucl Med,* Vol.27, No.1, (January 1997), pp.30-39, ISSN 0001-2998

Ohta, H; Yamamoto, K; Endo, K; et al. (1984). A new imaging agent for medullary carcinoma of the thyroid. *J Nucl Med,* Vol.25, No.3, (March 1984), pp.323-325, ISSN 0161-5505

Papantoniou, V; Christodoulidou, J; Papadaki, E; Valotassiou, V; Stipsanelli, A; Louvrou, A; Lazaris, D; Sotiropoulou, M; Pampouras, G; Keramopoulos, A; Michalas, S; Zerva, Ch. (2001). ^{99m}Tc(V)-DMSA scintimammography in the assessment of breast lesions: comparative study with ^{99m}Tc-MIBI. *Eur J Nucl Med,* Vol.28. No.7, (July 2001), pp.923–928, ISSN 1619-7070

Papantoniou, V; Christodoulidou, J; Papadaki, E; Valotassiou, V; Souvatzoglou, M; et al. (2002). Uptake and washout of ^{99m}TcV-dimercaptosuccinic acid and ^{99m}Tc-sestamibi in the assessment of histological type and grade in breast cancer. *Nucl Med Commun,* Vol.23. No.5, (May 2002), pp.461-467, ISSN 0143-3636

Papantoniou, VJ; Souvatzoglou, MA; Valotassiou, VJ; Louvrou, AN; Ambela, C; et al. (2004). Relationship of cell proliferation (Ki-67) to ^{99m}Tc-(V)DMSA uptake in breast cancer. *Breast Cancer Res,* Vol 6, No.2, (2004), pp.R56-R62, ISSN 1465-5411

Papantoniou, V; Tsiouris, S; Mainta, E; Valotassiou, V; Souvatzoglou, M; et al. (2005a). Imaging in situ breast carcinoma (with or without an invasive component) with technetium-99m pentavalent dimercaptosuccinic acid and technetium-99m 2-methoxy isobutyl isonitrile scintimammography. *Breast Cancer Res,* Vol.7, No.1, (January 2005), pp.R33-R45, ISSN 1465-5411

Papantoniou, V; Tsiouris S. (2005b). In vitro verification of the correlation of in vivo ^{99m}Tc(V)-DMSA uptake with cellular proliferation rate. *Eur J Nucl Med Mol Imaging,* Vol.32. No.10, (September 2005), pp.1240-1241, ISSN 1619-7070

Papantoniou, V; Ptohis, N; Tsiouris, S; (2006a). Diffuse tracer uptake in scintimammography: not as nonspecific or benign as originally believed? *J Nucl Med,* Vol.47, No.3, (March 2006), pp.554-555, ISSN 0161-5505

Papantoniou, V; Tsiouris, S; Koutsikos, J; Sotiropoulou, M; Mainta, E ; Lazaris, D; Valsamaki, P; Melissinou, M; Zerva, Ch; Antsaklis, A. (2006b). Scintimammographic detection of usual ductal breast hyperplasia with increased proliferation rate at risk for malignancy. *Nucl Med Commun,* Vol.27. No.11, (January 2006), pp.911-917, ISSN 0143-3636

Papantoniou, V; Tsiouris, S; Sotiropoulou, M; Valsamaki, P; Koutsikos, J; Ptohis, N; Dimitrakakis, C; Sotiropoulou, E; Melissinou, M; Nakopoulou, L; Antsaklis, A; Zerva, Ch. (2007). The Potential Role of Calcitonin Gene-Related Peptide (CGRP) in Breast Carcinogenesis and Its Correlation With ^{99m}Tc(V)-DMSA Scintimammography. *Am J Clin Oncol,* Vol.30. No.4, (August 2007), pp.420-427, ISSN 0277-3732

Papantoniou, V; Sotiropoulou, E; Valsamaki, P; Tsaroucha, A; Sotiropoulou, M; Ptohis, N; Stipsanelli, A; Dimitrakakis, K; Marinopoulos, S; Tsiouris, S; Antsaklis A. (2010a). Reduced uptake of the proliferation-seeking radiotracer technetium-99m-labelled pentavalent dimercaptosuccinic acid in a 47-year-old woman with severe breast epithelial hyperplasia taking ibuprofen: a case report. *Journal of Medical Case Reports,* Vol.4, (March 2010), pp89, doi:10.1186/1752-1947-5-598

Papantoniou V; Tsaroucha A; Valsamaki P; Fothiadaki A; Karianos T; Archontaki A; Marinopoulos S; Pappas V; Syrgiannis K; Liotsou T; Sotiropoulou M; Tsiouris S; Stipsanelli A; Dimitrakakis C; Antsaklis A. (2010b). Mixed invasive ductal associated with *in situ,* but not pure invasive breast carcinoma, correlates with neoangiogenesis, increased breast density, calcitonin gene related peptide positivity and cell proliferation seeking radiotracer ^{99m}Tc(V)DMSA uptake. *Eur J Nucl Med Mol Imaging,* Vol.37, Suppl.2, (October 2010), pp.417, ISSN 1619-7070

Papantoniou, V; Tsaroucha, A; Valsamaki, P; Tsiouris, S; Sotiropoulou, E; Karianos, T; Marinopoulos, S; Fothiadaki, A; Sotiropoulou, M; Archontaki, A; Syrgiannis, K; Dimitrakakis, K; Antsaklis (2010c). Ibuprofen induces reduction of the proliferation-seeking radiotracer ^{99m}Tc(V)-DMSA uptake in severe epithelial breast hyperplasia without atypia. *Mol Imaging,* Vol.9. No.5, (October 2010), pp.233-236, ISSN 1535-3508

Papantoniou, V; Sotiropoulou, E; Valsamaki, P; Tsaroucha, A; Sotiropoulou, M; et al. (2011a). Breast density, scintimammographic ^{99m}Tc(V)DMSA uptake and calcitonin gene related peptide (CGRP) expression in mixed invasive ductal associated with extensive in situ ductal carcinoma (IDC+DCIS) and pure invasive ductal carcinoma (IDC): correlation with estrogen receptor (ER) status, proliferation index Ki-67 and histological grade. *Breast Cancer,* Vol.18. No.4, (October 2011), pp.286-291, ISSN 1340-6868

Papantoniou, V; Valsamaki, P; Sotiropoulou, E; Tsaroucha, A; Tsiouris, S; Sotiropoulou, M; Marinopoulos, S; Kounadi, E; Karianos, T; Fothiadaki, A; Archontaki, A; Syrgiannis, K; Ptohis, N; Makris, N; Limouris, G; A. (2011b). Increased Breast Density Correlates with the Proliferation-Seeking Radiotracer ^{99m}Tc(V)-DMSA uptake in Florid Epithelial Hyperplasia and in Mixed Ductal Carcinoma In Situ with Invasive Ductal Carcinoma but not in Pure Invasive Ductal Carcinoma and in

Mild Epithelial Hyperplasia. *Mol Imaging,* Vol.1. No.10, (October 2011), pp.370-376, ISSN 1535-3508

Piccolo, S; Lastoria, S; Mainolfi, C; Muto, P; Bazzicalupo, L; Salvatore, M. (1995). Technetium 99m methylene diphosphonate scintimammography to image primary breast cancer. *J Nucl Med,* Vol.36, No.5, (May 1995), pp.718–724, ISSN 0161-5505

Rijks, LJM; Van Tienhoven, G; Noorduyin, LA; De Bruin, K; Boer, GJ; Janssen, AGM; Van Royen, EA. Imaging of primary breast cancer with the estrogen receptor specific radioligand Z-[I-123]MIVE. *Eur J Nucl Med,* Vol.23, (1996), pp.1096, ISSN 1619-7070

Rijks, LJM; Bakker, PJM; Veenhof, CHN; Boer, GJ; De Bruin, K; Janssen, AGM; Van Royen, EA. (1996). Imaging of recurrent or metastatic breast cancer with the estrogen receptor specific ligand Z-[I-123]MIVE. *Eur J Nucl Med,* Vol.23, (1996), pp.1226, ISSN 1619-7070

Scheidhauer, K; Muller, S; Smolarz, K; Brautigam, P; Briele, B. (1991). Tumour scintigraphy using ^{123}I-labelled estradiol in breast cancer-receptor scintigraphy. *Nuklearmedizin,* Vol.30, No.3, (1991), pp.84-99, ISSN 0029-5566

Spanu, A; Chessa, F; Meloni, GB; Sanna, D; Cottu, P; Manca, A; Nuvoli, S; Madeddu, G. (2008). The role of planar scintimammography with high-resolution dedicated breast camera in the diagnosis of primary breast cancer. *Clin Nucl Med,* Vol.33, No.11 (November 2008), pp.739-742, ISSN 1536-0229

Spanu, A; Chessa, F; Sanna, D; Cottu, P; Manca, A; Nuvoli, S; Madeddu, G. (2009). Scintimammography with a high resolution dedicated breast camera in comparison with SPECT/CT in primary breast cancer detection. *Q J Nucl Med Mol Imaging,* Vol.53, No.3 (June 2009), pp.271-280, ISSN 1824-4661

Stipsanelli, E; Valsamaki P. (2005). Monoclonal antibodies: old and new trends in breast cancer imaging and therapeutic approach. *Hell J Nucl Med,* Vol.8. No.2, (July 2005), pp.103-108, ISSN 1790-5427

Tamimi, RM; Byrne, C; Colditz, GA; Hankinson, SE. (2007). Endogenous hormone levels, mammographic density and subsequent risk of breast cancer in postmenopausal women. *J Natl Cancer Inst,* Vol.99, No.15, (August 2007), pp.1178 -1187, ISSN 0027-8874

Thompson, C; Stacker, S; Salehi, N. (1984). Immunoscintigraphy for the detection of lymph node metastases from breast cancer. *Lancet,* Vol.324, No.8414 (December 1984), pp.1245-1247, ISSN 0140-6736

Toda, M; Suzuki, T; Hosono, K; et al. (2008). Neuronal system-dependent facilitation of tumor angiogenesis and tumor growth by calcitonin gene-related peptide. *Proc Natl Acad Sci U S A,* Vol.105, No.36, (September 2008), pp.13550-13555, ISSN 0027-8424

Tsiouris, S.; Pirmettis, I.; Chatzipanagiotou, T.; Ptohis, N & Papantoniou, V. (2007). Pentavalent technetium-99m dimercaptosuccinic acid [^{99m}Tc-(V)DMSA] brain scintitomography--a plausible non-invasive depicter of glioblastoma proliferation and therapy response. *J Neurooncol,* Vol.85, No.3, (December 2007), pp.291-295, ISSN 0167594X

Uren, RF; Howman-Giles, RB; Thompson, JF; Malouf, D; Ramsey-Stewart, G; Niesche, FW; Renwick, SB. (1995). Mammary lymphoscintigraphy in breast cancer. *J Nucl Med,* Vol.36, No.10, (October 1995), pp.1775–1780, ISSN 0161-5505

Van Eijck, CH; Krenning, EP; Bootsma, A; Oei, HY; Van Pel, R; Lindemans, J; Jeekel, J; Reubi, JC; Lamberts, SWJ. (1994). Somatostatin-receptor scintigraphy in primary breast cancer. *Lancet,* Vol.343, (1994), pp.640–643, ISSN 0140-6736

Waxman, AD; Ramanna, L; Brachman, MB. (1989). Thallium scintigraphy in primary carcinoma of the breast: evaluation of primary and axillary metastasis. *J Nucl Med,* Vol.30, (1989), pp.844–848, ISSN 0161-5505

4

Digital Mammography

Cherie M. Kuzmiak
University of North Carolina
USA

1. Introduction

Full-field digital mammography has transformed mammography over the past decade. The technology has reached a level of maturity that has caused an increase in its utilization in hospitals and clinics world-wide. This chapter will discuss the advantages and disadvantages of the technology as compared to screen-film mammography, a discussion on the basic physics of digital mammography and the currently available detector technologies. In addition to the technical aspects, this chapter will explore the clinical trials published to date regarding the technology performed compared to screen-film mammography in both screening and diagnosis, and evaluate the various imaging process algorithms that have been applied to digital mammography. Finally, digital mammography's impact on daily clinical workflow will be discussed along with future directions for this technology.

Digital mammography has become part of everyday clinical practice across much of the developed world. However, I find it interesting that most of the radiologists in training (residents and fellows) have no concept of what "film" is and was to our practice of mammography. They are used to the digital age of computers, personal electronic devices and electronic social networking through the internet. To the present generation, softcopy display in some form is a way of daily life. To others who have devoted their medical career in screening and in the diagnostic evaluation of women for breast cancer, it has and continues to be a learning and transitional process. In order to understand and fully appreciate the advances in mammography technology, it is important to understand the natural history of breast cancer and the challenges and changes that our specialty has undergone and how it continues to evolve.

Cancer of the breast is not a new disease. It has been present since ancient times and was documented by the early Egyptians, Greeks, Babylonians and Chinese (Bland, 1998). If a woman presented to her local "healer/physician" with a lump in her breast, treatment may have stemmed from charms and chants to applied ointments or possibly intervention with a knife and hot irons for cauterization. For women, treatment for breast cancer was similar for centuries and prognosis was generally poor.

It was not until 1913, when Albert Salomon, a German surgeon, evaluated 3,000 mastectomy specimens in a radiology-histological study on comparing the x-ray findings with microscopic pathology that it became evident to evaluate radiography technology for breast cancer detection. In the 1920's and 30's, several attempts to implement radiography for the diagnosis of breast abnormalities were done by O. Kleinschmit, W. Vogel, J. Goyanes, and

Gershon-Cohen; however, it was not until four decades later that the use of x-rays for the diagnosis of breast became more established (Picard, 1998).

The modern era of mammography began in the late 1960's as the technique was refined with dedicated equipment, such as that developed by the physicist C. Gros (Van Steen & Van Tiggelen, 2007). During this time, the film industry began to develop dedicated mammography film with high-quality images, reliable capture parameters and reduced radiation dose to the patient. Previously, a general x-ray tube with industrial film (low sensitivity) with high radiation exposure to the patient was used to image the breast. By the late 1970's and 80's, dedicated mammography was established, and mammography was identified as the most reproducible and cost effective modality to screen the general population. In clinical studies with follow-up of patients, it was shown that early detection of breast cancer has led to a reduction of the mortality rate (range 18-30%) (Elmore, 2005; Hendrick, 1997; Nystrom, 1993; Strax, 1973; Tabar, 2011).

It is estimated that 1.38 million women were diagnosed with breast cancer worldwide in 2008. This accounted for approximately a tenth (10.9%) of all the new cancers and 23% of all female cancers (Ferlay, 2010). Female breast cancer rates vary. The highest rates are in Europe and the United States and the lowest are currently in Africa and Asia. Currently, breast cancer is the second leading cause of death in the women of the United States (Center of Disease Control, 2010) and the United Kingdom (Ferlay, 2010). Because of these cancer-related deaths and the continued incidence of the disease worldwide, further emphasis has been placed on using mammography as screening tool for early detection.

2. Physics of digital mammography

2.1 Comparison of screen film mammography

Screen-film mammography (SFM) has been (and continues to be in some countries) the standard imaging modality for detecting suspicious lesions at an early stage in the breasts of asymptomatic women. Film is a very useful medium that has been optimized over the past 50 years. SFM has a high sensitivity (100%) in detecting suspicious lesions in breasts composed primarily of fatty tissue (Dujm, 1997; Saarenmaa, 2000). However, that value is significantly decreased in breasts composed of dense glandular tissue because breast cancers are frequently similar in radiographic density to the fibroglandular tissue. Consequently, 10-20% of breast cancers are not visualized (Burrell et al., 1996). Also, part of this decrease in lesion conspicuity may be due to the film itself since it serves as the medium of image acquisition, display and storage. After the film is exposed and processed, the image cannot be significantly altered and portions of the mammogram may be displayed with suboptimal contrast. Only slight improvements can be made with a "hot light" or magnifying glass. If improvements cannot be made, the patient may need to undergo another mammographic image and consequently be exposed to more radiation dose.

Another limitation of film is that different regions of the breast image are represented according to the characteristic response of the mammographic film. There is a trade-off between the dynamic range (latitude) and contrast resolution (gradient). This is illustrated in Figure 1 by the sigmoid Hurter and Driffield (H&D) curve that is characteristic for a given type of SFM system under specific conditions. The H&D curve demonstrates the relationship between x-ray exposure, image density and contrast (Feig & Yaffe, 1998).

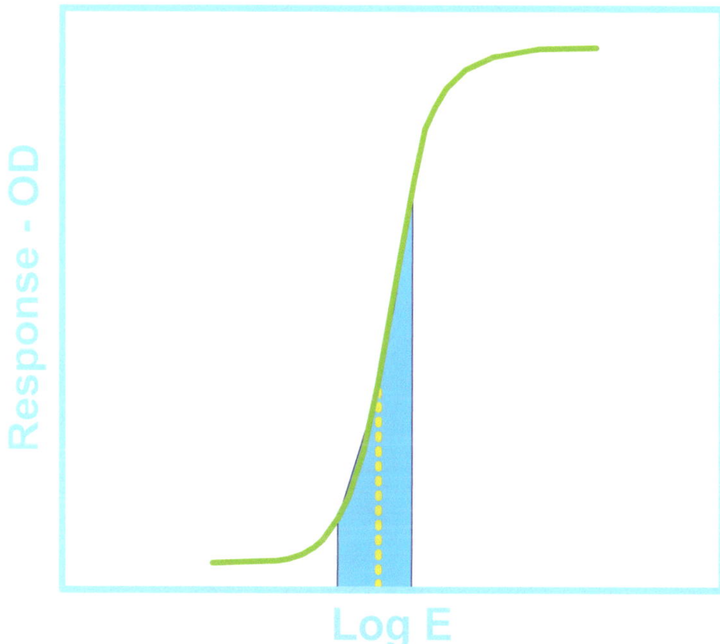

Fig. 1. Hurter and Driffield (H&D) curve for a SFM system where Log E represents the relative exposure and OD is the optical density.

With the limited range of soft-tissue densities in the breast, mammography requires high contrast. The fixed characteristics of an H&D curve mean that if high contrast is to be obtained in intermediate-density tissue, there must be lower contrast within the thicker, denser fibroglandular tissues represented at the toe of the curve and the fatty tissue represented at the shoulder of the curve (Feig & Yaffe, 1998). Consequently, mammographic film has a limited dynamic range.

Digital mammography offers several advantages over SFM. The digital system separates the process of x-ray detection from image display and storage. Since image acquisition and display are separated, each can be optimized. Digital detectors have a wider dynamic range (linear response) compared to film as seen in Figure 2. Digital detectors have increased efficiency at a lower radiation dose in the detection and depiction of the x-ray photons compared to film (Pisano, 1998; Feig, 1996). In addition, digital detectors (even with a lower spatial resolution than film) also appear to improve lesion conspicuity through their improved efficiency of absorption of x-ray photons, a linear response over a wide range of radiation intensities and low system noise (Feig & Yaffe, 1998). Plus, post-processing software can be utilized to assist the radiologist in evaluating the images for suspicious findings by altering contrast and brightness automatically or manually. With digital mammography, computer aided detection software can be utilized at a push of a button instead of waiting for someone to digitize the film images for each case. With digital mammography, the images can be displayed with hard and softcopy formats.

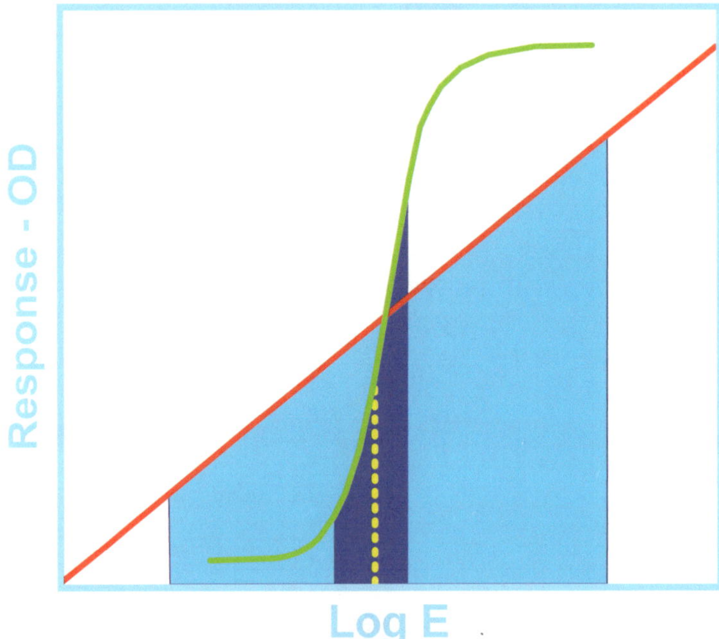

Fig. 2. Digital detectors have a linear response and wide dynamic range compared to SFM. The digital response is seen as the diagonal line. Log E represents the relative exposure and OD is the optical density.

2.2 Image acquisition

To obtain a mammographic image, x-rays must be generated from a target. A metal filter in the system will remove the majority of non-desirable energies of the beam before it enters the patient. In a SFM system, the automatic exposure control (AEC) will end the film exposure when the tissue above the AEC has transmitted a suitable number of x-rays to expose the film where its gradient (slope of the H&D curve) will be near or at its maximum value and there will be acceptable image brightness (Yaffe, in Bick & Diekmann, 2010). However, other areas of the breast may be suboptimally exposed - dense areas underexposed. In the SFM system, the intensifying screen produces light that is proportional to the amount of energy deposited by the x-rays. The now exposed film will be chemically processed to produce the permanent mammographic image of the different optical densities. The mammographic film serves the three roles of image acquisition, display and storage.

In digital mammography, a detector replaces the screen-film system. The detector will still be exposed to x-rays just as in a SFM system. The detector produces a signal that is linearly proportional to the intensity of the photons transmitted by the breast; therefore, it is possible to produce a better representation of the x-ray transmission of all parts of the breast (Feig & Yaffe, 1998). For digital mammography, AEC still plays a role. Unlike SFM where it was important in determining image contrast, in digital mammography the AEC aids in obtaining a predetermined signal-to-noise ratio and a reasonable radiation dose to the breast. After being exposed, the digital detector produces an electronic signal that is digitized and stored. With digital mammography, wet chemical processing is eliminated and the detector's only role is image acquisition. Another added benefit of a digital detector is the elimination of film granularity that adds noise to a system.

2.3 Properties of digital images

Spatial resolution in SFM is commonly based on the limiting resolution in terms of line-pairs/mm from a bar pattern, Figure 3. This test can be very subjective. Therefore, in order to evaluate spatial resolution more quantitatively, it can be evaluated with the modulation transfer function (MTF). The MTF describes how well the entire imaging system or one of its components is performing in the form of a sinusoidal shape (Bunch, 1987; Pisano, 2004). The MTF describes how well each spatial frequency is transferred through a system. The MTF of a system is the product of the MTFs of the components of each system. As seen in Figure 4, at low spatial frequencies the MTF value is at or near the value of 1.0 and the MTF value decreases with increasing spatial frequency. The MTF of SFM extends beyond 20 cycles/mm and it is predominately the result of the screen since film has a very high MTF (Pisano et al., 2004). In a digital system, the MTF will be based on the focal spot, patient motion, lateral spread of signal (light or electronic charges) in the detector, and spatial sampling.

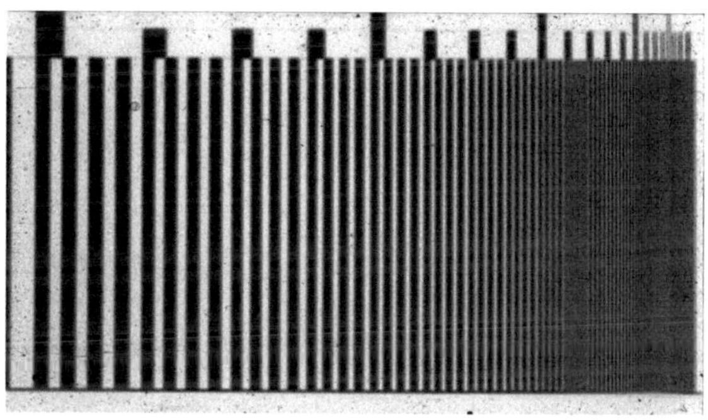

Fig. 3. Bar pattern of line-pairs/mm for determining spatial resolution for SFM.

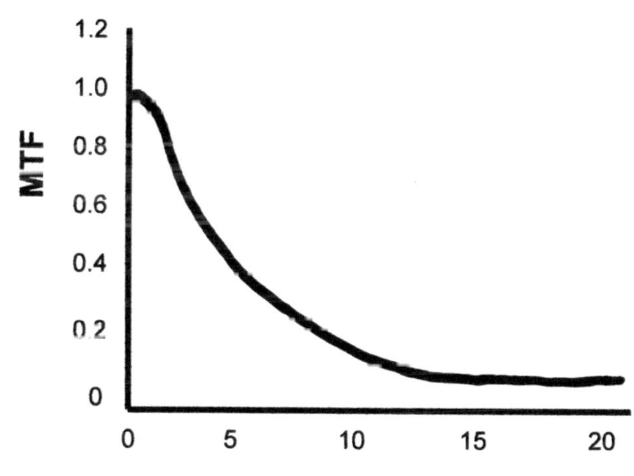

Fig. 4. Modulation Transfer Function (MTF) of a screen film system.

Spatial sampling is unique to digital mammography and affects resolution. The signal from each detector element (del) is averaged over the sensitive region or aperture (d). This will result in a decrease of the MTF of a detector (Pisano et al., 2004). The size of the del will supply the information displayed in one pixel. Dels can range from ~ 44 to 100 µm (0.04-0.1 mm). Dels are arranged with a specified center-to-center distance or pitch (p), Figure 5. If the pitch is too large, information will be lost in the sampling process.

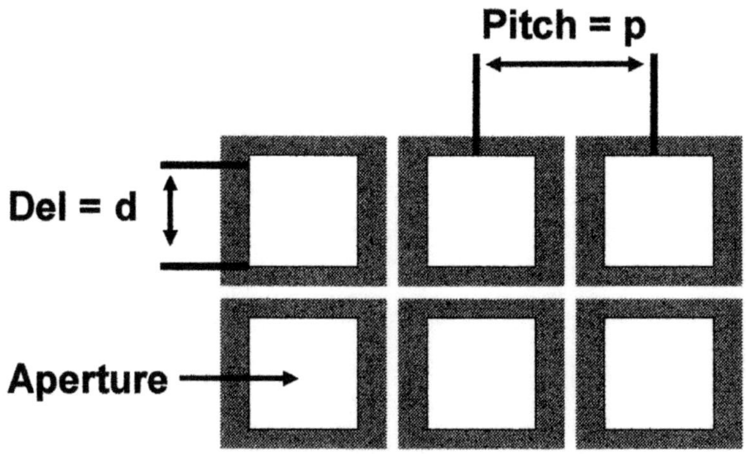

Fig. 5. Example of a detector composed of detector elements (d) that contain a sensitive region called the aperture. The distance between the centers of dels is the pitch (p).

2.4 Radiation dose

The flexibility of digital with decoupling allows for decreased radiation dose compared to SFM. Several factors account for this decreased dose. First, image brightness (display) is now independent of acquisition. Since brightness is not dependent on the amount of x-ray exposure needed to produce the image, it allows the user to determine the dose selection. Secondly, digital detectors have higher detective quantum efficiency with decreased signal-to-noise-ratios than a SFM image receptor (Pisano et al., 2004). Consequently, a more penetrating x-ray beam can be used with digital mammography, and this result in a lower patient dose. Currently, some digital mammography systems have dose reductions of 25-30% compared with SFM (Heddson, 2007; Hendrick, 2010; Yaffe, in Bick & Diekmann, 2010).

3. Digital mammography detectors

The detector is one of the key components of a digital mammography system. It produces an electronic signal that represents the pattern of x-rays transmitted by the breast. Optimally, a detector should include the entire range of x-ray intensities transmitted by different areas of the breast without loss of information. Besides the detector interacting with x-rays transmitted by the breast and absorption of the energy carried by the x-rays, it performs several other important functions. These other functions (in order) include: conversation of the transmitted and absorbed energy to a usable signal (light or electronic charge), collection of this signal, secondary conversion if needed (phosphor-based detectors), readout of the charge, amplification, and finally digitization of the information (Pisano et al., 2004; Yaffe, in

Bick & Diekmann, 2010). To provide high quality images, all of these steps need to be optimized. As a result, detectors are characterized by their quantum efficiency, sensitivity, spatial resolution, noise, dynamic range and linearity of response.

3.1 Quantum efficiency & noise

Quantum interaction efficiency describes the quantity of x-rays that reach the detector and interacts with it to produce signal. The quantum interaction efficiency of a detector can be increased by increasing the thickness of the detector. However, quantum interaction efficiency can be reduced by using higher energies since this will decrease the x-ray attenuation coefficient (Pisano et al., 2004). An exception to this is when the x-ray energy exceeds an absorption edge of the detector material, as in CsI. Thus, quantum detection efficiency will influence the sensitivity of detector. Detector sensitivity will also be dependent on the amount of energy required to produce an electron or light quantum to be measured¸ the efficiency of signal collection and measurement of the charge produced (Yaffe, in Bick & Diekmann, 2010).

Quantum noise (or mottle) is the result of random fluctuation in the x-ray beam. It is independent of breast density composition. Quantum noise can be statistically described by the Poisson distribution (Pisano et al., 2004). To decrease the quantum noise of an image (increase the signal-to-noise ratio), the amount of x-rays absorbed by the detector have to be increased. This can be performed by using a detector with better quantum detection efficiency or by increasing exposure (mAs).

Another source of fluctuation or noise that decreases image quality is structural noise. With the use of a detector, digital mammography has eliminated the structural noise of film granularity (random structure of the grains of silver halide) (Bunch, in Van Metter & Beutel, 1997) However, in digital mammography there is some structural difference across the detector and this is associated with spatial variations in detector sensitivity. Because these differences may remain constant over time, they do no represent traditional noise. In digital mammography this is referred to as "fixed pattern noise" or "structural noise". Through the use of image correction with flat-fielding or gain correction this can be removed as seen in Figure 6.

3.2 Detector systems

There are two main types of digital mammography imaging systems. One type uses a full-field detector to be imaged, Figure 7. The detector in this system is stationary and the system may utilize a grid to remove x ray scatter, thereby increasing the signal-to-noise ratio. The second major type of digital mammography system is a scanned-slot device that uses a detector rectangular in shape, Figure 8. The detector in this type of mammography system scans/moves across the inferior portion of the breast support at the same time a collimated x-ray beam moves during the image acquisition. The detector and the x-ray beam move in synchrony. In this latter type of system, no grid is needed since there is less scatter radiation from a narrower x-ray beam. Regardless of system type, it is important that the system is able to image as close to the chest wall as possible and for the system to accommodate all breasts sizes.

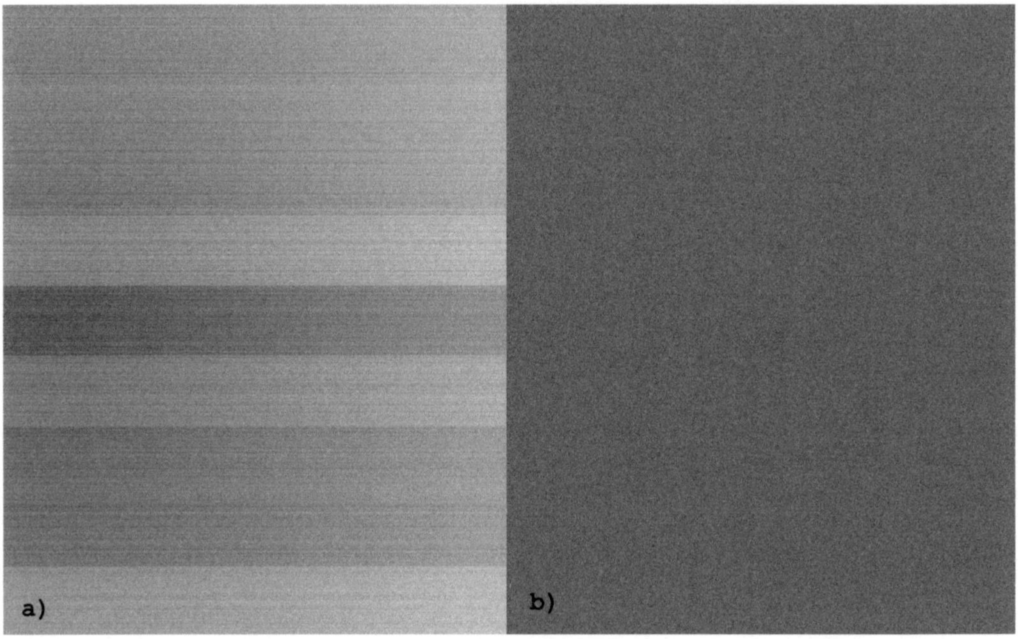

Fig. 6. Example of flat-field correction. a) Uncorrected image. b) Image after flat-field correction. Courtesy of Martin Yaffe, PhD; Sunnybrook Health Sciences Centre, Toronto, Canada. (from Digital Mammography, eds. ED Pisano, MJ Yaffe, CM Kuzmiak. Lippincott, Williams & Wilkins, a Walters Kluwer Company, 2004. With permission.)

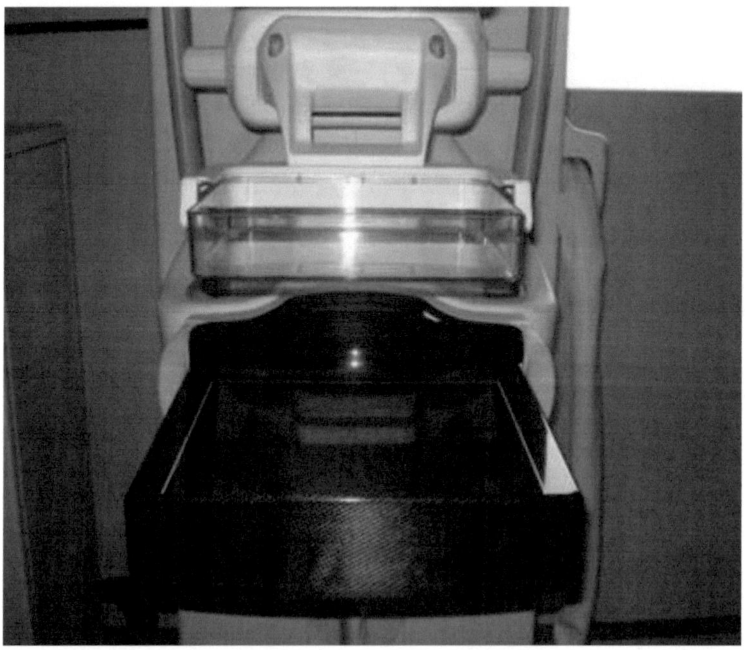

Fig. 7. Example of a FFDM detector system. Pictured is the General Electric Senographe Essential.

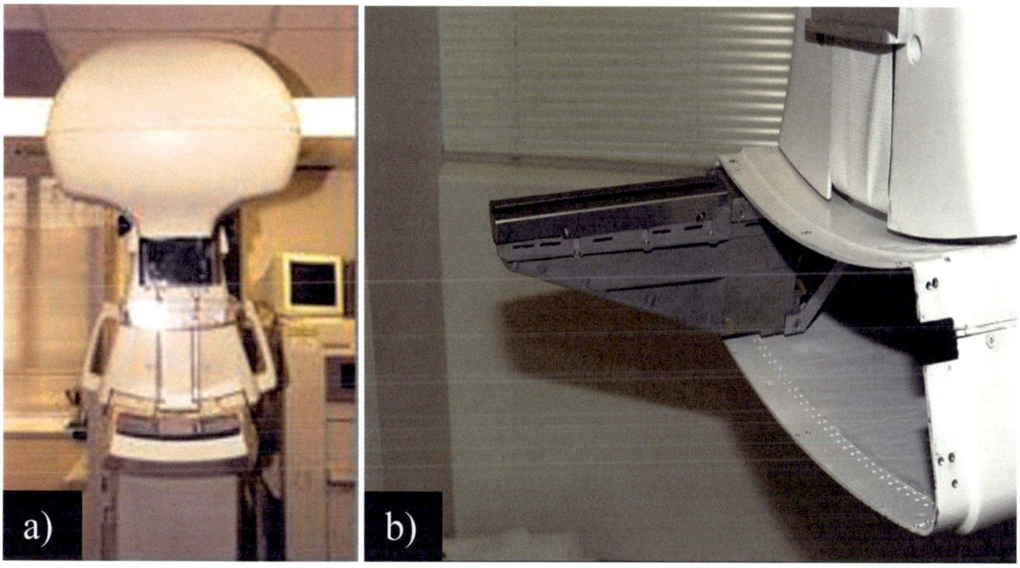

Fig. 8. Example of a scanned-slot digital mammography system. a) Pictured is a Fisher SenoScan mammography unit. b) Image of the detector.

3.3 Detector types

Many different types of detectors are used for digital mammography and these will be briefly described in this section. The first four discussed are used in direct radiography (DR) mammography systems and the last one is used in a computed radiography (CR) system.

3.3.1 Phosphor flat panel

A phosphor flat panel detector, Figure 9, is constructed of a plate of amorphous silicon. Through solid-state manufacturing, a rectangular array of light-sensitive photodiodes with a layer of thallium-activated cesium iodide phosphor, CsI (Tl) are deposited onto the plate. The photodiodes are the dels of the detector. These dels will detect the light emitted by the phosphor and create and store an electric charge.

Besides each del containing a photodiode, it also contains a thin film transistor (TFT) switch, and these are interconnected with an array of control and data lines. A readout line is present along each column of the detector, and when a control line is activated it activates all the TFTs in that row (Yaffe, in Bick & Diekmann, 2010). The signal from the row of activated dels is then transferred to an amplifier and digitizer. The digitized information from one del will represent the information corresponding to a pixel of the image.

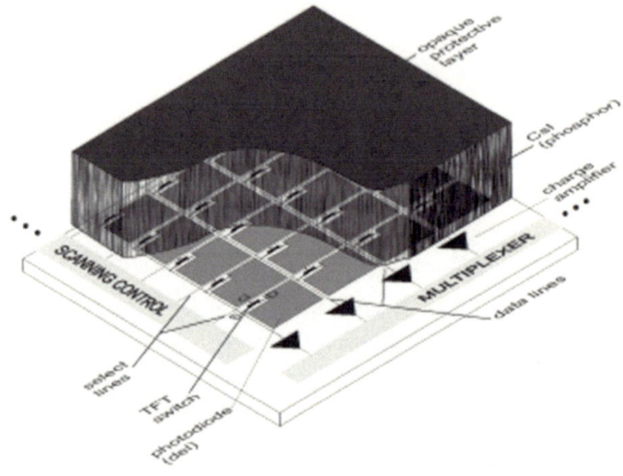

a)

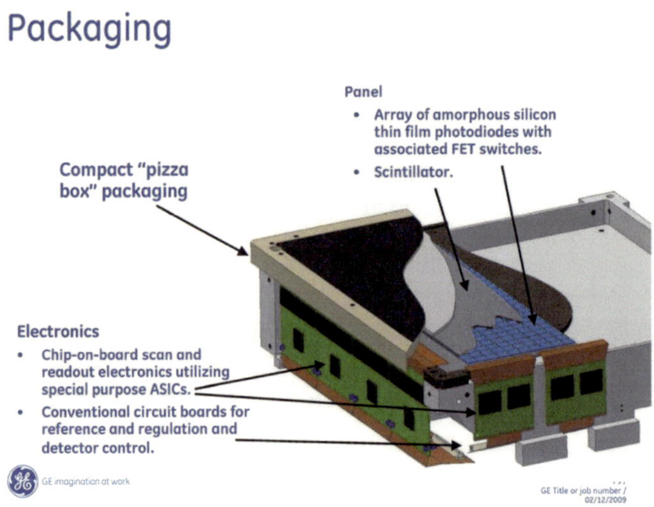

b)

Fig. 9. Illustrations of a CsI-amorphous silicon photodiode flat panel detector. a) Generic detector. Courtesy of Martin Yaffe, PhD; Sunnybrook Health Sciences Centre, Toronto, Canada (from Digital Mammography, eds. ED Pisano, MJ Yaffe, CM Kuzmiak. Lippincott, Williams & Wilkins, a Walters Kluwer Company, 2004. With permission. b) Commercial detector. (Courtesy of General Electric Medical Systems, Milwaukee, WI).

In this type of detector, CsI is used because of its crystal structure. These crystals can be commercially grown to form needle-like or columnar structures. Unlike granular phosphors that allow the produced light upon x-ray absorption to move laterally in the system leading to increased line-spread function in SFM, CsI crystals used in digital systems are more efficient at transferring the light produced (Pisano et al., 2004). This increase in efficiency is because the CsI crystals act as fiber optics. Consequently, the detector can be made thicker without loss of resolution.

An example of a commercial system with this detector is produced by General Electric Medical Systems (Milwaukee, WI), Figure 7. The field size is 24 cm x 31 cm, the del pitch is 100 µm, and the digitization is 14 bits (Ghetti et al., 2008). Of interest, to correct for inhomogeneous areas in the detector, flat-fielding or gain correction requires that an offset value and a gain be measured for each del (Pisano et al., 2004).

3.3.2 Phosphor-CCD system

A phosphor-CCD system also uses CsI(Tl) as the material for x-ray absorption to light conversion in the detector. However, the CsI(Tl) is deposited on a rectangular fiber-optic coupling plate. The fibers conduct the light from the CsI to a charge-coupled device (CCD) array. The CCD is an electronic chip containing rows and columns of light-sensitive elements. The CCD converts the light into an electronic signal that is digitized.

The phosphor-CCD system detector is long, narrow and rectangular in shape, approximately 1 cm x 24 cm as seen in Figure 8b. The x-ray beam is collimated into a narrow band since it and the detector scan across the breast in synchrony, Figure 10. The charge created in the CCD is transferred down the columns from row to row at the same rate, but in opposite direction to the physical motion of the detector. The bundles of charges are integrated, collected and read out corresponding to x-ray transmission on the detector for each x-ray path through the breast (Pisano et al., 2004). This is known as time-delay integration.

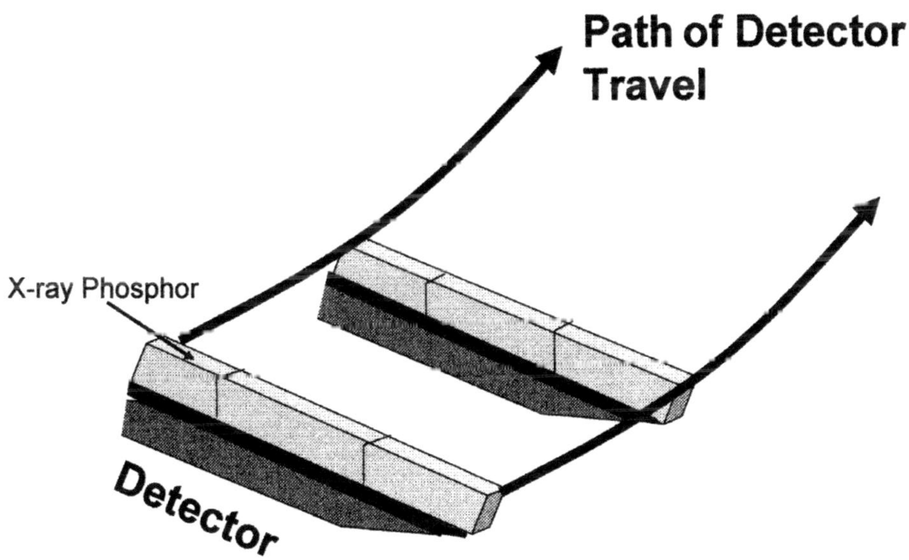

Fig. 10. Schematic of the path of detector travel in a scanned-slot detector system.

A major advantage of this scanned-slot system is the result of the x-ray beam being collimated and only part of the breast being imaged at a time. Consequently, the transmitted x-rays are not lost (scatter-to-primary ratio is reduced), resulting in a grid no longer being needed. Therefore, the dose should be reduced. A limitation of this type of system is that it requires a longer image acquisition time.

A commercial unit like this was originally marketed by Fischer Imaging Inc (Denver, CO) as seen in Figure 8. It has dels of 54 μm with digitization performed at 12 bits. Of interest, over a small area of the detector, data could be read out at 27 μm to provide a high-resolution mode.

3.3.3 Selenium Flat Panel

A selenium detector utilizes a thin layer (100-200 μm) of amorphous selenium for x-ray absorption. When an x-ray is absorbed by this material, it causes some electrons in the selenium to be liberated. The now "freed electron" and its corresponding "hole" from its departure create an electron-hole pair. This electron-hole pair creates the signal (Pisano et al., 2004). When electrodes are placed above and below the selenium and an electric field is applied, this causes the charges to move toward the electrodes. The signal is collected by one of the electrodes that are composed of a large matrix of dels. The dels act as capacitors to store the charge. At the corner of each del is a TFT switch. The readout of the charge is performed in the same manner as for the phosphor flat panel detector.

A detector of this kind is produced by Hologic (Danbury, CT). The Hologic detector dels are 70 μm with 14-bit digitization. Anrad (St Laurent Quebec, Canada) produces another selenium flat-panel system with 85 μm dels. To increase the geometric efficiency of this type of detector and to have a del of 50 μm, Fujifilm Medical has developed an amorphous selenium detector that has two separate layers of selenium as seen in Figure 11. In the Fuji system, the upper layer of selenium absorbs the x-rays and produces the electron-hole pairs. The charge is then stored in each del. The lower selenium layer will transfer the stored charge to a set of readout lines and then it will be transferred to an amplifier and digitized (Yaffe, in Bick & Diekmann, 2010). The information from one del will be used to create the information corresponding to a pixel of the image. This system has a bit depth of 14.

3.3.4 X-ray (Photon) Quantum Counting

The x-ray quantum counting detector is another example of a direct radiography mammography system. However, unlike the other detectors described above, it functions on the principle that each individual x-ray quantum is counted regardless of its energy. The unique design and concept of this detector allows each del to produce an electronic pulse every time an x-ray interacts with it (Pisano et al., 2004). The pulses are then counted and will create the signal for that pixel. Advantages of this type of detector are that no noise is associated with energy conversion and no analog-to-digital converter is needed.

Two quantum-counting systems have been developed. The detector in the Phillips Medical (Germany) [previously Sectra] system uses crystalline silicon in its multiple detectors. The detector and collimated x-ray beam move in synchrony across the breast. The x-rays are absorbed by the crystalline silicon. The electron-hole pairs are collected in an electric field and shaped into a pulse and counted (Aslund et al., 2007) as seen in Figure 12. The Phillips

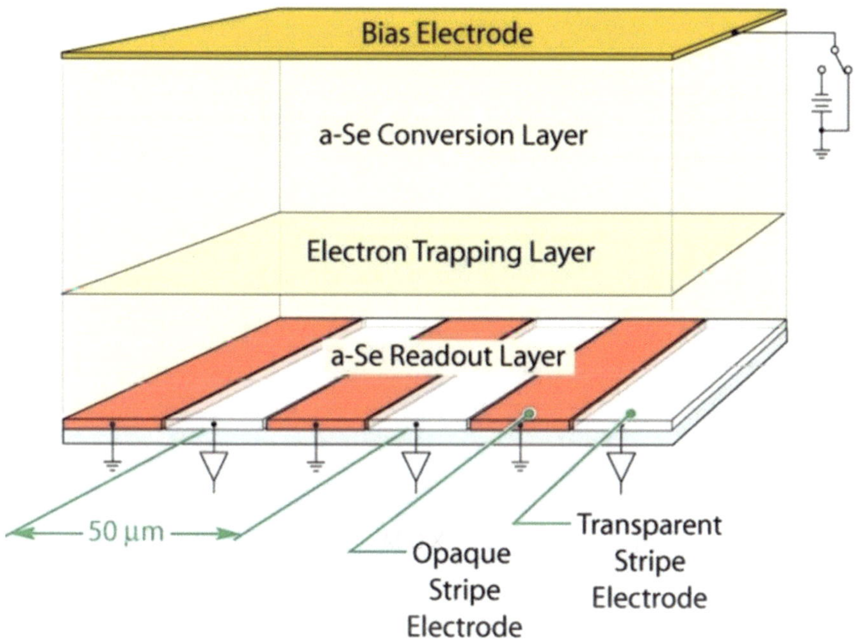

Fig. 11. An illustration of the Fuji FFDM system that uses two layers of selenium. (Courtesy of Fujifilm Medical, Stamford, CT).

system has a del size of 50 µm and a bit depth of 16. In the system by XCounter (Stockholm, Sweden), it uses a set of multiple linear detectors and scans across the breast in synchrony with a collimated x-ray beam similar to the Sectra system. However, it uses a pressurized gas as the x-ray absorber. The pulses of ions generated by the gas form the signal (Thunberg, in Antonuk & Yaffe, 2002). The XCounter system has the same del size and bit depth as the Sectra. Neither system uses a grid.

3.3.5 Photostimulable Phosphor (PSP) System

The last detector to be discussed is the PSP system which is a computed radiography (CR) system. CR systems have been in use in general radiography for many years and are based on the principle of photostimulable luminescence. More recently they have been developed and used in mammography. The CR mammography systems utilize a phosphor screen. Energy from x-ray absorption causes electrons in the phosphor crystal to be liberated from the matrix and captured and stored in "traps" in the crystal lattice (Pisano et al., 2004), as seen in Figure 13. The number of traps filled is proportional to the amount of absorbed x-ray signal.

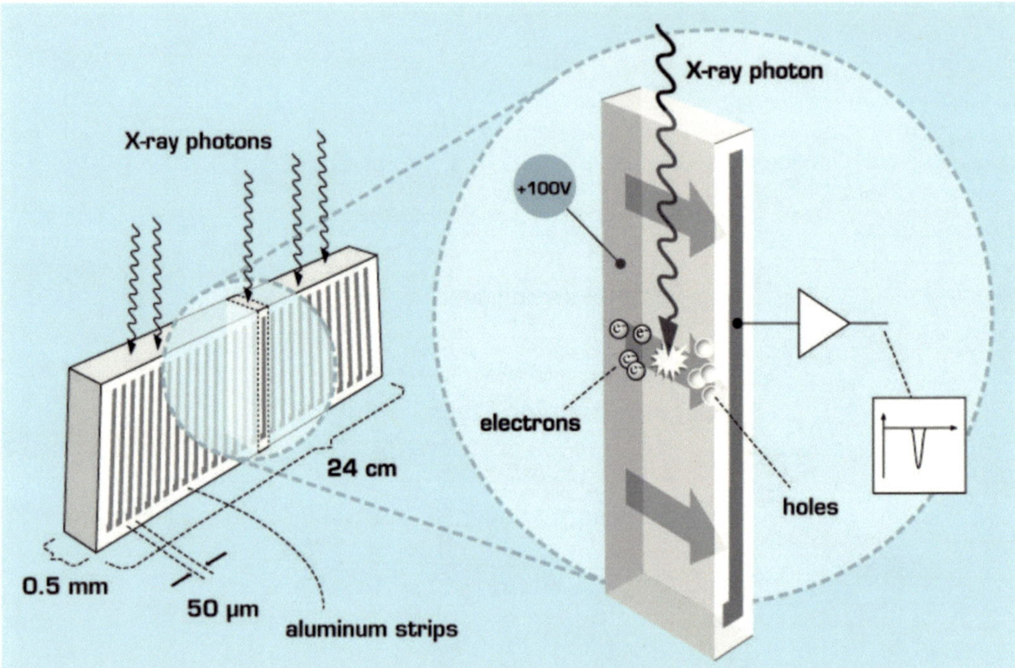

Fig. 12. X-ray (Photon) quantum counting detector. Schematic of a silicon based photon counting detector. (Courtesy of Phillips Medical, Germany)

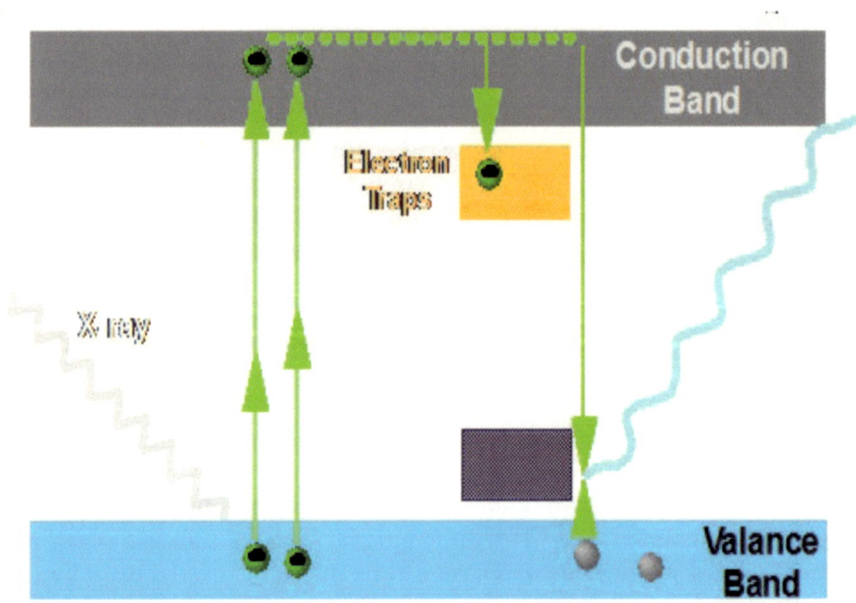

Fig. 13. Schematic demonstrating energy from x-ray absorption liberates electrons from the phosphor crystal and are captured and stored in "traps" in the crystal.

The CR image, which is analog, is then read out by placing the screen in a reading device. The reading device will scan it with a red laser beam in one dimension as it moves through the reader in the orthogonal direction. The red laser beam will free the electrons from the traps and cause them to return to their original resting state in the crystal lattice. As they return to their original state, the electrons will pass between energy levels created in the crystal with certain materials. The selected materials incorporated into the crystal typically emit blue light that is proportional to the x-ray energy absorbed by the phosphor (Yaffe, in Bick & Diekmann, 2010). The emitted blue light is measured with a light-collecting system composed of a photomultiplier tube, selected optical filter to eliminate the red light from interfering with the measurement, and a photomultiplier tube. Because the PSP is not composed of physical dels, spatial resolution of the system is the result of the size of the laser spot (del size) and the distance between sampling measurement (pitch) (Pisano et al., 2004). To decrease scan time while increasing light collection efficiency, SNR and sensitivity, some PSP vendors utilize a double-sided (read from the top and bottom surface of the PSP) reading device as seen in Figure 14.

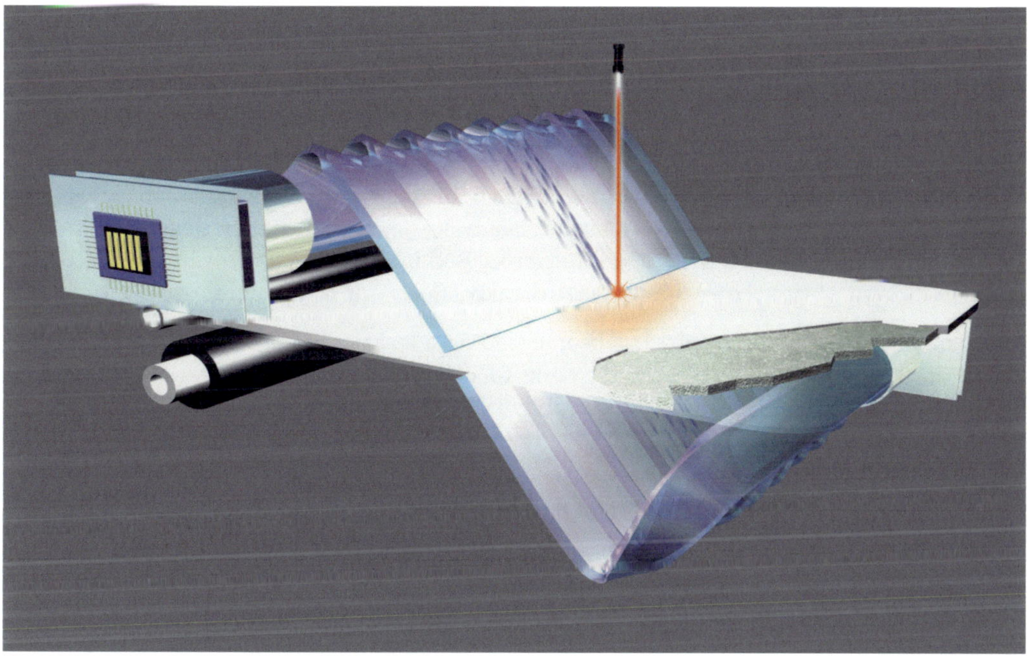

Fig. 14. CR mammography dual optical collection system scanned with a red laser beam. (Courtesy of Fujifilm Medical, Stamford, CT)

A system of this type was developed by Fujifilm Medical Systems (Stamford, CT). Its del size is 50 μm and has a bit depth of 12. There are other PSP systems developed and used throughout the world that have similar del and bit depths.

Unlike the DR systems, the CR system uses removable cassettes that are placed into a bucky tray. This system can be a cost saver to some institutions since they may be able to convert their current SFM machine to CR. For work-flow, there may be little change in daily routine for technologists. For some mammography technologists, CR systems have a similar "feel" as SFM. Cassettes with the PSP are still placed into the bucky tray, the patient is positioned and imaged the same, and then the plate is placed into a reading device without having to go into a darkroom. The mammographic image obtained can be printed to hard copy or displayed on softcopy just like the DR systems.

3.4 Quality Control (QC)

Mammography must be of high image quality in order for radiologists to detect the subtle changes of breast cancer. This can be difficult since breast cancer can present as a mass of the same density as normal breast parenchyma or be obscured by it. To ensure optimal performance from a system, the equipment must be properly set up and maintained. In the United States, the Mammography Quality Standards Act (MQSA) was established in 1992 to establish a federal mandated quality control program for screen film mammography. It now includes digital mammography. In Europe, as countries began to develop a breast cancer screening program, each began to develop their own national program. To standardize quality assurance and quality control, the European Commission published guidelines in 2006. Now in its 4th edition, the published guidelines include digital mammography (Perry et al., 2006). However, there is no single international source on QC procedures. In the United States, it is required that users follow the manufacturers' QC procedures for their systems.

Digital imaging allows the decoupling of acquisition, processing and display. In order to have meaningful QC of a digital system, each of the components must be evaluated separately. To evaluate acquisition (detector, beam, scatter, and radiation dose), quantitative measures are performed on the "raw" or unprocessed images. The QC for image processing is still in its early stages. To evaluate image display, electronic test patterns are used.

Image quality for mammography has been based on a test phantom, with objects imbedded within it. This test is subjective and prone to observer error. In the future, automated software may be useful for solving this problem (Young et al., 2008). Instead of a phantom, a more reliable measurement for verifying the consistency of image contrast in a digital system is the contrast-to-noise ratio (CNR). It is sensitive to changes in dose, object contrast and beam quality for each digital machine (Young, in Bick & Diekmann, 2010). The CNR object imaged is made of different materials that simulate the attenuation coefficient of breast tissue.

As with SFM, digital mammography can have artifacts. The artifacts may arise from detector non-uniformities. Over time, there can be degradation of the homogeneity of the detector leading to image degradation. To correct for this, an algorithm can be applied to all the images. The procedure is called "flat-field" or "gain correction" and is based on the principle that the detector responds linearly to radiation exposure. The first step in this test is to record the receptor response for the same amount of time of an image, but without any x-ray exposure. The values from this "dark" image are stored in the dels. In a subsequent image acquired using x-rays, the values stored are subtracted from the measurement from each corresponding del resulting in an image where it appears that the dark signals from all dels are zero (Yaffe, in Bick & Diekmann, 2010). Figure 15 is an example of flat-field correction.

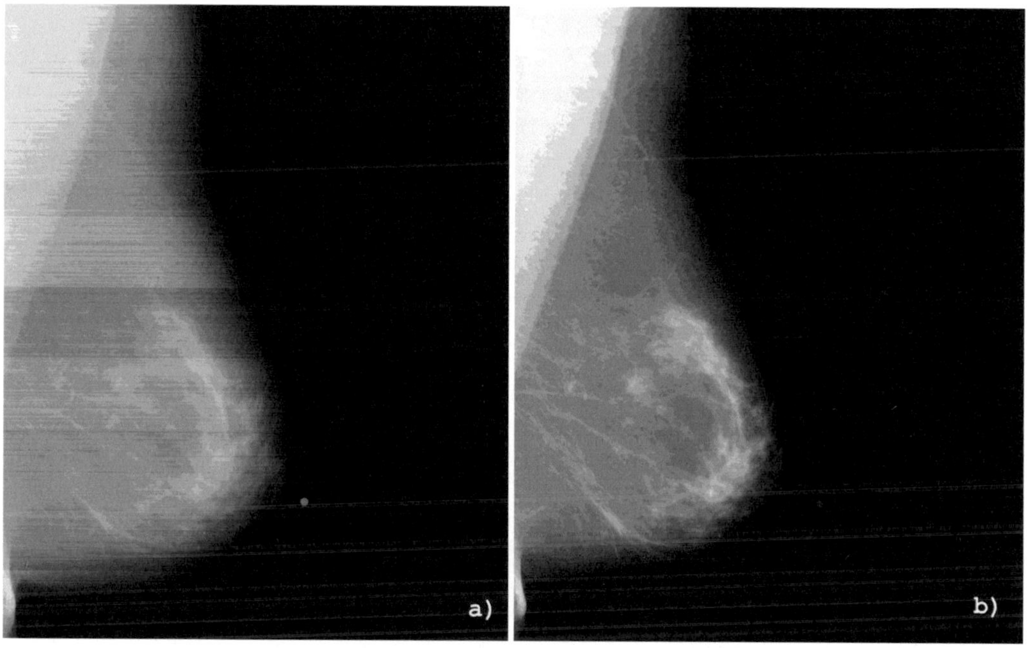

Fig. 15. Digital mammogram a) before and b) after flat-filed correction. Courtesy of Martin Yaffe, PhD; Sunnybrook Health Sciences Centre, Toronto, Canada. (from Digital Mammography, eds. ED Pisano, MJ Yaffe, CM Kuzmiak. Lippincott, Williams & Wilkins, a Walters Kluwer Company, 2004. With permission.)

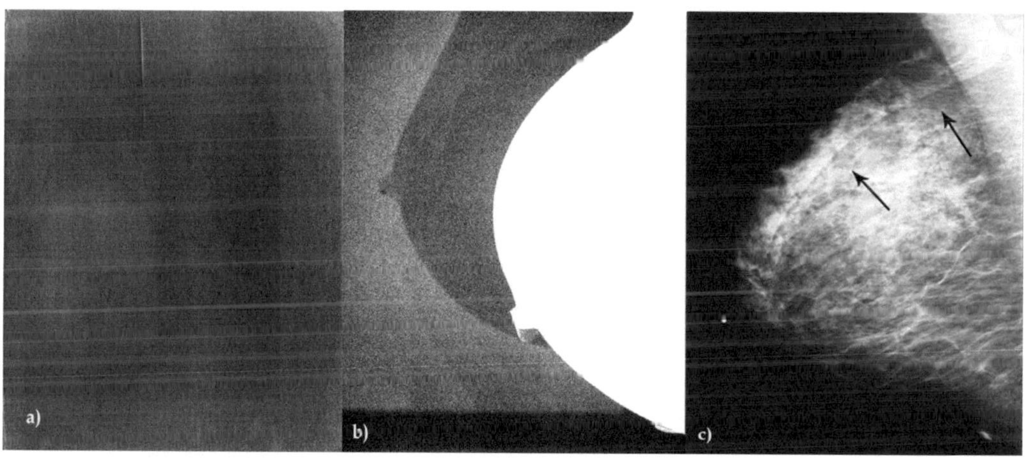

Fig. 16. Ghost or lag artifact. a) Artifact seen on a detector. b) Another example of ghosting. c) Clinical image with the appearance of a second breast (arrows). (Images **b** & **c** are courtesy of Elizabeth Franklin of Carolinas Medical Center, Charlotte, North Carolina, USA)

Other digital artifacts can be attributed to the digital detector. A single non-functioning pixel may not be noticed or even affect clinical images, but if the numbers of non-functioning pixels are too many it will impact clinical images. The non-functioning pixel can appear as a white dot and may simulate calcifications. If a pixel discharges too early it may result in a bloom artifact, a white spot with a black halo secondary to the increase in charge of the neighboring dels (Van Ongeval, in Bick & Diekmann, 2010). If there is crystallization of the selenium of the detector, the images may become blurred over time (Marshall, 2006). Figure 16 are examples of ghost or lag artifact and are the result of incorrect electron clearing. Electronic interference can result in a zigzag artifact as seen in this CR image, Figure 17. Artifacts can be the result of image processing in which there is significant edge artifact between dense and fatty tissue, Figure 18. Also, artifacts can be related to the patient, i.e. chin, nose, finger, or hair artifact as seen in Figure 19.

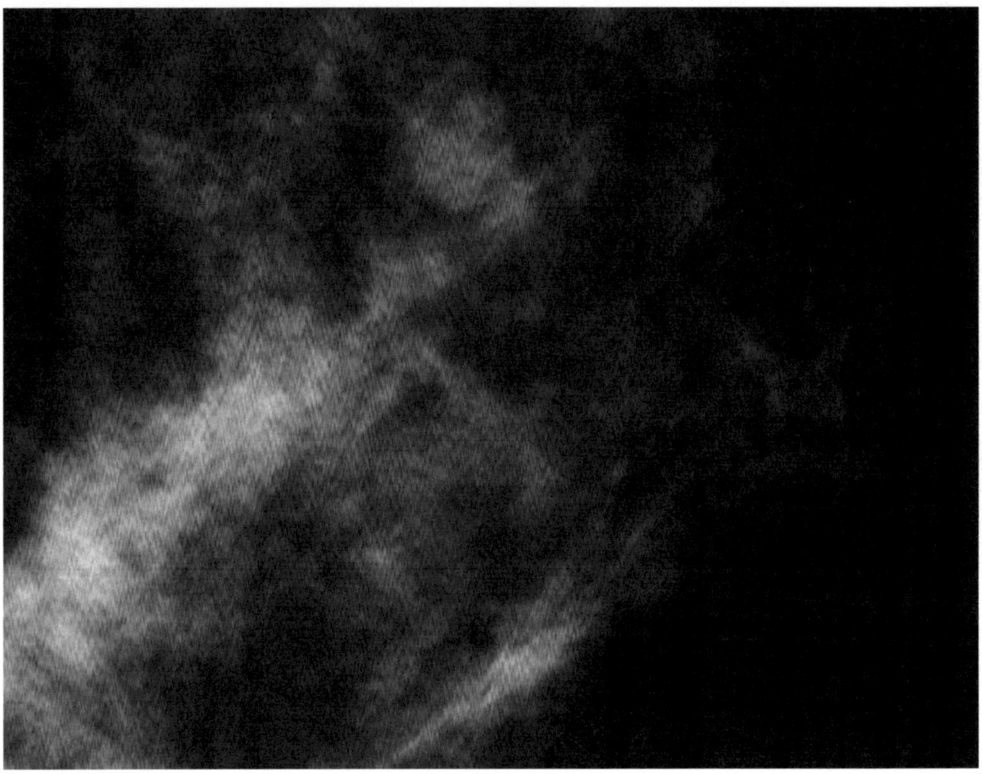

Fig. 17. Electronic interference in a CR system resulting in a "zigzag" black line artifact.

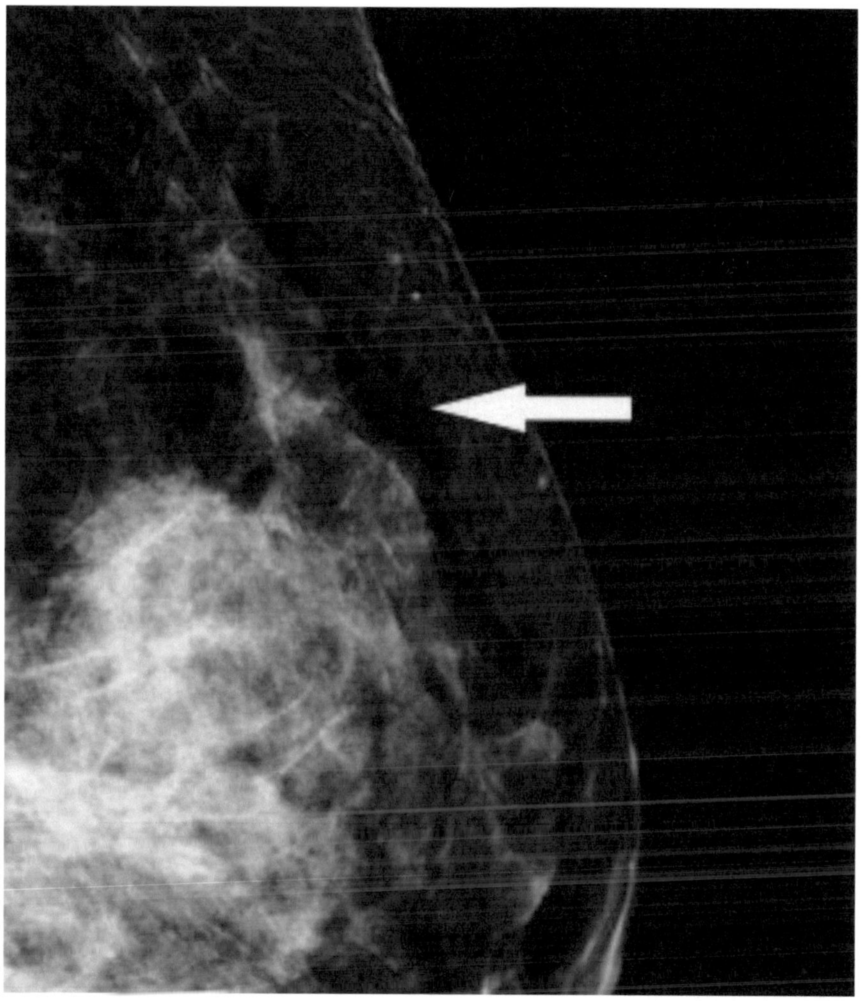

Fig. 18. Processing artifact. Significant edge enhancement between the white breast tissue and black fat. This results in significant "blackness" of the image adjacent to the black white interface (arrow).

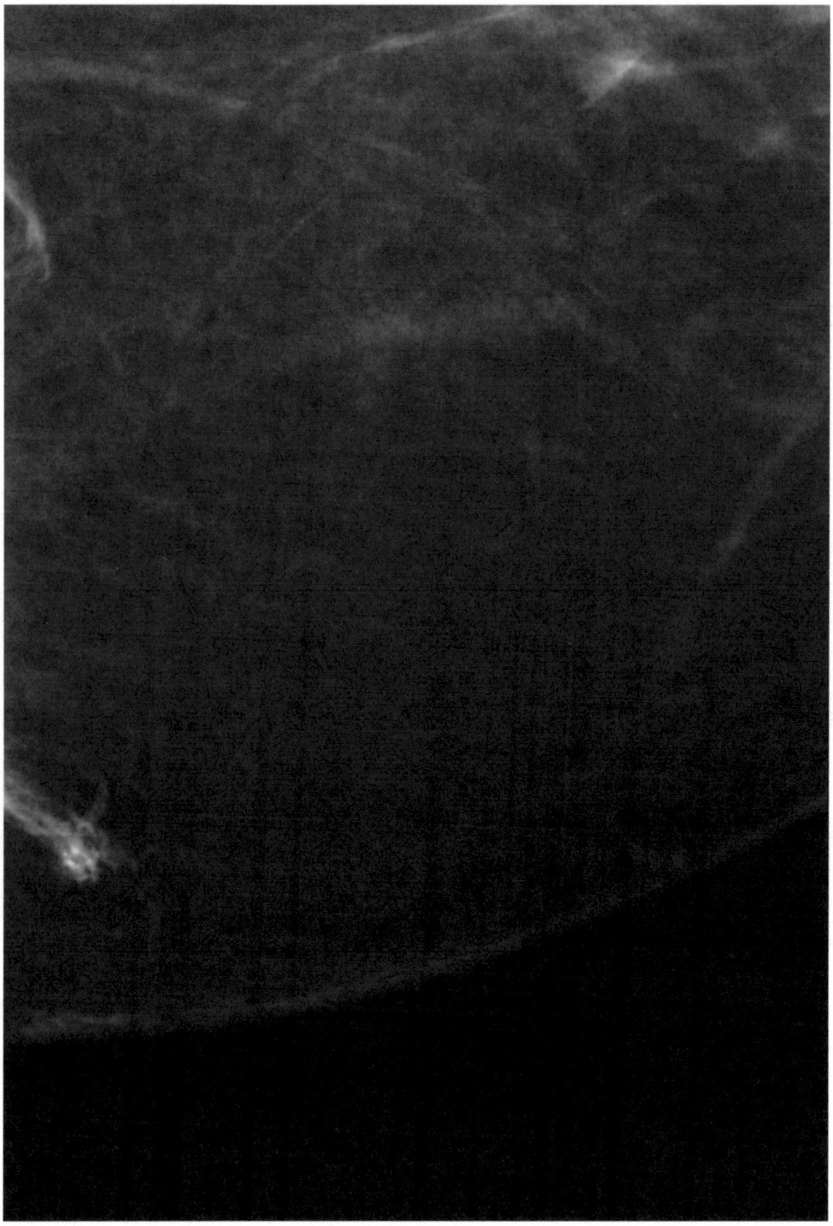

Fig. 19. Hair artifact. White swirling lines representing the patient's hair are seen projecting over the medial portion of the breast.

4. Clinical trials

4.1 United States

In 1996 in the United States, the Federal Food and Drug Administration (FDA) published the *Information for Manufacturers Seeking Marketing Clearance of Digital Mammography Systems* (Food and Drug Administration, 1996; Pisano, 2004). For manufacturers of digital mammography equipment seeking FDA-approval through 510(k) or Premarket Approval, the document required that each manufacturer demonstrate through a designed clinical trial that digital mammography equipment was equivalent to SFM. However, this was not without some challenges. The original FDA guidelines required manufacturers to demonstrate a higher rate of inter-reader agreement with FFDM than was obtainable between readers of SFM when SFM was compared to itself (Beam, 1996; Elmore, 1992; Howard, 1993). There was no requirement that manufacturers determine the truth about the presence or absence of breast cancer, only that the mammogram interpretations agree.

After an Advisory Panel met to discuss the "flawed" guidelines, the FDA released its revised guidelines on February 8, 1999. The guidelines now required approval trials to be based on breast cancer status truth. Consequently, sensitivity and specificity as measured by a Receiver Operating Characteristic (ROC) analysis was to be used with the goal of the studies to demonstrate that the difference in the areas under the ROC curve between digital and film was no greater than 0.1 (Pisano et al., 2004). This was now the FDA's standard for proving "substantial equivalence" of the two technologies.

Several minor clinical trials studies have been published in the US comparing digital mammography versus SFM, and these demonstrated promising results for digital mammography (Cole, 2001; Hendrick 2001; Pisano, 2004). One of the first major published clinical trials was the Colorado-Massachusetts Screening Trial (Lewin et al., 2001, 2002). The goal of this two-site study was to prospectively compare full-field digital mammography (FFDM) and SFM for cancer detection in a screening population. The design of the study was simple. All women at least 40 years old presenting for a screening mammogram were eligible to undergo both a SFM and a FFDM. A FFDM prototype system made by General Electric Medical (Milwaukee, WI) with a 18 cm x 23 cm amorphous silicon detector with a CsI crystal and a commercial SFM unit (DMR: General Electric Medical Systems, Milwaukee, WI) were used for imaging. A prototype softcopy display workstation was also used.

Final results by Lewin et al. were published in 2002 (Lewin et al., 2002). A total of 6,736 paired exams were performed on 4,521 women over a 30-month period. In these patients, 2,048 findings were detected in 1,467 of the studies with film, digital, or both imaging modalities. Additional work-up of the findings led to 183 biopsies and 42 were positive for cancer. The cancer detection rate was not statistically significant ($p > 0.1$). The difference between the ROC area for digital (0.74) and SFM (0.80) were not significant ($p > 0.1$). FFDM had fewer recalls than SFM ($p < 0.001$); however, the positive predictive values of both modalities were similar (3.3% SFM, 3.4% FFDM) (Lewin et al., 2002). Although FFDM did not lead to a higher cancer detection rate, it did lead to fewer recalls with a study that used a prototype unit and display workstation. This study becomes the foundation for the next major screening clinical trial, Digital Mammography Imaging Screen Trial.

The Digital Mammography Imaging Screening Trial (DMIST) was sponsored by the American College of Radiology Imaging Network (ACRIN) and the National Cancer Institute (NCI) (Pisano et al., 2005). It was a cooperative venture by 33 sites in two counties led by Dr. Etta Pisano. A total of 49,528 asymptomatic women presenting for a screening mammogram underwent both a digital mammogram and SFM in a random order by the same technologist on the same day. A total of five digital systems were used: Senographe 2000D (General Electric), SenoScan (Fischer Medical), Selenium Full-Field Digital Mammography System (Hologic), Digital Mammography System (Hologic) and Computed Radiography System for Mammography (Fuji Medical). The images were read independently by radiologists, one radiologist for each exam. The radiologist scored each study on a 7-point malignancy scale for ROC analysis and a BIRADS (American College of Radiology, 2003) final impression to guide clinical work-up. The patient was recalled for additional diagnostic imaging whether the film, digital and/or both screening modalities demonstrated an abnormality. Standard work-up at each institution was performed that may have led to a biopsy. Breast cancer status was based on a breast biopsy within 15 months of study entry or a follow-up mammogram acquired at least 10 months after study entry.

Of the total patients recruited to DMIST over its 2-year accrual period, data was complete for 42,760 (86.3%) patients. A total of 335 breast cancers were diagnosed. Of these, 254 (75.8%) were diagnosed within 365 days and 81 (24.2%) were diagnosed between 366 and 455 days after study entry. The results demonstrate that for the entire population, the diagnostic accuracy of digital and film mammography was similar with a mean AUC of 0.78+/-0.02 for digital and 0.74+/-0.02 for film (difference in AUC, 0.03; 95 percent confidence interval, -0.02 to 0.08; P = 0.18). However, for certain subgroups, the accuracy of digital mammography was significantly higher than that of film mammography. The subgroups include women under the age of 50, women with heterogeneously dense or dense breasts, and premenopausal or perimenopausal women (P values of P =0.002, P = 0.003, P =0.002, respectively) (Pisano et al., 2005). Although the overall diagnostic accuracy of digital was similar to film, this large prospective, multicenter center study showed advantages for younger women with dense breasts.

4.2 European clinical trials

The first prospective digital screening study in Europe was performed in Norway in 2000 (Skaane et al., 2003, 2005). The Oslo I trial was a prospective study to compare SFM and FFDM with soft-copy reading in a population-based screening program. By invitation from the Norwegian Breast Cancer Screening Program (NBCSP), women aged 50-69 years of age were invited to participate. The women who agreed to participate in the study underwent two standard views of each breast with each modality (similar to the US studies). The FFDM studies were performed with Senographe 2000D (General Electric Healthcare, Buc, France) and interpreted on a GE softcopy display system with 2K x 2.5K monitors. Eight radiologists performed independent double readings for both modalities and used a 5-point malignancy scale. All images deemed positive (score of 2 or higher) were reviewed in a consensus meeting for each technique used. It was the consensus conference that decided whether the patient should be called back for additional imaging or scheduled for follow-up screening in 2 years.

The Oslo I study resulted in 3,683 women participating and a total of 31 cancers detected (detection rate 0.84%). Twenty-eight cancers were seen with SFM (detection rate 0.76%) and 23 by FFDM (detection rate 0.62%). The cancer detection rates were not significant (P= 0.23). The PPV for SFM was 46% and FFDM 39%. The recall rate after the consensus meeting was 3.5% (128 cases) for SFM and 4.6% (168 cases) for FFDM (Skaane et al., 2005). The recall rate was not significant. The authors concluded that there was no statistically significant difference in cancer detection rate; cancer conspicuity was equal between the modalities and soft-copy reading is comparable to SFM in a population based screening (Skaane et al., 2005).

Other data to come out of the Oslo I study was a retrospective review of the cancers (Skaane et al., 2003). In this retrospective review, a side-by-side feature analysis of conspicuity of the cancers was performed and there was no difference between the modalities. In 2005, Skaane et al. published follow-up information on the missed FFDM cancers from the Oslo I study (Skaane et al., 2005). They concluded that inexperience of the readers with softcopy, improper viewing conditions and rapid interpretations might have contributed to the lower detection rate.

Within a few months after completion of the Oslo I trial, patient enrollment for the Oslo II screening trial began. The aims of this study were to prospectively compare cancer detection rates, recall rates and positive predictive values of SFM versus FFDM in a screening program in Norway (Skaane & Skjennald, 2004). Women 50-69 years old were invited to the NBCS and women 45-49 years old were invited to the Oslo screening program. The patients were randomized for age and residence to undergo SFM or FFDM. Due to the physical location of the mammography equipment, the study investigators decided to have 70% of the patients undergo SFM and the other 30% to undergo FFDM (Skaane & Skjennald, 2004). The same radiologists who participated in the Oslo I trial participated. All images were again independently double-read (now with appropriate viewing conditions in the room) and scored using a 5-point malignancy scale. The potential "call back" cases were again reviewed at a consensus conference.

Results of the Oslo II study demonstrated a total of 64 cancers (cancer detection rate 0.38%) detected in 16,985 women who underwent SFM and 41 cancers (cancer detection rate 0.59%) in 6, 944 women who underwent FFDM (Skaane et al., 2007). The difference was in support of FFDM and was statistically significant (p = 0.03). The sensitivity was 77.4% for FFDM and 61.5% for SFM (P =0.07). The specificity was 96.5% and 97.9% respectively for the imaging modalities (P<0.005). The PPV was 15.1% for SFM and 13.9% for FFDM and this difference was not significant. The recall rate for SFM was 2.5% and 4.2% for FFDM (P < 0.001) (Skaane et al., 2007). The higher recall rate of this study confirmed the higher recall rate in the Oslo I trial. However, it is important to know that recall was based on a consensus conference, and it was only at the conference where comparison mammograms were made available for review. The study concluded that FFDM with softcopy interpretation is well suited for breast cancer screening programs.

Unlike the prior studies, the Swedish Helsingborg Study by Heddson et al. was a retrospective study that compared SFM, photon counting DR (PC-DR), and CR mammography from January 2000 to February 2005 (Heddson, et al., 2007). The goals were to evaluate cancer detection rates, recall rates, and PPV values in a screening population. A total of 52,172 screening mammograms were performed on 24,875 women during the study.

Fifty percent of the studies were performed with SFM, 19% with photon counting DR system (Sectra, Sweden), and 31% with a CR system (Fujifilm, Japan). The age range of the patients was 46-74 years of age. Forty percent of the SFM cases and 65% of the FFDM cases were double read by two radiologists. Recall of the patient was based by consensus of the radiologists.

Results of Helsingborg study demonstrated a statistically significant difference in the cancer detection rate for PC-DR versus SFM (P= 0.01) (Heddson et al., 2007). The cancer detection rates were 0.31% (81/25,901) for SFM, 0.49% (48/9841) for PC-DR, and 0.38% (63/16,430) for CR. In contrast to the Oslo studies, this study demonstrated a significantly higher recall rate for SFM than digital. The recall rate was for SFM, PC-DR, and CR were 1.4%, 1.0%, and 1.0%. As a result of the higher cancer detection rate and lower recall rate, the PPV for digital was higher than film [(P< 0.001): PC-DR = 47%, CR = 39% and film = 22%] (Heddson et al., 2007).

In addition to the above results, the Helsingborg Study demonstrated that digital mammography provided a dose reduction compared to film mammography as expected by its linear response to x-ray (Heddson et al., 2007). PC-DR provided a 75% dose reduction and CR a 16% dose reduction. The average glandular dose was 0.28 mGy, 0.92 mGy, 1.1 mGy, for PC-DR, CR, and SFM, respectively. The authors concluded that given the advantages of digital mammography, it is a valid alternative to screen film mammography.

Study	Study Design	SFM Exams	FFDM Exams	Recall Rate (%) SFM	Recall Rate (%) FFDM	Cancer Detection Rate (%) SFM	Cancer Detection Rate (%) FFDM	PPV (%) SFM	PPV (%) FFDM
Oslo I	Prospective, paired	3,683	3,683	3.5	4.6	0.71	0.54	20.2	11.8
Oslo II	Prospective, randomized	16,985	6,944	2.5	4.2	0.38	0.59	15.1	13.9
Helsingborg	Retro-spective	25,901	9,841	1.4	1.0	0.31	0.49	21.8	47.1
Florence	Retro-spective	14,385	14,385	3.5	4.3	0.58	0.72	14.7	15.9
Vestfold	Retro-spective	324,763	18,239	4.2	4.1	0.65	0.77	15.1	18.5
CELBSS	Retro-spective	31,720	8,478	4.4	4.8	0.65	0.68	14.6	14.3
Barcelona	Retro-spective	12,958	6,074	5.5	4.2	0.42	0.41	7.5	9.7

CELBSS = Central East London Breast Screening Service Study.

Table 1. Published European studies comparing screen film mammography (SFM) and full field digital mammography (FFDM) for recall rate, cancer detection rate, and positive predictive value.

Three of the European studies have been discussed above to give examples of designs and results. In total, there have been seven published European population-based screening studies comparing SFM and FFDM (Del Turco, 2007; Heddson, 2007; Sala, 2009; Skaane, 2005, 2007; Vigeland, 2008; Vinnicombe, 2009). Table 1 compares the results. It is important to keep in mind when reviewing the data that each of the studies is of different design. Only the Oslo studies were prospective studies. The Oslo I was a paired-designed as were the US studies. Double reading was performed in the European studies followed by consensus or arbitration meetings for positive studies. In the US studies, each modality was interpreted using an independent reader blinded to the results of the other modality. The Colorado-Massachusetts Screening Trial by Lewin et al. used a consensus conference, DMIST did not. In DMIST, if a single reader, regardless of modality, noted an abnormality then the patient was recalled. The recall rates reports vary in the studies; four of the European studies show a higher recall rate with digital (Del Turco, 2007; Skaane, 2005, 2007; Vinnicombe, 2009). In five of the studies, the cancer detection rate was greater for digital (Del Turco, 2007; Heddson, 2007; Skaane, 2007; Vigeland, 2008; Vinnicombe, 2009). Two were statistically significant: Oslo II and Helsingborg Study (Skaane, 2007; Heddson, 2007). From these results, the utilization of digital screening mammography in the Western European Countries and the United States continues to increase.

5. Image processing

Image processing is the application of applying mathematical operations to the "raw" digital image with the aim to visualize subtle abnormalities so that they can be perceived by the radiologist as seen in Figure 20. Image processing should be robust and reproducible. The need for extra manipulation of the images should be none or very minimal for the radiologist. In addition, the radiologist should feel confident in reviewing the images. The unique property of digital is that each component of the system can be optimized. A few of the basic methods used will be discussed.

Intensity windowing algorithms are based on the principle that each acts on individual pixels in the image. A small portion of the full intensity range of the image is selected and then remapped to the full intensity range of the display (Pisano et al., 2000). With this process, it allows for the selection of specific intensity values of interest. Consequently, dense normal tissue and abnormal tissue values are exaggerated to accommodate for their small differences. This may result in increased lesion conspicuity.

Manual Intensity Windowing (MIW) is one of the versions of intensity windowing. It is operator dependent. The radiologist manually windows and levels the images on a display system. Several examples are demonstrated in Figure 21. This can be quite variable depending on the radiologist's image reading preference and experience. Another version is histogram-based. In this version, it allows the system to select a window to allow the full range of contrast across the part of the histogram representing any fatty, mixed, or dense portion. The advantage of HIW is that it can adapt to individual breast types. The third version is Mixture-Model Intensity Windowing (MMIW). It provides region-specific window settings: background, compressed and non-compressed fat, dense tissue, and muscle (Pisano et al., 2000). Examples of these are demonstrated in Figure 22.

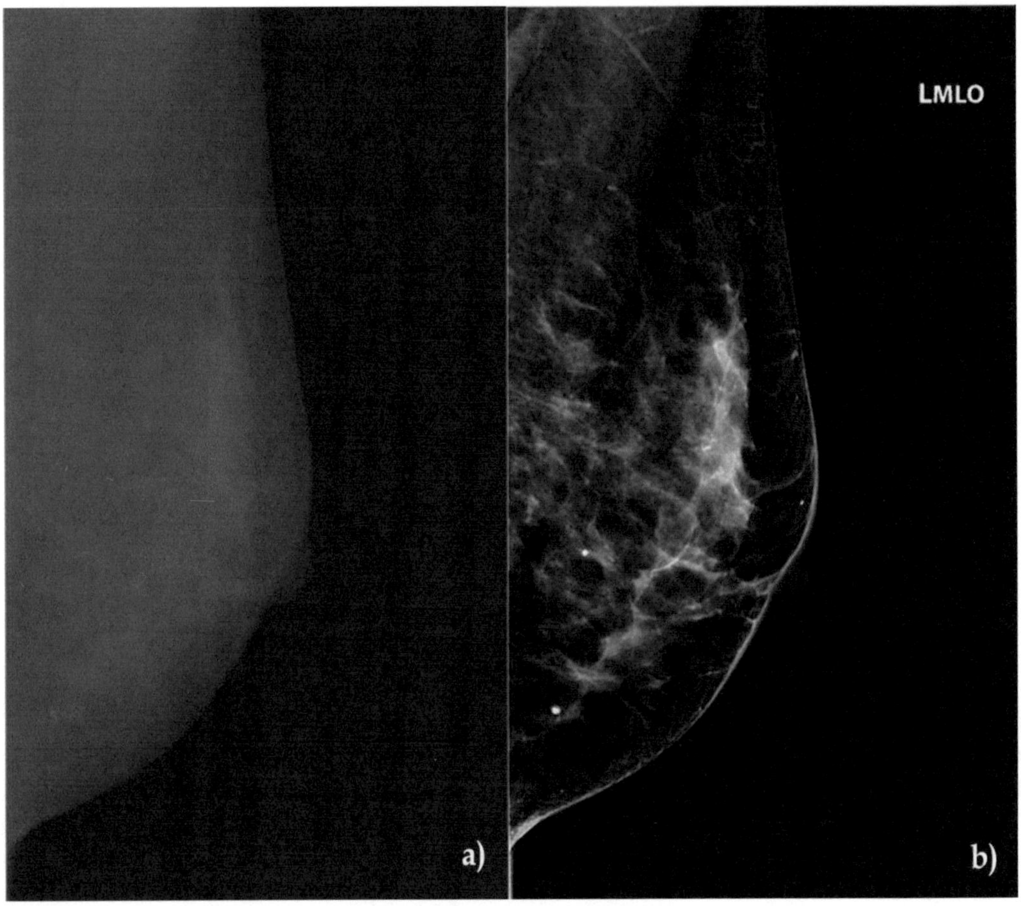

Fig. 20. Digital mammogram. a) Raw image. b) Processed image. (Courtesy of Fujifilm Medical, Stamford, CT)

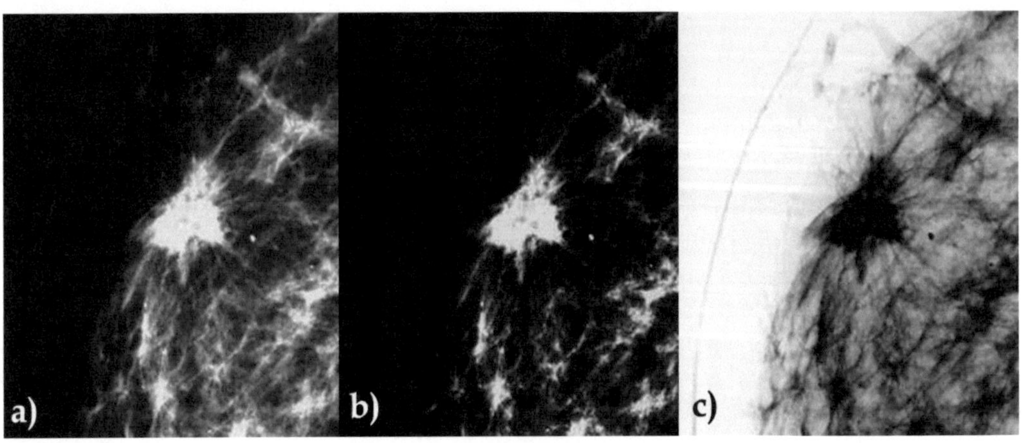

Fig. 21. Examples of different manual windowing and leveling of a digital mammogram that contains a spiculated mass. a) Initial. b) Manipulated image. c) Inverted image.

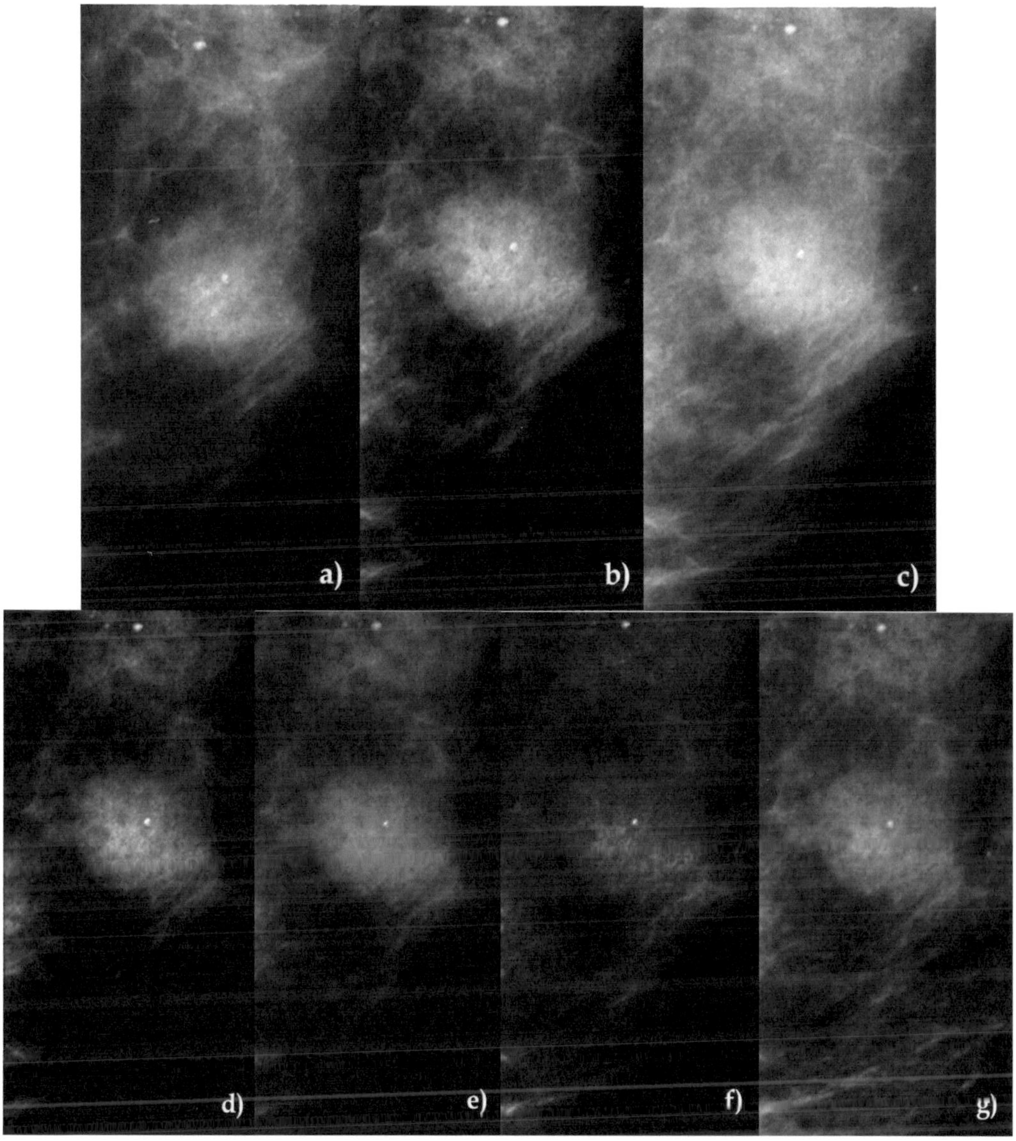

Fig. 22. Different post-processing algorithms (a) SFM of a cyst. (b-g) Photographic magnifications of a digital mammogram process with MIW (b), HIW (c), MMIW (d), CLAHE (e), unsharp masking (f), and peripheral equalization (g) (from *RadioGraphics*. Pisano et al. 2005. With permission).

Adaptive Histogram Equalization (AHE) is a spatial enhancement method that changes pixel value based on spatial content. When applied to an image, there is enhancement of each pixel in relation to its local area. In doing so, all the gray values occur at an equal frequency in the image and consequently, the contrast of the background may be enhanced at the loss of contrast in the breast tissue (Karssemeijer, in Bick & Diekmann, 2010). In addition to the tissue contrast being increased in the image, so is noise. To limit noise, Contrast-Limited Adaptive Histogram Equalization (CLAHE) was developed. It limits the maximum contrast adjustments by clipping and renormalizing the histogram (Pisano, 2000; Karssemeijer, 2010).

Unsharp Masking (UM) is a post-processing technique that is created by subtracting a low-pass filtered version of the original image from the original image (Chan et al., 1987). This process enhances high frequencies in the image such as calcifications and mass edges. A disadvantage of UM is that it also adds noise to the images. Also, it may falsely enhance a margin of a mass (i.e. an indistinct mass may appear more circumscribed and lead to inappropriate classification and follow-up of a mass instead of the need for a biopsy) (Pisano et al., 2000).

Peripheral Equalization or Peripheral Enhancement (PE) is a post-processing technique developed to improve the visualization of the less compressed (and over penetrated) outer edges of the breast. A filter is used to obtain a blurred version of the mammogram representing tissue thickness. This blurred image "mask" is scaled from 0 to 1, and the mammogram is divided by means of the mask values on a pixel-by-pixel bases (Byng et al., 1997). The applied algorithm acts on the pixels in the breast and where there is a thickness change. The result is that the pixels near the periphery are changed so the image becomes "flatter" across the mammogram and the periphery appears less black.

Image processing is a vital component of digital mammography. We may find that it may take more than one algorithm and not necessarily "film-like display" to evaluate for masses, distortion and calcifications. Image processing algorithms are currently not assessed as part of QA protocols. However, they should be to ensure the image chain is working optimally. Automated systems may be of great importance for efficient use of technologist and physicist time in QA and QC. There is a great need to continue to develop and evaluate this area of digital mammography.

6. Image display

Image display of digital images can be performed with a laser printer onto hard copy "film-like" medium or viewed on high-resolution computer monitors. Regardless of display type, it is important to know how the image is being seen relative to its full spatial resolution. Commercial laser printers for digital mammography can support spatial resolutions, grey scale and optical density similar to mammographic film. If the images are printed with a laser printer, it may be done with 8, 10, or 12 bits per pixel displayed. If a digital mammography system uses larger bits than the printer, there will be loss of the dynamic range of digital image and the contrast scale will be compressed (Pisano et al., 2004). Consequently, not all the shades of grey can be displayed. If more than one version of the image is needed to display a finding, another image may need to be printed and this is a disadvantage. However, an advantage of laser-printed film is that it allows radiologists to use the same reading and workflow protocols as SFM.

Softcopy display is performed with high-resolution mammography monitors that allow the flexibility of image display and contrast. An early study by Pisano et al. compared the speed and accuracy of the interpretation of Fischer digital mammograms on softcopy versus those on laser-printed film (Pisano et al., 2002). In the study, 8 radiologists interpreted 63 digital mammograms both on a prototype softcopy display system and on laser-printed film per the manufacturer's recommendation. All studies had comparisons for review. All radiologists read both conditions with at least one month between reads. Six cancers, 13 biopsy-proven benign lesions, 23 probably benign findings and 20 normal cases were included. The results demonstrated that softcopy display interpretations tended to be faster than film: mean time 34 seconds versus 40.5 seconds. In contrast, the ROC curve and sensitivity favored film (0.67:0.71 for film and 0.65:0.69 for softcopy). Specificity was slightly higher with softcopy (0.563 versus 0. 528), but not significant (Pisano et al., 2002).

With specificity of softcopy as a concern, a retrospective study comparing the specificity for calcifications in digital mammograms using softcopy versus film was performed by Kim et al. in 2006 (Kim et al., 2006). Eight radiologists reviewed 130 biopsy-proven cases of calcifications on softcopy and screen film. For each condition, the radiologists were asked to rate the probability of malignancy on a 5-point scale. For film, the radiologists could use a magnifying glass for further evaluation of the images, and for softcopy they could "roam and zoom" to manually window for contrast. The study concluded that there was no statistically significant difference in specificity achievable using softcopy digital versus screen-film mammography.

For radiologists using softcopy display for interpretations, appropriate room ergonomics and viewing conditions are absolutely necessary to minimize radiologist distractions and fatigue. Vendors need to continue developing hanging protocols and other tools that allow the radiologists to view all digital images with little manipulation of buttons or clicks of the mouse.

7. Digital imaging and clinical workflow

7.1 Clinical workflow

Digital mammography has transformed our everyday working environment. For many, gone are the days of darkrooms with wet chemical processing and the challenges associated with them. Film screen mammography view boxes are being used less each day as softcopy display becomes more familiar to the radiologist. Digital mammography images can be viewed from anywhere, and the trend for comparisons to be on softcopy is becoming apparent. Also, with prior studies being in digital format, the number of lost or missing priors has decreased. Files rooms with overcrowded shelves and stacks of folders piled on the floor are starting to disappear as picture archiving systems (PACS) with electronic storage are used.

Digital mammography has also had a large impact on patient throughput. Technologist image acquisition and processing time with direct radiography (DR) digital mammography has been significantly decreased in both screening and diagnostic mammography (Berns, 2006; Kuzmiak, 2010). In the DR FFDM digital screening study by Berns et al., they studied the timed comparison of 183 hard-copy SFM cases and 181 FFDM softcopy display cases. Their results demonstrated a 7.5 min/case (35%) time savings over SFM (Berns et al., 2006).

Results were similar in the diagnostic timed mammography study by Kuzmiak et al. (Kuzmiak et al., 2010). This prospective study consisted of 3 phases: 1st Phase, 100 patients imaged with SFM; 2nd Phase, 100 patients imaged on DR FFDM and interpreted on a recently installed softcopy display mammography system; 3rd Phase, same as 2nd Phase but 3-months after installation of the softcopy display system. Their results showed the diagnostic mammographic acquisition times with processing were 13.02 min/case for SFM (Phase 1), 8.16 min/case for digital (Phase 2), and 10.66 min/case for digital (Phase 3). All phases also included the measured time for additional imaging that was requested by the interpreting study radiologists. Compared to SFM, acquisition time for Phase 2 and 3 digital were significantly less ($P < .001$ and $P < .0001$, respectively). For Phase 2 & 3 digital, there was a 4.86 min/case (37.3%) and 2.36 min/case (18.1%) time savings compared to SFM (Kuzmiak et al., 2010).

Regardless of reason for the mammogram, the main reason for the time savings is the elimination of processing time with DR mammography. The technologist no longer has to leave the exam room with SF cassettes to develop. With SFM, each film takes approximately 90 seconds to develop. This time is now saved. The technologist now can review the images on a 1-megapixal monitor after exposure while the patient is still in the room. After initial review by the technologist for positioning and technique, the images are sent to PACS with a push of a button or touch of a screen.

As part of the clinical workflow, there has been the concern of radiologist interpretation time with digital mammography. Berns et al. published average interpretation times, interpreted by seven radiologists, for their screening study of 1.2 minutes for SFM and 2.0 minutes for DR FFDM (Berns et al., 2006). Study results by Haygood et al. showed similar results in longer interpretation times with digital (Haygood et al., 2009). Haygood's study included 4 radiologists who were timed in clinical interpretation of 457 screening mammograms consisting of 189 SFM and 268 digital mammograms. They reported increased interpretation times for digital ranging from 1.27 to 3.37 minutes. The average interpretation time for all readers for SFM was 2.12 minutes and 4.0 minutes for digital (Haygood et al., 2009).

In contrast to the above screening studies, Kuzmiak et al. found the radiologist interpretation time for digital mammography on softcopy display was not significantly different from that for film mammography in a diagnostic mammography setting (P = .2853 and P = .2893, respectively) (Kuzmiak et al., 2010). The mean interpretation times were 3.75 min/case for screen film (Phase 1), 2.14 min/case for digital (Phase 2), and 2.26 min/case for digital (Phase 3). The results provide support to radiologists for conversion to direct radiographic digital mammography for clinical use and that radiologists planning on using softcopy display systems must have appropriate training to optimize throughput. In addition, softcopy display manufacturers should continue to improve the functionality and ergonomics of their products to make softcopy interpretation more efficient.

7.2 Electronically generated report

With softcopy display systems an electronically generated reporting system can be integrated with it. Numerous vendors are available and each has different functions depending on radiologist preference. With these systems, mammograms and other imaging reports can be dictated (generated) and electronically signed off. Thus, it decreases the time from the initiation of the patient's exam to the exchange of information to the patient's referring physician.

8. Conclusion

Digital mammography decouples the process of image acquisition, processing and display so that each component can be optimized. The digital format has allowed the development of additional software to aid the radiologist in lesion detection - computed aided detection. We are now able to view mammography images and interpret them from other clinical sites in different parts of the city, state, or country through televideo. Other emerging technologies such as three dimensional tomosynthesis are now entering clinical use. Digital technology has changed mammography over the last decade, and it will continue to change it for decades to come. It will be interesting to see what the future holds for our patients and us.

9. Acknowledgement

Dr. Kuzmiak is grateful for the inspiration and guidance provided over the years by her friend and colleague, Etta Pisano, MD. She would like to express her gratitude to Martin Yaffe, PhD, and Elodia Cole, MS, for their clinical insights and outstanding work. Finally, she would also like to thank Shiela Kuzmiak for the many hours of support during this project.

10. References

Aslund M, Cederstrom B, Lundqvist M, et al. Physical characterization of a scanning photon counting digital mammography system based on Si-strip detectors. *Med Phys* 2007; 34(6):1918-1925

Beam CA, Layde PM, Sullivan DC. Variability in the interpretation of screening mammograms by US radiologists. Finding from a national sample *Arch Intern Med* 1996; 156(2):209-213.

Berns EA, Hendrick RE, Solari M, et al. Digital and screen film mammography: comparison of image acquisition and interpretation times. *AJR* 2006; 187:38-41.

Bland KI, Copeland EM. *The Breast Comprehensive Management of Benign and Malignant Diseases. 2nd edition*. W.B. Saunders Company, Philadelphia, 1998.Bunch PC, Huff KE, Van Metter R. Analysis of the detective quantum efficiency of a radiographic screen film combination. *J Opt Soc AM* 1987; A4:902-909.

Bunch PC. The effects of reduced film granularity on mammographic image quality. In: Van Metter R, Beutel J (eds) Medical imaging 1997; Physics of medical imaging. Proc. SPIE 3032, 302-317.

Burrell HC, Sibbering DM, Wilson AR, et al. Screening interval breast cancers: mammographic features and prognostic factors. *Radiology* 1996; 199:811-817.

Byng JW, Critten JP, Yaffe MJ. Thickness equalization processing for mammographic images. *Radiology* 1997; 203:564-568.

Chan HP, Vyborny CJ, MacMahon H, et al. Digital mammography ROC studies of the effects of pixel size and unsharp mask filtering on the detection of subtle microcalcifications. *Invest Radiol* 1987; 22:581-589.

Cole EB, Pisano ED, Hanna LG, et al. Multicenter Clinical Assessment of the Fischer SenoScan Digital Mammography System. (abstract). Radiology (supplement) 2001; 221 (P):285.

Del Turco MR, Mantellini P, Ciatto S, et al. Full field digital versus screen film mammography: comparative accuracy in concurrent screening cohorts. *AJR* 2007; 189:860-866.

Dujm LEM, Guit GL, Zaat JOM, et al. Sensitivity, specificity, and positive predictive values of breast imaging in the detection of cancer. *BJR* 1997; 76:377-381.

Elmore JG, Wells CK, Lee CH, et al. Variability in radiologists' interpretations of mammograms. *N Engl J Med* 1992; 331(22):1493-1499.

Elmore JG, Armstrong K, Lehman CD, Fletcher, SW. Screening for breast cancer. *JAMA* 2005; 293(10), 1245-56.

Feig SA, Yaffe MJ. Current status of digital mammography. *Semin US CT MRI* 1996;17(5):424-443.

Feig SA, Yaffe MJ. Digital Mammography. *Radiographics* 1998; 18(4):893-901.

Ferlay J, Parkin DM, Steliarova-Foucher E GLOBOCAN 2008, Cancer Incidence and Mortality Worldwide: IARC CancerBase No. 10 [Internet] Lyon, France: International Agency for Research on Cancer; 2010. http://globocan.iarc.fr. Accessed Aug 1, 2011.

Food and Drug Administration. Information for manufacturers seeking marketing clearance of digital mammography systems.www.fda.gove/cdrh/ode/digmammo.html. Accessed Aug 1, 2011.

Ghetti C, Borrini A, Ortenzia O, et al. Physical characteristics of GE Senographe Essential-DS digital mammography detectors. *Med Phys* 2008; 35:456-463.

Haygood TM, Wang J, Atkinson EN, et al. Timed efficiency of interpretation of digital and film screen screening mammograms. *AJR* 2009; 192:216-220.

Heddson B, Roennow K, Olsson M, et al. Digital versus screen-film mammography: a retrospective comparison in a population-based screening program. *Eur J Radio* 2007; 64: 419-425.

Hendrick RC, Smith RA, Rutledge KH, Smart CR. Benefit of screening mammography in women ages 40-49: a new meta-analysis of randomized controlled trials. *J Natl Cancer Inst Monogr* 1997; 22:87-92.

Hendrick RE, Lewin JM, D'Orsi CJ, et al. Non-inferiority study of FFDM in an enriched diagnostic cohort: comparison with screen-film mammography in 625 women. In Yaffe MJ (ed) IWDM 2000; 5th International Workshop on Digital Mammography. Madison, WI: Medical Physics Publishing 2001:475-481.

Hendrick RE, Pisano ED, Averbukh A, et al. Comparison of acquisition of parameters and breast dose in digital mammography and screen-film mammography in the American College of RadiologyImaging Network Digital Mammography Imaging Screening Trial. *AJR* 2010; 194:362-369.

Howard DH, Elmore JG, Lee CH, et al. Observer variability in mammography, *Trans Assoc Am Physicians* 1993; 106:96-100.

Lewin JM, Hendrick RE, D'Orsi CJ, et al. Comparison of full field digital mammography to screen film mammography for cancer detection: results of 4945 paired examinations. Radiology 2001; 218:873-880.

Lewin JM, D'Orsi CJ, Hendrick RE, et al. Clinical comparison of full field digital mammography for breast cancer detection. AJR 2001;179:671-677.

Karssemeijer N, Snoeren P. Image Processing. In Bick U, Diekmann F (eds), *Digital Mammography*. Springer, Berlin, 2010.

Kim HH, Pisano ED, Cole EB, et al. Comparison of calcification specificity in digital mammography using softcopy display versus screen film mammography. *AJR* 2006; 187:1-4.

Kuzmiak CM, Cole EB, Zeng D, et al. Comparison of image acquisition and radiologist interpretation time in a diagnostic mammography center. *Acad Radiol* 2010; 17:1168-1174.

Marshal NW. Retrospective analysis of a detector fault for a full field digital mammography system. *Phys Med Biol* 2006; 51(21):5655-5673.

Nystrom L, Rutqvist LE, Wall S, et al. Breast cancer screening with mammography: overview of Swedish randomized trials. *Lancet* 1993; 342:973-978.

Perry N, Broeders M, de Wolf C et al (eds). European guidelines for quality assurance in breast cancer screening and diagnosis. 2006. 4th ed. European Communities. European Commission, Luxembourg.

Picard, JD. History of mammography. *Bull Acad Natl Med* 1998; 182(8):1613-20.

Pisano ED, Yaffe MJ. Digital mammography. *Breast Dis* 1998; 10(3,4):127-136.

Pisano ED, Cole EB, Hemminger BM, et al. Image Processing: Algorithms for digital mammography: a pictorial essay. *RadioGraphics* 2000; 20:1479-491.

Pisano ED, Cole EB, Kistner EO, et al. Interpretation of digital mammograms: comparison of speed and accuracy of softcopy versus printed film display. *Radiology* 2002; 12:1378-1382.

Pisano ED, Yaffe MJ, Kuzmiak CM. *Digital Mammography*. Lippencott, Williams & Wilkins, Philadelphia, 2004.

Pisano ED, Gatsonis C, Hendrick E, Yaffe MJ, et al. Diagnostic performance of digital versus film mammography for breast cancer screening. JAMA 2005; 353:1773-1783.

Saarenmaa I, Salminen T, Geiger U, et al. The effect of age and density of the breast on the sensitivity of breast cancer diagnosed by mammography and ultrasonography *Breast Cancer Res Treat* 2000; 67:117-123.

Sala M, Commas M, Macia F, et al. Implementation of digital mammography in a population-based breast cancer screening program: Effect of screening round on recall rate and cancer detection. *Radiology* 2009; 252:31-39.

Skaane P, Young K, Skjennald A. Population-based mammography screening: comparison of screen film mammography and full field digital mammography using soft copy reading: the Oslo I study. Radiology 2003; 229:877-884.

Skaane P, Skjennald A. Screen film mammography versus full field digital mammography with softcopy reading: randomized trial in a population-based screening program – The Oslo II study. *Radiology* 2004; 232:197-204.

Skaane P, Skjennald A, Young K, et al. Follow-up and final results of the Oslo I study comparing screen film mammography and full field digital mammography with softcopy reading. *Acta Radiol* 2005;46:679-689.

Skaane P, Hofvind S, Skjennald A. Randomized trial of screen film versus full field digital mammography with softcopy reading in population-based screening program: follow-up and final results of Oslo II study. *Radiology* 2007; 244:708-717.

Strax PS, Venet L, Shapiro. Value of mammography in reduction of mortality from breast cancer in mass screening. AJR 1973; 117(3):686-689.

Tabar L, Vitak B, Chen T, et al. Swedish Two-County Trial: Impact of mammographic screening on breast cancer mortality during 3 decades. *Radiology* 2011; 206(3):658-670.

Thunberg S, Francke T, Egerstrom J, et al. Evaluation of a photon counting mammography system. In: Antonuk LE, Yaffe MJ (eds) *Medical Imaging* 2002: physics of medical imaging. Proceeding of SPIE vol 4682.

Van Ongeval C, Jacobs J, Bosmans H. Classification of artifacts in clinical digital mammography. In Bick U, Diekmann F (eds), *Digital Mammography*. Springer, Berlin, 2010.

Van Steen a, Van Tiggelen R. Short History of Mammography: A Belgian Perspective. *JBR-BTR* 2007; 90:151-153.

Vigeland E, Klaasen H, Klingen TA, et al. Full field digital mammography compared to screen film mammography in the prevalent round of a population-based screening program: the Vestfold County study. *Eur Radiol* 2008; 18:183-191.

Vinnicombe S, Tinto Pereira SM, McCormack VA, et al. Full field digital versus screen film mammography: comparison within the UK breasts screening program and systematic review of published data. *Radiology*2009;251:347358.

www.acr.org/SecondaryMainMenuCategories/quality_safety/BIRADSAtlas/BIRADSAtlas excerptedtext/MammographyFourthEdition.aspx. Accessed August 2,2011.

www.cdc.gov/cancer/breast/statistics/Accessed Aug 1, 2011.

Yaffe MJ. Basic physics of digital mammography. In Bick U, Diekmann F (eds), *Digital Mammography*. Springer, Berlin, 2010.

Yaffe MJ. Detectors for Digital Mammography. In Bick U, Diekmann F (eds), *Digital Mammography*. Springer, Berlin, 2010.

Young KC, Alsager A, Oduko JM, et al. Evaluation of software for reading images of the CDMAM test object to assess digital mammography systems. Proc SPIE *Med Imaging* 2008; 69131C:1-11.

Young KC. Quality control in digital mammography. In Bick U, Diekmann F (eds), *Digital Mammography*. Springer, Berlin, 2010.

5

Image Quality Requirements for Digital Mammography in Breast Cancer Screening

Margarita Chevalier[1], Fernando Leyton[2,3], Maria Nogueira Tavares[3], Marcio Oliveira[3], Teogenes A. da Silva[3] and João Emilio Peixoto[4]
[1]*Complutense University of Madrid*
[2]*Diego Portales University*
[3]*Centro de Desenvolvimento da Tecnologia Nuclear*
[4]*Instituto Nacional do Câncer*
[1]*Spain*
[2]*Chile*
[3,4]*Brazil*

1. Introduction

Mammography is currently considered to be the best tool for early detection of breast cancer. The target groups of most of the population-based screening programmes are women aged between 50 and 65 years. A recent study has also shown mortality benefit in the age group 40-49 (Hellquist, et al, 2010). Screen-film mammography has been to date the traditional test for breast screening having been shown its efficacy in reducing breast cancer mortality in large randomised trials (Duffy, et al, 2006). The potential advantages of digital mammography over screen-film techniques have been the subject of several investigations which provides an improved diagnosis in dense breasts and an increase in breast cancer detection rate (Pisano et al, 2006; Hendrick et al, 2010).

Breast screening using X-ray mammography only confers a benefit on the screened population if it is able to detect breast cancer at an early stage, whereby the prognosis is improved. This can only be achieved by having high quality breast images to assure as much as possible the detection of small and subtle lesions in the breast (Muller, 1997;Karellas, 2004; Lewin, 2004; ICRU, 2009). High quality mammography must be achieved and maintained by applying rigorous and comprehensive quality assurance and control programmes.

The quality of the breast images depends critically on the design and performance of the radiographic unit, the image receptor, and on how that equipment is used to acquire and process the mammogram. The type of display and the conditions under which the image is viewed have an important effect on the ability of the radiologist to extract the information recorded in the mammogram. The diagnostic information is integrally related to the quality of the image and higher image quality will result in more accurate diagnosis (Nishikawa, 2004). The systematic monitoring of both image quality and radiation dose is needed to guarantee a constant high quality of the mammography examination (ICRU, 2009; Ng, 2005). Conventional film/screen mammography is being gradually substituted by digital technology in most countries. Consequently, there is an important activity related with developing quality control protocols adapted to this new digital technologies (CEC,2006; SEFM, 2008;NHSBSP, 2009; IAEA, 2011).

Data retrieved from programmes in the Netherlands (Beckers, 2003), Sweden (Leitz, 2001), Norway (Pedersen, 2000) and the UK (NHSBSP, 2003) show that the levels of DG in screen-film mammography range between 0.8 and 2.5 mGy for a 5.3 cm compressed breast thickness. Thus, several national and international protocols have established an accepted DG limit of 2.5 mGy for a 5.3 cm standard breast thickness. Data from a European survey (Report EUR 14821, 2001) on radiation doses developed in 56 mammography institutions showed DG values ranging from 1.0 to 3.0 mGy for 6.0 cm thick breasts. This value was established from measurements using an acrylic simulator.

This chapter is devoted to describe the relevant parameters and procedures for the quality control of digital mammography systems making the necessary distinctions among the two technologies (computed radiography (CR) and flat panel detectors (DR)).

2. Detectors for digital mammography

2.1 Flat panel Systems – DR

Flat panel systems (DR) have an active matrix of electronic detectors where each element absorbs the radiation transmitted through mammary tissue, producing an electrical signal proportional to the intensity of the X-rays.

2.1.1 Indirect capture of an image

In the indirect capture of an image, a flat screen scintillator, a photodiode circuitry layer, and a TFT array are used (Fig. 1). Caesium iodide crystals (CsI(Tl)) are the scintillators usually employed. CsI(Tl) crystals are structured in an array of thin needles that guide the light photon reducing the light diffusion within the scintillator layer. The light is captured by the elements of the photodiode matrix (amorphous silicon), which converts the light into electrical current. These amorphous silicon sensors (a-Si) are connected to a matrix of thin-film transistors (TFT) which store the information of each pixel up to the moment of its reading by the scan circuit in the detector (Vedantham, 2000; Suryanarayanan, 2004; Peixoto, 2009).

2.1.2 Direct capture of an image

In the direct capture mode, an amorphous selenium plate (a-Se) photoconductor is used to convert the incident X-ray photons into electron-hole pairs (Yaffe, 1997, Peixoto, 2009). Each charge of the electron-hole pair created is attracted by the corresponding electrode under the action of the strong electric field applied between the electrodes. The created charge is accumulated and stored by a TFT matrix (Fig. 2).

2.2 Computed radiography system – CR

Computed radiography (CR) is a process comparatively similar to the conventional screen-film system. The film is replaced by a plate (IP) made up of photostimulable phosphorus

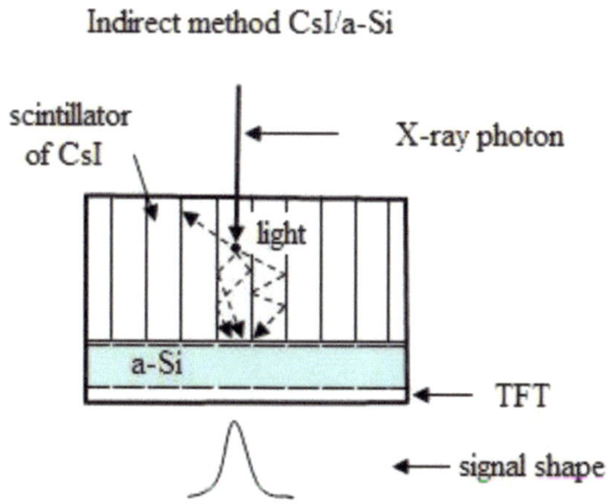

Fig. 1. Indirect method of image acquisition with CsI(Tl)/a-Si. The CsI scintillators hold needle structures and work as channels which guide the light perpendicularly to the surface of the photodiodes (Peixoto, 2009).

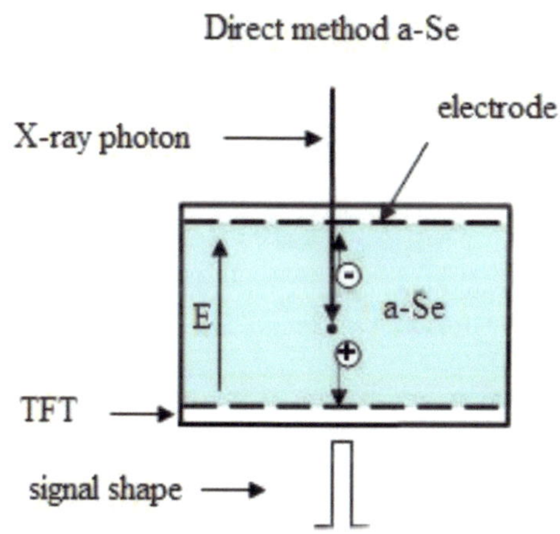

Fig. 2. Method of direct acquisition of an image with a-Se (Peixoto, 2009)

(PSP) which is introduced into a cassette of similar characteristics than the one used with the film.

Inside the cassette, the photostimulable phosphorus plate is used to absorb and store the energy of the X-ray transmitted through the breast, thus producing a 'latent image'. The energy stored in the phosphorous plate is associated to the electrons raised to excited levels of energy in which they hold trapped ("F-centre"). This is the non-observable electronic latent image, where the number of electrons trapped is proportional to the number of incident X-ray photons (Marcelino V.A. Dantas., 2010). As follows, the cassette is inserted into the reading unit (Fig. 3). Inside this unit, the plate is scanned with a low energy intense laser light (~ 2 eV) which is highly focused. The electrons trapped in the phosphorus photostimulable matrix (PSP) are stimulated by the laser energy, and a significant fraction returns to the lowest energy level with a simultaneous emission of a higher energy photo-stimulated luminescence (PSL) (~ 3 eV). The intensity of the PSL, proportional to the number of electrons emitted, is captured by a light guide system near the IP (Fig. 4). A photomultiplier tube (PMT) at the output of the light guide amplifies and converts the PSL into a corresponding output voltage (Rowlands, 2002; Dantas, 2010).

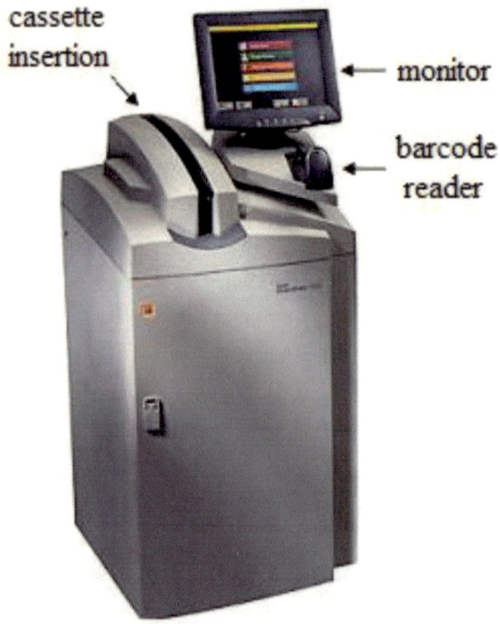

Fig. 3. Image digitiser for CR Systems (Alvarenga, 2008).

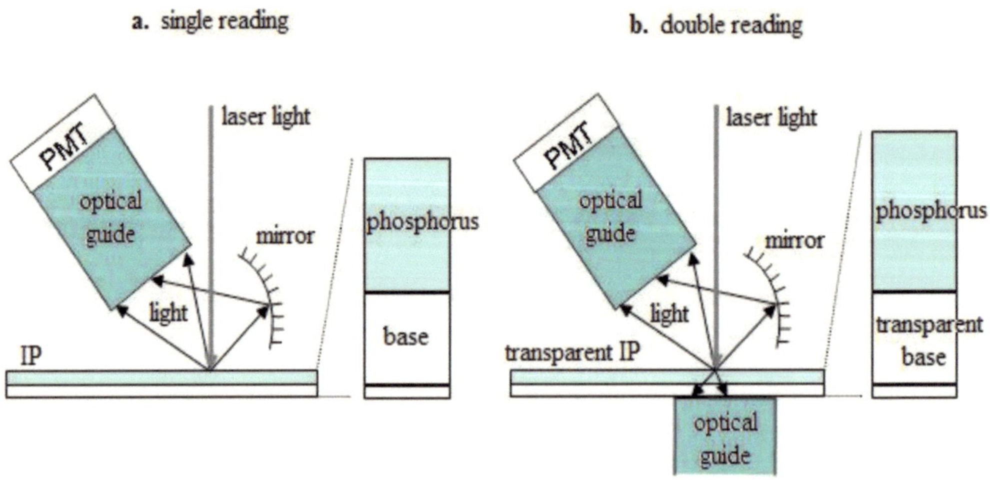

Fig. 4. Image acquisition for the CR system: (a) single reading; (b) double reading (Peixoto, 2009).

The residual latent image information is erased through an intense light which removes the electrons not released by the laser stimulation, and the IP returns to the cassette "reset" and ready to be reused.

The diagram of the whole process involving the image acquisition with a CR system is shown in Fig. 5 (left).

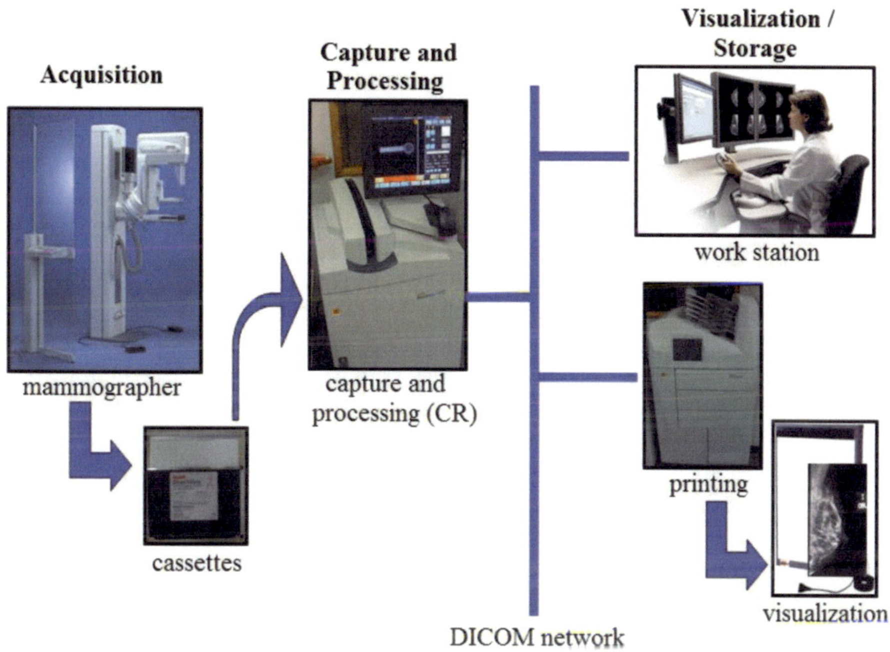

Fig. 5. Acquisition process, processing and visualisation of mammography images CR (Alvarenga, 2008).

3. Parameters with the greatest impact on dose and image quality

The objective of mammography is to provide the early detection of cancer, and therefore the image quality is a fundamental aspect. The image with a suitable diagnostic-quality has to be acquired with a radiation dose as low as possible. Nowadays, it is widely accepted that mean glandular dose (D_G) is the best indicator to estimate the risk associated with breast irradiation in mammography (see definition in SectionV). Both factors, image quality and D_G, are depending on breast characteristics (glandularity and thickness), exposure factors (beam quality, exposure time and compression force), detector features and mammography system performance (automatic exposure control) and characteristics (geometry, focal spot size).

3.1 Characteristics of the breast

Breast composition varies among women due to different proportion of glandular, fibrous and adipose tissue. The composition also changes with the age of the woman such that the proportion of adipose tissue increases with age.

Differences among the x-ray attenuation properties of the different breast tissues can be observed at the breast images. Glandular and fibrous tissues are visualised in mammography as radio-opaque whereas the adipose tissues are observed as radio-lucent (dark). Therefore, given the same compressed breast thickness a dense breast (having a higher proportion of glandular tissues) absorbs a higher amount of radiation than an adipose breast.

The lesions of interest for diagnosis are microcalcifications, masses, asymmetries and distortions of the breast architecture. Microcalcifications are small (100 μm) and "easily" detected regardless of breast density. The masses tend to have low contrast, making it difficult to detect. Therefore, mammography must have - besides optimal resolution - good contrast, which makes visible those anatomic structures and pathological signs which have very similar densities.

3.2 The compression system

A proper compression of the breast is fundamental to provide a good quality image. Breast compression brings the structures close to the detector enhancing sharpness, prevents breast movement, reduces the breast thickness penetrated by X-rays and reduces the scattered radiation. All these factors improve the contrast and even reduce the absorbed dose (Karellas, 2004). In addition, the exposure factors in modern mammography systems are automatically selected in base of the compressed breast thickness. Quality control programmes have to include procedures to verify the compression force and the accuracy of the breast thickness determined by the system.

3.3 Automatic exposure control

In mammography, the automatic exposure control (AEC) (also known as "photo timer") cuts off the exposure when arrives to the AEC radiation sensor, which lies below the anti-scatter grid and the image receptor, the necessary dose resulting in optimum optical density or pixel value. The sensor can be placed at several positions (3 in most of the units) between the thorax and the nipple in depending of the breast size.

Flat panel detectors of digital mammography units operate as AEC sensors. In this case, the information can be derived from the whole area of the detector or from predefined regions.

The AEC of most modern mammography units uses the information associated with a pre-exposure to determine the attenuation of the breast. This information along with the breast thickness automatically detected (compressor) determines all the exposure factors (anode/filter, kV, mAs).

The AEC is committed to provide images with an appropriate optical density, independently from the beam quality and the characteristics of the breast. Thus, there is a guarantee that the information will be registered in the linear region of the characteristic curve of the film.

In digital systems, the main role of the AEC is to assure that signal noise ratio (SNR) and contrast noise ratio (CNR) are adequate throughout the image and that the dose values comply with recommendations.

3.4 X-ray spectrum

For both digital and screen-film detection techniques, the energy spectrum of the X-ray beam (including their filtering) is of a great concern when evaluating the performance of the mammographic systems, demanding careful and accurate quality controls in a clinical environment.

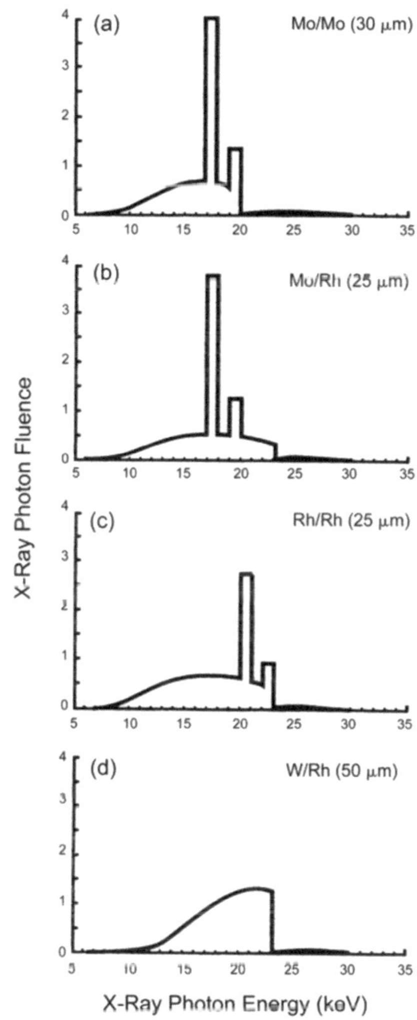

Fig. 6. X-ray spectra for 30 kVp operating potential for Mo/Mo (a), Mo/Rh (b), Rh/Rh (c), and W/Rh (d) source/filter assemblies (NCRP 149, 2005).

The attenuation coefficient of the glandular tissue is similar to that of the tumour tissue which makes difficult the visualization of smaller tumours; low energy X-ray beam is needed to demonstrate the subtle density differences between non-calcified normal and abnormal tissues. X-ray tubes of mammography systems are equipped with special anode/filter combinations, such as Mo/Mo or Mo/Rh, operating in the 25-35 kVp range. The spectra of several anode/filter combinations (Fig. 6) show the important proportion of of X-rays characteristics (17.5 and 19.7 keV) from the molybdenum target and the strong suppression of the spectrum at energies >20 keV because of the k-shell absorption edge of the molybdenum filter (Fig. 6a) or else higher than 23 keV because of the Rh filter (Fig. 6b). The characteristics of the new digital detectors make it possible to use other anode/filter combinations such as Rh/Rh (Fig. 6c), W/Rh (Fig. 6d), W/Ag and W/Al which have some advantages for imaging dense or thick breasts. In addition, the breast doses associated with these combinations are lower than those delivered with Mo/Mo or Mo/Rh.

The adequate selection of the spectrum (beam) may reduce the dose values above 20% (Young, 2006; Dance, 2000; Riabi, 2010). The threshold value for breast thickness where the spectrum is changed depends on the AEC calibration which is performed by technical services who install the equipment (which should be done together with those medical staff who use the equipment). The correct selection of the X-ray beam will strongly influence the dose and image quality.

4. Image quality in mammography

Image quality is a fundamental concept for the control and optimisation of mammography; it aims to improve the early detection of cancer and other pathological lesions in the breasts. The image quality can be quantified by measuring the contrast noise ratio, the signal noise ratio, the modulation transfer function (MTF) (spatial resolution), the noise, the uniformity and various artefacts such as the ghost image. In order to assess these physical parameters, phantoms and more specific devices are needed to perform quality control in mammography. The current trend is to utilise a contrast-detail phantom (CDMAM) which permits the assessment of the image quality as a function of the contrast threshold associated with the circular objects of different diameters and thickness (SEFM, 2008). The "clinical "assessment of the image quality is better performed by means of the receiver operating curve (ROC) methodology. Unfortunately, this type of analysis is far too complex and is time consuming. In addition, it is required a database with too many images, which makes its application difficult in the clinical practice of routine image quality control (NCRP, 2005).

4.1 MTF

The modulation transfer function (MTF) is a quantitative and objective measurement of the image quality that can be provided by a system. MTF gives information about the magnitude of the object contrast which is transferred to the image as a function of the spatial frequency. The low spatial frequencies correspond to rough details, whereas the high ones define the fine details or the edges of the structures. For example, an MTF with a value of 0.5 for a determined frequency means that the inherent modulation (contrast) of the object will diminish at 50% given the limitations of the image system (ICRU, 2009) (Fig. 7).

In practice, the MTF is determined through the Fourier transform of the line spread function (LSF), which is obtained through the differentiation of the edge response (ESF).

Spatial resolution is expressed in terms of spatial frequency, which in turn is associated with a MTF value.

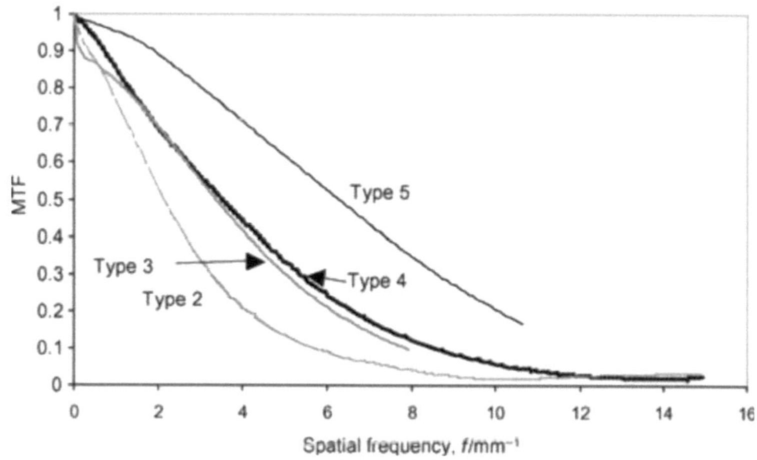

Fig. 7. Modulation transfer function of mammography systems (ICRU, 2009).

4.2 Noise

The main component of noise in radiographic images is the quantum noise, which is associated with the statistical fluctuations in the photons' fluence on the detector and with the random variations in the absorption. The simplest way to define the noise is through a measurement of the standard deviation (sd) of the number of photons absorbed (N) in a region of the detector. This figure complies with Poisson statistics, and therefore sd = $N^{0.5}$ (i.e., the sd is related to the square root of the Kerma) (Chevalier, 2010).

The structural noise in the digital detectors emerges mainly from the lack of homogeneity in the sensitivity of the elementary detectors (i.e., from the fixed spatial variation of the image detecting structure), which means that it is also proportional to the dose. Moreover, this noise causes the appearance of a structured background in the image, which is usually removed through the flat field techniques. These techniques include the creation of a corrective mask from a direct and uniform image of the X-ray beams (Chevalier, 2010).

In digital systems, what has to be added to these two types of noise is the electronic one, which emerges from the electronic readout outside the pixels and in the amplification of the signal and which does not depend on the dose. The electronic noise owes essentially to the dark noise in the detectors and decreases if the temperature of the surroundings is lowered or reduced. Therefore, the digital equipment has to operate in temperatures at intervals between 20-30 °C.

4.3 Uniformity

The initial operation which usually occurs is a "flat-field", a correction of the uniformity of gain. The non-uniformity of the sensitivity of the detector is corrected through a gain map and is also used to correct all the images acquired. Moreover, if an element of a single (pixel) detector is defective its signal can be replaced with a reasonable combination of adjacent detector signals. This is acceptable if the defective detectors are isolated and only few of them are faulty. Detectors of the CR type presents a lack of uniformity due to the heal effect that is very depending on the X-ray unit.

4.4 Artefacts

Artefacts are undesirable characteristics which are not related to the mammary anatomic structures of a radiographic image. They can hinder the image by hiding or simulate a lesion on detection.

Artefacts can be caused by the source of X-rays, the beam filter, the compression device, breast support, grid, and flaws in processing, amongst others. In digital mammography, besides the sources just cited, the non-uniformity in the response of the elemental detectors may also generate artefacts, owing to the results of an inadequate flat-fielding. Another drawback in the digital system is the presence of reminiscent images (ghost images), resulting from previous exposures (ICRU, 2009). The latest appears more often with CR systems or aSe based flat panel detectors.

5. Dosimetry in mammography

One of the pillars underpinning the analysis of the risks-benefits of mammography is the accurate knowledge of the imparted doses, since it is well-established that there is an association between breast dose and the increased incidence of breast cancer. Assessments of breast doses are particularly important in breast screening programmes in which large groups of asymptomatic women undergo mammographic examinations. As in other radiological examinations, dose values are indicative of the diagnostic adequacy of the mammography technique selected in clinical practice. In addition, knowledge of dose values is essential for optimisation strategies developed to minimise doses while maintaining the necessary image quality.

The X-ray spectrum in mammography is of low energy and the depth dose within the breast decreases rapidly. Due to this, it is important to use a dosimetric quantity which gives a measure of the dose to the whole organ. Glandular tissue is the most vulnerable in the breast as compared to adipose, skin and areolar (nipple) tissues (Hammerstein et al., 1979). At present, it is widely accepted that mean glandular dose (D_G) is the most appropriate dosimetric quantity to predict the risk of radiation carcinogenesis. Therefore, this quantity has been recommended by several national and international organisations (NCRP, 1986; IPSM, 1989; IAEA, 2007) and it is the quantity used in many national protocols for mammographic quality assessment (CEC, 1996, 2006; ACR, 1999; IAEA, 2007). The factors that affect D_G are the X-ray beam quality and breast thickness and composition. These two latter parameters have a larger variability than the former, varying both within and between populations, and the latter with women's age as well. Even when the average glandularity would be the same, its distribution is unpredictable and changes from breast to breast.

Direct measurements of D_G are not possible for individual breasts and, therefore, D_G is derived from the entrance surface dose (or a related quantity) using adequate conversion factors (ICRU, 2005; NCRP, 2004). These factors were initially measured (Hamerstein, 1979; Stanton, 1984) and further calculated by means of Monte Carlo techniques (Rosenstein, 1980; Dance, 1990, 2000, 2009; Wu et al, 1991, 1994; Klein et al., 1997; Boone et al., 2002). This latter approach allows for the possibility of estimating conversion factors for a wide range of input spectra and breast features. Differences among the conversion factors (c_G) obtained by several authors mainly arise from differences in breast model geometry, mammographic X-ray spectral data, photon interaction cross-sections and Monte Carlo codes. Other important factors affecting the calculations are the mammography system's characteristics and the imaging system components and geometry. The differences in c_G values quoted by different authors were as high as 15-16% (Klein, 1997; ICRU, 2005; Dance 2000).

The breast model most commonly adopted (Fig. 8) has a central region consisting of a homogeneous mixture of adipose and glandular tissue surrounded by a layer at all sides, except for the one corresponding to the chest wall representing the skin. It is assumed that the breast is firmly compressed by a polycarbonate compression paddle. The percentage of breast glandularity is defined as the fraction by weight of glandular tissue at the central region (without skin). Most authors employ the elemental tissue composition published by Hammerstein et al. (1979).

Initially, it was assumed that a 50:50 mixture of adipose and glandular tissues was representative of a typical breast (Hammerstein, 1979). On this basis, phantoms of several thicknesses were constructed assuming this "standard" composition with the aim of facilitating D_G estimates in the practice. This assumption implied that the fraction of glandular tissue was independent of compressed breast thickness. On the basis of this data, the standard "phantom" was defined as a 4.5 cm thickness of PMMA, representing the "standard breast" (4 cm thick and 50%/50% glandular/adipose tissue) (IPEM, 1989; CEC, 1996). Data indicating that the composition of the average compressed breast deviates from the 50:50 composition has been published (Geise, 1996; Klein et al., 1997; Young et al., 1998; Chevalier, 1998; Beckett, 2000; Zoetelief et al., 2006). In addition, it was found that breast glandularity decreases when the compressed breast thickness increases. In some of these works it is also determined that the equivalent thickness of PMMA gives the same incident air kerma at its upper surface as for that of a breast of a specified thickness and composition (Geise, 1996; Dance et al., 2000, 2009; Kruger, 2001; Argo, 2004).

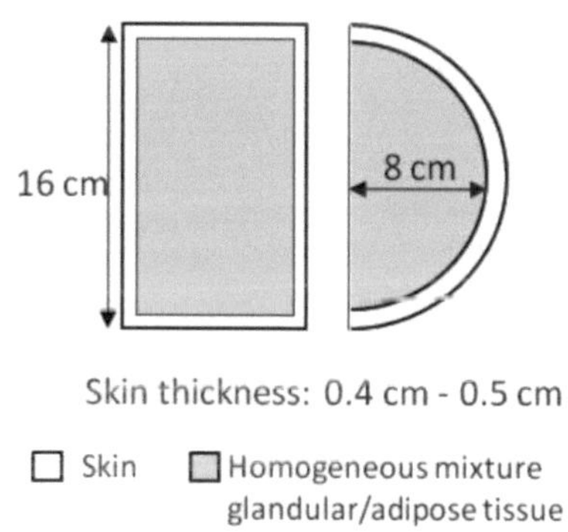

Fig. 8. Breast model geometry. The rectangular section represents a vertical cross section through the breast coplanar with the focal spot of the X-ray tube. The D-shape section represents the breast in craniocaudal projection. The shaded and outer regions represent, respectively, the breast parenchyma and the skin (0.5 cm of adipose tissue). In the work of Dance (2009) it is used as a voxelised breast model.

5.1 Practical issues

D_G is generally calculated through the following relationship (ICRU, 2005):

$$D_G = c_G \cdot K_{a,i} \tag{1}$$

where $K_{a,i}$ represents the incident air kerma (without backscatter) and c_G is the appropriate conversion factor. The incident air kerma is the air kerma free in the air (without backscatter) at the central axis of the incident X-ray beam at the skin-entrance plane which yields the desired image optical density (screen-film mammography) or signal:noise ratio (digital mammography).

5.1.1 Determination of the incident air kerma

Two approaches have been used to determine the incident air kerma, Ka,i. In the European and IAEA approach (CEC, 1996, 2006; IAEA, 2007), this quantity is calculated from the measured value of the X-ray tube output, Y(d), in terms of air kerma per tube-current-exposure-time product (mGy/mAs), measured at a distance d from the focal spot of the mammography unit. The value of Ka,i at the focus to surface distance for the phantom or for compressed breast (d') is determined as follows:

$$K_{a,i} = Y(d) P_{it} \cdot \left(\frac{d}{d'}\right)^2 \tag{2}$$

Where P_{it} is the mAs employed for a given exposure of the compressed breast or phantom, which is determined from the AEC post-exposure readout. The tube output has to be measured using an ionisation chamber with a flat energy response (CEC, 1996; ICRU, 2009) and conveniently calibrated for the mammography beam qualities. The ionisation chamber is placed at 6 cm from the chest wall and laterally centre. The distance d is usually fixed at 4.5 cm above the breast support. The compression plate should be about 10 cm above the chamber so as to avoid backscatter effects.

	Wu, 1991	Wu, 1994	Dance, 1990	Dance, 2000	Dance, 2009
c_G	D_GN	$\overline{D_GN}$	p·g	g·c·s	g·c·s
Units	mrad/R	mrad/R	mGy/mGy	mGy/mGy	mGy/mGy
Breast composition (% glandular tissue)	Homogeneous mixture. 100%; 50%; 0%		Homog. mixture. 50%	Homog. mixture 0% - 100%	Homog. mixture 0% - 100%
Breast thickness (cm)	3 - 8		2 - 8	2 - 11	2 - 11
Spectra	Mo/ Mo	Mo/Rh; Rh/Rh	Mo/Mo; W/Mo; W/Rh; W/Pd; W/Al	Mo/Mo; Mo/Rh Rh/Rh; W/Rh	W/Ag W/Al
Tube voltage (kV)	10 - 35		23 - 50	25, 26, 28, 30, 32	25 - 40
Source image distance	60 cm				65
Compressor	In place compressing the breast				
Grid	-----		-----	In place	In place
Image receptor	-----		Yes (screen)	Yes (screen)	Yes (screen)

Table 1. Important parameters considered by Dance and Wu for the calculation of the conversion factors using Monte Carlo techniques.

In the ACR approach (ACR, 1999), $K_{a,i}$ is directly measured by placing the ionisation chamber adjacent to the ACR phantom at the level of the entrance surface of the phantom. The chamber is positioned at 4 cm from the chest wall. The compressor plate is located above the phantom and the chamber. The exposure conditions are those used clinically for a 4 cm compressed breast.

Ka,i can be also measured using TLD dosimeters (ACR, 1999; CEC, 1996) placed on the entrance surface of the phantom or breast. The TLDs have to be calibrated in terms of air kerma free-in-air against a suitable ionisation chamber and dosimeter. Hence, the entrance dose measured by TLDs placed on the phantom or patient surface includes backscatter. Measurements performed with TLD dosimeters are influenced by many factors, including the performance of the instrument and those related to procedure of dosimeter preparation and handling. In addition, TLDs' response dependence of scatter gives rise to underestimations of $K_{a,i}$ in a magnitude that is dependent on the dosimeter's thickness and the relative amount of backscatter radiation (Dance at al., 1999). Another factor that limits the use of TLD dosimeters is related with its visibility in the breast image. It is recommended that they be positioned on the upper inner quadrant of the breast so as to minimise interference with breast tissues.

5.1.1.1 Mean glandular dose (D_G) estimates

The ACR protocol adopted the c_G values calculated by Wu (1991, 1994; Sobol, 1997). The European and the IAEA protocols (CEC, 1996, 2006; IAEA, 2007) recommended the use of the c_G values from Dance (1990; 2000; 2009). Fig. 8 and Table 1 summarise the details used by both authors to perform the Monte Carlo calculations. The c_G values depend on the beam quality (half value layer (HVL)), breast thickness and breast composition. It is important to measure HLV and compressed breast thickness with accuracy in order to minimise the errors in the D_G estimate. Narrow beam geometry is recommended for HVL measurements with the aim of reducing the influence of scattered radiation (IPEM, 2005; IAEA, 2007). In addition, Al filters of high purity (>99%) should be used and the compressor plate should be in place during the measurements. Errors in the compressed breast thickness measurement are due to the compressor plate which can bend and deform considerably. Several authors have proposed methods to gain accuracy in these measurements (Burch, A, 1995; Maria S. Nogueira., 2011).

D_G values derived from phantom measurements are useful for 1) simplifying the follow-up of the mammography system's performance, 2) comparing with references or limiting values allowing the checking of the compliance of the equipment with recommendations, 3) checking if the exposure factors selected by the mammography system are suitable in terms of radiation dose, 4) for developing optimisation strategies.

The evaluation of the mean glandular dose with large patient's samples enables a more direct evaluation of the risk of radiation induced cancer. However, it is difficult to know the composition of individual breasts needed to determine the conversion factors. A fairly widespread method is to determine the composition of the breast from its image. To avoid bias or subjective criteria the BI-RADS criteria are used (ACR, 1998) so that the individual breasts are classified by the radiologist into one of four possible groups according to its ascribed glandularity (0%, 25%, 75% and 100%).

5.1.1.2 The European and the IAEA approach: measurements of phantoms

Dose assessment in mammography initially (CEC, 1996) relied on the estimation of D_G for a 4.5 cm thick standard breast model with 50% glandularity in a central region by using a 4.0 cm thickness PMMA phantom. D_G was estimated using the c_G from Dance (1990) given in Table 1. It was recommended that patient dosimetry be performed by recording the exposure data and compressed breast thickness of at least 50 patients. Ka,i and D_G were calculated for each patient using the c_G factors tabulated by Dance (1990) for the corresponding HVL value and compressed breast thickness. The main problem associated with this methodology was firstly due to the fact that the average compressed breast thickness of a typical population is 5.5 cm. Secondly, several works showed a breast composition for the standard breast different to that of 50% glandularity. In addition, modern X-ray systems select different spectra as a function of both breast thickness and composition. In order to take into account all these factors, Dance et al. (2000) modify the definition of c_G according to the expression given in Table 1. In this expression, the g-factor (unchanged from that initially used) corresponds to a glandularity of 50% and is tabulated for different breast thicknesses and HVL. The c-factor corrects for any difference in breast composition from 50% glandularity and is tabulated for different HVL, breast thicknesses and breast glandularities. The factor s makes a correction for the use of an X-ray spectrum other than that for a Mo/Mo target–filter combination. The value for s depends only on the anode/filter combination, except in the case of W/Al which depends also on the kVp (Dance, 2009).

The equivalence between a range of PMMA thickness (2 - 8 cm) and compressed breast thickness has also been determined (Dance, 2000). According to the resulting equivalences, Ka,i delivered for a 4.5 cm thick PMMA phantom is equivalent to that for a 5.3 cm thick breast with 29% glandularity. This result was deduced from a sample of women in the age range 50-64 (Young, 1998; Becket, 2000). The mean glandular dose for different PMMA thicknesses is estimated using the relationship:

$$D_{G,PT} = K_{PT} \cdot g_{CBT} \cdot c_{CBT} \cdot s \quad (3)$$

K_{PT} is the air kerma at the entrance surface of a phantom of $_{PT}$ thickness and the g_{CBT} and c_{CBT} factors are the values tabulated for the equivalent compressed breast thickness.

The D_G limits proposed by the European (CEC, 2006) and IAEA (2011) protocols are given in Table 2 for a range of PMMA thickness. These values have been derived from screen/film mammography, since the cost associated with the transition to digital mammography should not imply an increase in the doses.

Thickness of PMMA (mm)	Thickness of equivalent breast (mm)	Acceptable level for D_G to equivalent breast (mGy)	Achievable level for D_G to equivalent breast (mGy)
20	21	1.0	0.6
30	32	1.5	1.0
40	45	2.0	1.6
45	53	2.5	2.0
50	60	3.0	2.4
60	75	4.5	3.6
70	90	6.5	5.1

Table 2. Acceptable and achievable limits for mean glandular dose (D_G).

5.1.1.3 Measurements on patients

The method followed for patient dosimetry relies on the results obtained in two studies (Young et al 1998; Beckett et al., 2000) that have each independently estimated the breast composition of women attending for screening. As a result, the average breast composition as a function of breast thickness was established for two age groups. One age group (aged 50 to 64) corresponds to the ages of women currently invited for breast screening in most of the programmes. The second age group corresponds to women aged between 40 and 49. D_G is calculated for each breast thickness by using the c-factors for the corresponding average composition of each age group.

The impact of the new factors c and s on D_G values obtained through the patients sample was analysed by recalculating the dose values obtained in previous studies (NHSBSP, 2003). It was found that, for the largest breasts (thickest on compression), the use of the c-factor increases doses by approximately 30%. For the smallest breasts, the dose estimates are decreased by 11%. The overall effect is to increase the average doses by about 11% for craniocaudal views and by about 14% for mediolateral oblique views.

6. Acknowledgments

This work took place within the framework of the Centre of Development of Nuclear Technology in Brazil through the project "Avaliação da Qualidade e Requisitos de Proteção Radiológica em Mamografia Digital e Monitoramento Dos Serviços de Mamografia de Minas Gerais - apoiado pela FAPEMIG e PCI-CNPq."

7. References

ACR. American College of Radiology (1998). Illustrated Breast Imaging Reporting and Data System (BI-RADS®), 3rd ed. *American College of Radiology*, Reston, Virginia, USA

ACR. American College of Radiology. (1999). Mammography Quality Control Manual, *American College of Radiology*, Reston, Virginia, USA

Alvarenga, FL and Nogueira MS. (2008). Análise de Parâmetros e Controle da Qualidade de Sistemas de Radiologia Computadorizada para Mamografia. *Centro de Desenvolvimento da Tecnologia Nuclear,* Belo Horizonte, 2008. Available from http://www.dominiopublico.gov.br/pesquisa/DetalheObraForm.do?select_action=&co_obra=125026

American Association of Physicists in Medicine. (2006). Acceptance testing and quality control of photostimulable storage phosphor imaging systems. *AAPM Report n° 93*, October 2006. ISSN:0271-7344

Argo WP, Hintenlang K, and Hintenlang DE. (2004). A tissue-equivalent phantom series for mammography dosimetry. *JACMP*. vol 5, N°4: 112-119. ISSN : 1526-9914

Beckers, S.W. et al. (2003). Results of technical quality control in the Dutch breast cancer screening programme(2001-2002). (Nijmegen, The Netherlands). Proc. EFOMP Congress.

Beckett J and Kotre C J. (2000). Dosimetric implications of age related glandular changes in screening mammography. *Phys Med Biol,* 45 (2000): 801–813. ISSN 1361-6560

Boone, JM. (2002). Normalized glandular dose (DgN) coefficients for arbitrary x-ray spectra in mammography: Computer-fit values of Monte Carlo derived data. *Med. Phys.* 29(2002):869–875. ISSN: 0094-2405

Brazil Ministry of Health. Report nb. 453 of June 1, (june 1998). Guidelines for Radiological Protection in Medical and Odontological Radiodiagnostic. *Ministry of Health*, Official Press, Brasília, Jun 2, 1998.

Burch A, and Law J. (1995). A method for estimating compressed breast thickness during mammography. *Br J Radiol*. 68: 394–399. ISSN: 1748-880X

CEC. European Commission. (1996). European Protocol on Dosimetry in Mammography, Report EUR 16263. *European Commission*. Office for Official Publications of the European Communities, Luxembourg

CEC. European Commission. European Guidelines for Quality Assurance in Mammography Screening. (2006). Report EUR 14821 4th ed. *European Commission*. Office for Official Publications of the European Communities, Luxembourg

Chevalier M, Morán P, Pombar M, Lobato R, Vañó E. (1998). Breast Dose Measurements on a Large Group of Patients: Results from a Four Years Period. *Radiat Prot Dosimetry*. (1998) 80 (1-3): 187 - 190. ISSN 1742-3406

Chevalier and Torres R. (2010). Mamográfica digital. Rev Fis Med 11(1):11-26 (SEFM, Madrid)

Dance DR. (1990). Monte-Carlo calculation of conversion factors for the estimation of mean glandular breast dose. *Phys Med Biol*. 35: 1211–1220. ISSN 1361-6560

Dance DR, Skinner CL, Young KC, Beckett J R and Kotre CJ. (2000). Additional factors for the estimation of mean glandular breast dose using the UK mammography dosimetry protocol. *Phys Med Biol*. 45: 3225–3240. ISSN 1361-6560

Dance DR., Thilander Klang A, Sandborg M, et al. (2000). Influence of anode/filter material and tube potential on contrast, signal-to-noise ratio and average absorbed dose in mammography: a Montecarlo study. *Br J Radiol* 73: 1056-1067. ISSN: 1748-880X

Dantas MVA and Nogueira MS. (2010). Dose glandular e controle de qualidade da imagem em serviços de mamografia com sistema de radiografia computadorizada. Comissão Nacional de Energia Nuclear, *Centro de Desenvolvimento Da Tecnologia Nuclear*, Programa de Pós-Graduação em Ciência e Tecnologia das Radiações Minerais e Materiais, Belo Horizonte, Brasil, 2010. (Available from, http://www.dominiopublico.gov.br/pesquisa/DetalheObraForm.do?select_action=&co_obra=181971)

Duffy SW, Tabar L, Chen THH, Smith RA, Holmberg L, Jonsson H, Lenner P, Nyström L, and Törnberg S. 2006. Reduction in breast cancer mortality from organized service screening with mammography:1.Further consideration with extended data. Cancer Epidemiol. Biomarkers Prev 15: 45–51

Geise RA, and Palchevsky A. (1996). Composition of mammographic phantom materials. *Radiology*. 198: 347–350. ISSN 1527-1315

Riabi HA, Mehnati P, Mesbahi A. (2010). Evaluation of mean glandular dose in a full-field digital mammography unit in Tabriz, Iran. *Radiat Prot Dosimetry* 142, 22-227. ISSN 1742-3406

Hammerstein GR, Miller DW, White DR, Masterson ME,Woodard HQ and Laughlin JS. (1979). Absorbed radiation dose in mammography. *Radiology*. 130, 485–491. ISSN 1527-1315

Hellquist BN, Duffy SW, Abdsaleh S, Björneld L, Bordás P, Tabár L, Viták B, Zackrisson S, Nyström L, and Jonsson H, (2010) Effectiveness of Population-Based Service Screening with Mammography for Women Ages 40 to 49 Years. Evaluation of the Swedish Mammography Screening in Young Women (SCRY) Cohort. *Cancer* 117: 714–722. doi: 10.1002/cncr. 25650

Hendrick RE, Pisano ED, Averbukh A, Moran C, Berns EA, Yaffe MJ, Herman B, Acharyya S, and Gatsonis C. 2010. Comparison of Acquisition Parameters and Breast Dose in Digital Mammography and Screen-Film Mammography in the American College of

Radiology Imaging Network Digital Mammographic Imaging Screening Trial. *Am. J. Roentgenol* 194:362–369. ISSN: 1546-3141

IAEA. International Atomic Energy Agency. (2007). Dosimetry in Diagnostic Radiology: An International Code of Practice, Technical Reports Series No. 457. *International Atomic Energy Agency*, Vienna ; Austria

IAEA. International Atomic Energy Agency. (2011). Quality Assurance Programme For Digital Mammography. IAEA Human Health Series No 17. *International Atomic Energy Agency*, (Vienna, Austria). ISBN 978–92–0–111410–5

ICRU. International Commission on Radiation Units and Measurements. (2005). Patient Dosimetry for X Rays Used in Medical Imaging, ICRU Report 74. *J. ICRU.* 5(2), University Press, Oxford, UK

ICRU. International Commission on Radiation Units and Measurements. (2009). Mammography- Assessment of Image Quality. ICRU Report 82. *J. ICRU* 9(2), University Press, Oxford, UK

IPEM. Institute of Physical and Engineering in Medicine. (1989). The commissioning and routine testing of mammographic x-ray systems. Report 59 1st ed. *IPEM,* ISBN : 1 903613 21 3, York, UK

Lewin JM, D'Orsi CJ, Hendrick RE. 2004. Digital mammography. *Radiol Clin N Am.* 42:871 – 884. ISSN 1557-8275

Karellas A and Giger M L. 2004. Advances in Breast Imaging: Physics, Technology, and Clinical Applications. *The Radiological Society of North America* (RSNA 2004), Presented at the 90th Scientific Assembly and Annual Meeting of the Radiological Society of North America, November 28–December 3, 2004, Chicago, USA. ISSN 0271-5333

Klein R, Aichinger H, Dierker J, Jansen J T M, Joite-Barfuss S, Säbel M, Schulz-Wendtland R and Zoetelief J. (1997). Determination of average glandular dose with modern mammography units for two large groups of patients. *Phys Med Biol.* 42:651–671. ISSN 1361-6560

Kruger R L and Schueler B A. (2001). A survey of clinical factors and patient dose in mammography. *Med. Phys.* 28:1449-1454. ISSN 0094-2405

Leitz, W and Jönsson H (2001). Patientdoser från röntgenundersökningar i Sverige. SSI Rapport 2001:1. *Swedish Radiation Protection Authority.* (Sweden)

Maria S. Nogueira; Luciana de J. S. Pinheiro; Danille S. Gomes, William José de Castro, Katiane Costa; Marcio A. de Oliveira; Margarita Chevalier del Rio (2011). Development of methodology for estimating thickness of compressed breast in mammography. *International Conference on Medical Physics ICMP*, April 17-20, 2011. Porto Alegre, Brazil

Muller S (1997). Full field digital mammography designed as a complete system. *European Journal of Radiology* 31: 25–34. ISSN: 0720-048X

NCRP. National Council on Radiation Protection and Measurements. (1986). Mammography – A User's Guide. NCRP Report 85. *National Council on Radiation Protection and Measurements,* Bethesda, Maryland, USA. ISBN-10: 0913392790

NCRP. National Council on Radiation Protection and Measurments. (2004). A Guide to Mammography and Other Breast Imaging Procedures, NCRP Report 149. *National Council on Radiation Protection and Measurements.* Bethesda, Maryland, USA. ISBN 0-929600-84-3

NG, KH, Jamal, N, Dewerd, L. (2006). Global quality control perspective for the physical on technical aspects of screen-film mammography-image quality and radiation dose. *Radiat Prot Dosimetry* 121(4): 445-451. ISSN 1742-3406

NHSBSP. National Health Service Breast Screening Programmes. (2003). Review of Radiation Risk in Breast Screening. NHSBSP Publication No 54. *NHS Cancer Screening Programmes*. ISBN 1 871997 99 2. Sheffield, UK

NHSBSP. National Health Service Breast Screening Programmes. (2009). Commissioning and Routine Testing of Full Field Digital Mammography Systems. NHSBSP Equipment Report 0604. (London, UK).

Nishikawa R M. (2004). Advances in Breast Imaging: Physics, Technology, and Clinical Applications. *The Radiological Society of North America* (RSNA 2004), Presented at the 90th Scientific Assembly and Annual Meeting of the Radiological Society of North America, November 28–December 3, 2004, Chicago, USA. ISSN 0271-5333.

Pedersen, K Nordanger J (2000). Mammografiscreening. Teknisk kvalitetskontroll - resultater og evaluering etter fire års prøveprosjekt. StrålevernRapport 2000:2. Østerås: Norwegian Radiation Protection Authority (Norway).

Peixoto, J. E. (2009). Controle de Qualidade em Mamografia. In Aguillar VLN, Bauab SP, Maranhão NM. Mama: diagnóstico por Imagem. *Revinter*, 2009. p. 83-106. ISBN-10: 8537202444. Rio de Janeiro, Brazil

Pisano ED, Gatsonis C, Hendrick E, Yaffe M, Baum JK, Acharyya S, et al. 2005. Diagnostic Performance of Digital versus Film Mammography for Breast-Cancer Screening, New England Journal of Medicine. 353: 1-11.

Rosenstein M, Andersen LW and Warner GG. (1985). Handbook of Glandular Tissue Doses in Mammography, *HHS Publication FDA* 85-8239. Center for Devices and Radiological Health, Rockville, Maryland, USA

Rowlands JA. (2002). The physics of computed radiography. Phys Med Biol;47: R123–R166.

SEFM. Sociedad Española de Física Médica. (2008). Protocolo de Control de Calidad en Mamografía Digital. Edicomplet (Madrid, Spain)

Sobol WT and Wu X. 1997. Parametrization of mammography normalized average glandular dose tables. *Med Phys* 24:547–554. ISSN: 0094-2405

Stanton L, Villafana T, Day JL and Lightfoot DA. (1984). Dosage evaluation in mammography. *Radiology*.150: 577–584. ISSN :0033-8419

Vedantham S, Karellas A, Suryanarayanan S, Albagli D, Han S, Tkaczyk EJ, Landberg CE et al. (2000). Full Breast Digital Mammography with an Amorphous Silicon-based Flat Panel Detector: Physical Characteristics of a Clinical Prototype. Med Phys 27:558-567

Suryanarayanan S, Karellas A and Vedanthama S. (2004). Physical characteristics of a full-field digital mammography system. *Nuclear Instruments and Methods in Physics Research A*. 533:560–570. ISSN: 01689002

Wu X, Barnes G T, and Tucker D M. (1991). Spectral dependence of glandular tissue dose in screen-film mammography. *Radiology* 179:143–148. ISSN : 1527-1315

Wu X, Gingold E L, Barnes G T, and Tucker D M. (1994). Normalized average glandular dose in molybdenum target-rhodium filter and rhodium target-rhodium filter mammography. *Radiology* 193:83–89. ISSN : 1527-1315

Yaffe MJ, Rowlands JA. (1997) X-ray detectors for digital radiography. Phys Med Biol;42:1–39.

Young KC, Ramsdale ML and Bignall F. (1998). Review of dosimetric methods for mammography in the UK breast screening programme. *Radiat Prot Dosim*etry. 80: 183–6. ISSN : 0144-8420

Young KC, Oduko JM, Bosmans H, Nijs K and Martinez L. (2006). Optimal beam quality selection in digital mammography. *Br J Radiol* 79: 981-990. ISSN: 1748-880X

Zoetelief J, Veldkamp W J H, Thijssen M A O, and Jansen J T M. (2006). Glandularity and mean glandular dose determined for individual women at four regional breast cancer screening units in the Netherlands. *Phys Med Biol*. 51:1807–1817. ISSN 1361-6560

6

Contrast Enhancement in Mammography Imaging Including K Edge Filtering

George Zentai
Ginzton Technology Center of Varian Medical Systems
USA

1. Introduction

To understand how we can optimize the spectrum of an X-ray beam to obtain the maximum contrast using the minimum dose for a given x-ray exam we need to know a little about how the X-rays are generated, how an x-ray tube works, how the energy spectrum of the output X-ray beam will look and how the X-rays interact with the human body and with the imager.

A general X-ray tube has two electrodes, the cathode and the anode, with a high voltage applied between them. Electrons are generated at the cathode. After the electrons are emitted from the cathode they are accelerated by the high voltage toward the anode (positive) electrode. The high speed electrons hitting the anode material then generate invisible radiation i.e. X-rays. The energy spectrum of the output X-rays is dependent on the anode-cathode voltage difference and on the material of the anode and is measured in electronvolts. The energy spectrum is a so called Brehmstrahlung radiation meaning that it is continuous over a wide range of energies and has more photons emitted at the lowest energies. The photon flux decreases to zero at the anode-cathode voltage difference level.

When the Brehmstrahlung radiation of the X-ray beam passes into the human body, some photons are absorbed while others pass through. The ones that have passed through are available for imaging. Because the absorption of the human body is higher at lower energy X-rays, the beam exiting the body has a higher average energy than the beam had when it entered the body. This effect is called beam hardening and it causes a decrease in the contrast of images and difficulties in CT reconstruction. Furthermore, the dose the patient receives from the very low energy X-rays serves no purpose; it does not contribute to the final image in any way.

Figure 1 demonstrates the difference between input and exit X-ray beams showing that the very low energy X-rays do not penetrate the human body at all and only add extra (unwanted) dose to the patient (Sutton 2009). Three cases are shown in the figure. The original input beam, an 80kVp X-ray beam from a W anode filtered through a 2 mm Al filter, is shown in blue and has the highest photon flux and widest energy spectrum. The red series shows the energy of the beam after having passed through simulated soft tissue (150 mm soft tissue and 50 mm water). This exit beam shows that only X-ray photons with >25keV energy will contribute to the image. The green series shows the energy of the beam after having passed through simulated tissue and bone (150mm soft tissue + 50 mm water + 30 mm bone). This exit beam now shows that only X-ray photons with >37 keV are available to contribute to the image. The very low energy input photons are completely absorbed in the body, adding extra patient dose, because there is no exit photon for imaging[1].

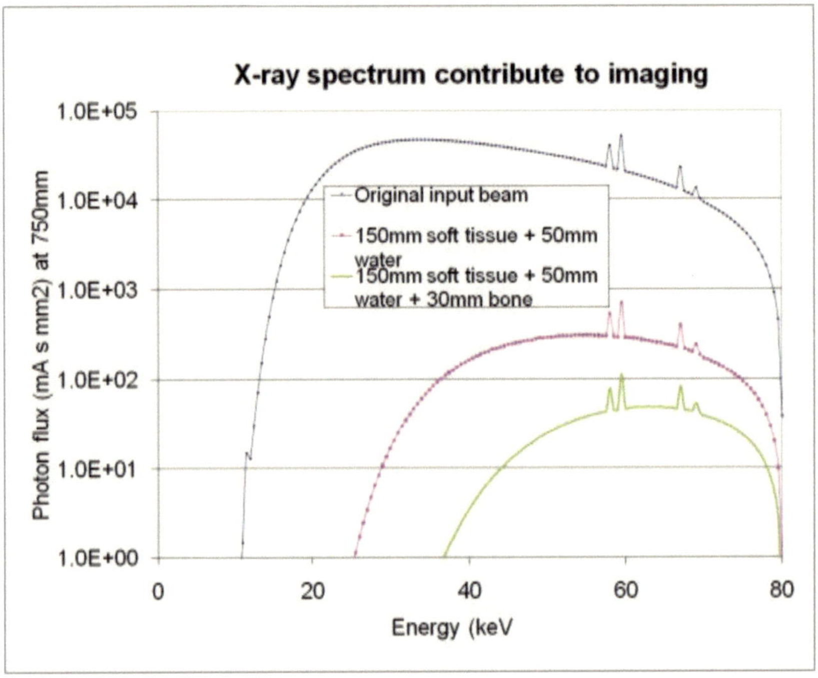

Fig. 1. Comparison of the ratio of the incident photons (original beam) to the exit photons after going through different body tissues including water. Only the exit photons contribute to the imaging.

So, how can we optimize contrast of the x-ray image using the minimum dose?

2. Using the right x-ray energy range

Figure 1 implies that the spectrum of the input x-ray beam has to be optimized for each imaging modality for minimum patient dose. For instance, a thicker body part such as the pelvis, which contains lots of bony structures, absorbs most of the low energy X-ray beams below 30 keV so we need to use higher X-ray beam energies to get a reasonable number of exiting x-ray photons for imaging while avoiding overdosing the patient with low energy X-rays which would be completely absorbed in the thick pelvis.

By contrast, imaging of the breast, which is smaller (thinner) relative to the pelvis and does not contain any bony structure, requires much lower X-ray energy to get sufficient X-ray

[1] Note that some low energy X-rays are removed by the inherent filtration of the X-ray tube. In many cases the exit window of the X-ray tube is made of 2mm Aluminum which removes most of the X-ray radiation below 15 keV.

photons for good imaging. Figure 2 shows the contrast/dose relationship for mammography. From the diagram, the optimum X-ray energy for imaging the breast is in the range of 18-21 keV (mean energy).[2]

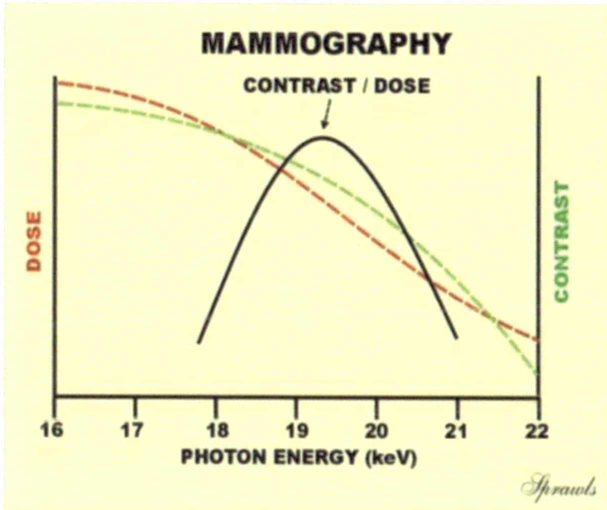

Fig. 2. The general relationship of contrast and dose to photon energy in mammography (Sprawls).

There are several methods for limiting the input X-rays to an optimum range. They include dual energy imaging, monochromatic X-ray imaging, and quasi-monochromatic X-ray imaging.

3. Dual energy imaging

In many cases X-ray images must capture both hard (bony) structures and soft tissues, which may be overlapping, in the same picture. A method to separate two different tissues, and optimize the contrast between them, is to acquire two images at different x-ray energies and do a weighted subtraction. This is called dual energy imaging. Taking images at low and high energies and doing a subtraction can remove either the soft or the bony structure depending on the techniques used.

3.1 Brief theory of dual energy imaging

The data processing methods that make use of dual energy data are referred to as decomposition techniques and are divided into three classes based on the type of information returned by the technique. The three types of information about the object being imaged that may be returned by decomposition techniques are: (1) effective atomic number and density; (2) attenuation due to Compton scattering and electron density; or (3) the physical densities of two known components (Walter, Wu et al. 2004).

[2] This range will vary depending on the size and density of the breast.

The ability to determine material composition from dual energy techniques fundamentally results from the fact that the linear attenuation coefficient of X-ray absorption, ($\mu(E)$), for an element has a unique functional dependence on photon energy. Over the range of x-ray photon energies used, the attenuation coefficient is dominated by two major attenuation processes: the photoelectric effect and Compton scattering. A major simplifying factor of the analysis is that each of these two processes has a fixed and unique functional dependence on energy that can serve as a linear basis set for any material. That is,

$$\mu(E) = x\mu_p(E) + y\mu_c(E) \tag{1}$$

where $\mu_p(E)$ is the linear attenuation as a function of energy due to the photoelectric effect and $\mu_c(E)$ is the linear attenuation as a function of energy due to the Compton scattering effect and x and y are material specific constants.

A consequence of this relationship is that the energy dependence of any material's attenuation coefficient can be expressed as the linear combination of any two other materials. Therefore, each material can be characterized by two density values, p_A p_B, which are derived from the attenuation measured at two different kVp spectra, $\mu_A(E)$, $\mu_B(E)$. As in,

$$\mu(E) = x\mu_p(E) + y\mu_c(E) = p_A\mu_A(E) + p_B\mu_{Bc}(E) \tag{2}$$

The important consequence for image formation is that these two material density values are available to encode the pixel values apart from or in combination with Hounsfield units in the case of CT imaging. Materials with similar density can now be differentiated based on average atomic number. Of particular interest is the use of contrast agents with atomic numbers significantly different from the usual materials present in the body as these agents will show up on images in high contrast to the normal materials of the body. Moreover, because the dual energy analysis makes explicit use of the energy dependence of the attenuation, the beam hardening artifacts are absent here, a distinct advantage over conventional CT. Also, in the dual energy technique as opposed to the conventional approach, the accuracy of the CT number associated with pixels is not affected by the beam hardening corrections which must approximate the energy dependent attenuation with data from a single energy value.

3.2 Dual energy imaging applications

Dual energy imaging was used in CT scanning as long ago as 1976 (Alvarez and Macovski 1976) when it was also being used for the exact determination of the atomic number of elements (Rutherford, Pullan et al. 1976). It has been used for mammography as well. Johns et al. described the first applications of dual energy imaging to mammography (Johns, Drost et al. 1983). Later work optimized the method to get the best SNR with minimum dose (Johns and Yaffe 1985). Since that time, several articles were published about optimization of parameters in dual energy breast imaging. Boone at al. (Boone, Shaber et al. 1990) analyzed detector parameters, effects of X-ray parameters and filtrations and the effect of scatter on the quality of the dual energy images. Kappadath et al. (Kappadath, Shaw et al. 2004) used digital subtraction techniques and a method they developed called DEDM (Dual Energy Digital Mammography) to improve the visibility of micro calcifications.

Dual energy techniques have also been used to improve Computed Tomography (CT) imaging. While 3D CT scans and the use of Iodine (I) as a contrast agent have, on their own, greatly improved the visibility of malignant cancerous tissues (Chen, Jing et al. 2006; Arvanitis, Royle et al. 2007; Puong, Bouchevreau et al. 2007), the combination of dual energy CT and Iodine contrast together offers yet more improvements to our ability to separate different tissues from one another in an image (Carton, Lindman et al. 2007), (Puong, Patoureaux et al. 2007; Saunders, Samei et al. 2008).

Dual energy imaging is used in many fields of medical imaging, such as for lung imaging when we need to separate (or suppress) the overlapping rib shadows from the soft lung tissues to enhance visualization of lung nodules (Kashani, Varon et al. 2010), or, similarly, for digital angiography to visualize the heart behind the ribs (Ersahin, Molloi et al. 1994). In many cases dual energy angiography is used in combination with Iodine (I) or Gadolinium (Gd) contrast agents (Fiedler, Elleaume et al. 2000).

Dual energy imaging is an important technique for performing bone densitometry tests (Shimura, Nakajima et al. 1993) and specialized systems have been developed and sold by GE and Hologic (GE ; Hologic).

3.3 Dual energy imaging methods

Generally dual energy imaging is implemented by use of X-ray tube voltage switching to obtain two images; one at low and one at high kVp values. To avoid motion artifacts between the two images quick changes in tube voltage are necessary.

Different methods and detectors have also been developed for dual energy imaging. Coello et al. (Coello, Dinten et al. 2007) built a system where, instead of switching voltages, a filter wheel containing multiple filter materials is rotated in front of the X-ray tube, providing different X-ray spectra. This paper also provides an excellent overview of the theory of dual energy imaging and its optimization for best signal to noise ratio and image contrast.

4. Monochromatic X-ray imaging

Beam hardening has a significantly deleterious effect on the precision of CT reconstruction. It can be avoided by using monochromatic X-ray beams. Furthermore, for each imaging object there is an ideal energy at which enough X-ray photons make it through the object to allow for low noise imaging while still using a low enough X-ray energy to provide the best contrast ratio. Synchrotrons are ideal sources of monochromatic beams of high flux. Some experiments on breast imaging with synchrotrons were made and compared to normal mammographic images (Fiedler and et al. 2004). A further advantage of monochromatic imaging is that it allows for phase contrast imaging, which greatly improves the contrast even between different soft tissues. However, the size and price of a synchrotron make it impractical for general radiographic use. X-ray tubes with monochromators can provide monochromatic x-ray beams but the flux is too low for practical applications (Donath, Pfeiffer et al. 2008).

5. Quasi monochromatic X-ray beam imaging

5.1 Generation of quasi monochromatic beams using diffraction

Different methods have been developed to approximate monochromatic beams i.e. to provide quasi monochromatic beams, which consist of not a single X-ray energy but a narrow range of X-ray energies.

One method utilizes mosaic crystals to produce quasi-monochromatic X-ray beams. When an X-ray hits the crystalline structure of a material, constructive interference takes place in accordance with the Bragg equation:

$$2d \times \sin\theta = \lambda \times n \tag{3}$$

where, λ is the exiting X-ray photon wavelength, d is the spacing between atomic planes of the crystal and θ is the diffraction angle and n is an integer. The d-spacings are substance-specific and like the λ have an inverse relationship with the energy of the output beam. At different θ, different X-ray energy photons are reflected back from the crystal. This is called Bragg reflection and this method was proposed by Baldelli et al. (Baldelli, Taibi et al. 2003) to generate monochromatic X-rays. However, this method has some drawbacks. First of all, because it is a Bragg reflection from a plain surface it provides only a monochromatic fan beam and not a cone beam; furthermore, the intensity of the diffracted beam is very low because only a very small portion of the total incoming X-ray spectrum is reflected back. Moreover, because of the variation of crystal angle in the mosaic crystal and the finite width of the slits the X-ray beam is only quasi monochromatic with an energy bandwidth of ~ΔE.

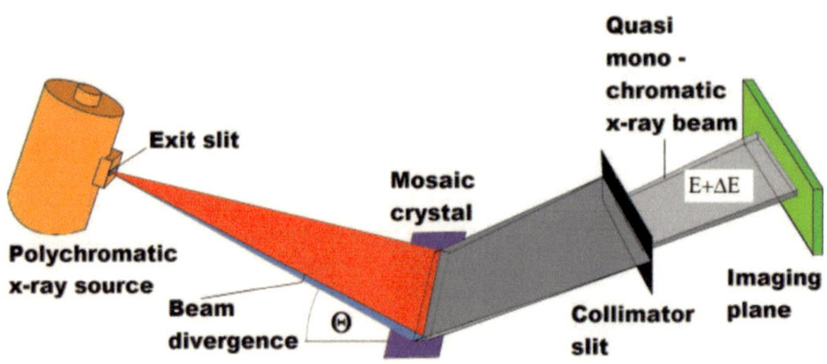

Fig. 3. Quasi monochromatic X-ray beam by X-ray diffraction.

A prototype of a quasi monochromatic diffraction system has also been developed for mammography (Baldelli and et al. 2005). Advantages of the system are that it is tunable in the range of 18-24keV, and according to the authors, the dose can be decreased by half. Disadvantages are that it uses little of the available X-ray flux and requires scanning, as it produces only a sheet beam, so the scanning time is a few seconds long (possible motion blur). The resolution of the system is also lower than the best digital mammo systems can produce.

5.2 Applications for quasi monochromatic beams

A similar system to that of Baldelli's (Baldelli and et al. 2005) was developed for a combined breast SPECT - CT system (Gambaccini, Fantini et al. 2001). It had the same advantages and disadvantages as the mammography system.

The spatial resolution of such a system was analyzed by Gambaccini et al. (Gambaccini, Tuffanelli et al. 2001) who found that along the direction perpendicular to the diffraction plane the resolution properties of the imaging system mainly depend on the x-ray tube focal spot size and position. Along the diffraction plane the spatial resolution depends on mosaic crystal characteristics and on the geometry of the setup.

6. K edge filters

6.1 Theory of K edge filters

There is another method of generating small energy bandwidth X-ray radiation. It is known that in addition to the Brehmstrahlung radiation, materials bombarded with electrons produce characteristic radiation which increases the intensity of the X-ray radiation at energy levels specific to each material. For instance, a typical X-ray radiation spectrum for a Tungsten (W) anode using 100 kV anode-cathode potential and a 2 mm Al window is shown in Figure 4. As before, the lowest energy X-rays are absorbed by the Al output window. The sharp peeks in the X-ray spectrum are characteristic for the anode material. These peeks are the result of the electron structure of a given material and they show the energy differences between electron shells of the atomic structure.

For example, W has 3 electron shells that play a role in its use as a K edge filter. The 3 innermost electron shells are designated "K", "L", "M", where K is the innermost shell, and M the outermost. For W, K has an energy of 70keV, L has an energy of 11keV, and M has an energy of 3keV. The characteristic peaks for W will occur at "L minus K" and "M minus K" or at 59keV (designated the K_{α} peak) and 67keV (designated the K_{β} peak). W also has a second electron in its K shell with a slightly different binding energy which explains the doublets in Figure 4.

The same phenomenon works in the opposite way; materials absorb X-ray photons which are above their binding energy. This is the basis of the K edge filters. Generally at these (energy) levels the X-ray absorption of the material jumps (increases) when the material is used as an X-ray filter. Figure 5 shows the X-ray spectrum for the same W anode and the same X-ray tube voltage as in Figure 4 but with an added 0.2 mm W sheet as a filter. This

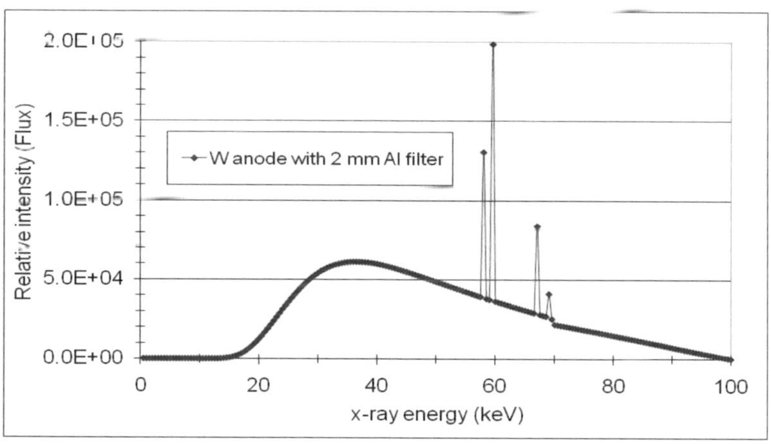

Fig. 4. W anode spectra with low energy filter of 2 mm Al.

added tungsten sheet filters out not only the low energy X-rays but the X-ray spectrum also shows a huge drop in intensity (the absorption increases dramatically) above the tungsten K edge. Please note that the total intensity decreased as well. The scale of Figure 5 is different from that of Figure 4 for better visibility. The total intensity after K edge filtering is always lower than without it for the same energy range but the characteristic K edge radiation peaks are still present. This example shows that material K edge absorption can be used to suppress both low and high energy portions of the original X-ray spectrum to produce narrow bandwidth X-ray radiation or so called quasi-monochromatic X-rays.

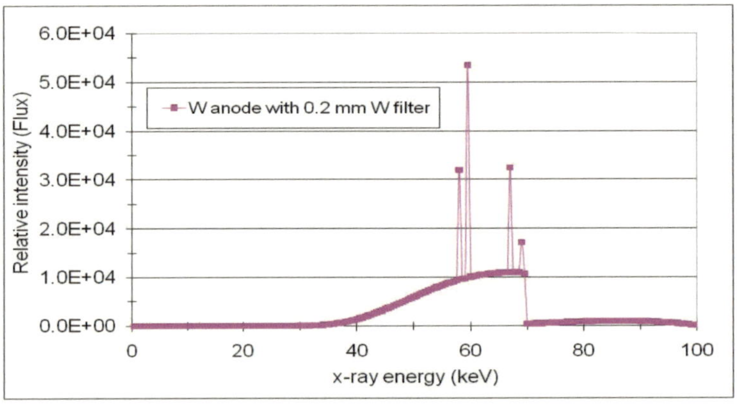

Fig. 5. Tungsten (W) anode with 0.2 mm W (K edge) filter.

The absorption spectra of K edge filters can be calculated. If there are no K-edge discontinuities, then the energy dependence of the linear attenuation coefficient $\mu(E, \vec{x})$ of materials can be described by a linear combination of the photo-electric and the Compton cross-sections $f_{ph}(E)$ and $f_{KN}(E)$(Alvarez and Macovski 1976)

$$\mu(E,\vec{x}) = a_{ph}(\vec{x})\frac{1}{E^3} + a_{Co}(\vec{x})f_{KN}(E/E_e) \tag{4}$$

Here E_e = 510.975 keV denotes the rest mass energy of the electron, and the vector $\vec{x}$ describes the space dependence of the attenuation and $1/E^3$ approximates the energy dependence of the photoelectric interaction. The energy dependence of the Klein-Nishina cross-section (Compton scattering) is given by:

$$f_{KN}(\alpha) = \frac{1+\alpha}{\alpha^2}\left[\frac{2(1+\alpha)}{1+2\alpha} - \frac{1}{\alpha}\ln(1+2\alpha)\right] + \frac{1}{2\alpha}\ln(1+2\alpha) - \frac{1+3\alpha}{(1+2\alpha)^2} \tag{5}$$

Where α = E/510.975 keV, and a_{ph} and F_{KN} are given as:

$$a_{ph} \approx K_1 \times \frac{\rho}{A} \times Z^n \qquad n \approx 4 \tag{6}$$

$$a_{Co} \approx K_2 \times \frac{\rho}{A} \times Z \tag{7}$$

where K_1 and K_2 are constants, ρ is mass density, A is atomic weight and Z is atomic number. When a material with high atomic number Z is present, the above description of the attenuation properties of the matter has to be modified. To correctly describe the attenuation of a sample containing a single element with K edge discontinuity inside the relevant energy range, the decomposition (4) has to be extended by the energy dependent attenuation function of this particular element as a third component (Sukovic and Clinthorne 1999). The decomposition for a high Z element with K edge in the diagnostic energy range becomes:

$$\mu(E,\vec{x}) = a_{ph}(\vec{x})\frac{1}{E^3} + a_{Co}(\vec{x})f_{KN}\left(\frac{E}{E_e}\right) + a_K(\vec{x})f_K(E) = \sum_{a=1}^{3} a_a(\vec{x})f_a(E) \quad (8)$$

where the values a = 1, 2, 3 represent the photoelectric, Compton and the K edge components, respectively. In the above formula, $a_K(\vec{x})$ and $f_K(E)$ denote the local density and the mass attenuation coefficient of the K edge material. The latter includes the photoelectric effect, Compton effect and K edge contributions of the material.

6.2 K edge materials, energies, and applications

Table 1 provides a list of some K edge filters whose K edge energies (except for Al and Cu filters) fall into the region where they are or could be applied to X-ray imaging. From the table it is clear that the K edge energy increases with increasing atomic number.

K edge filtering has been used for mammography for some time where different Rhodium (Rh) and Molybdenum (Mo) anode and filter combinations are used to generate energy peaks in the 15- 23 keV energy range.

Material	Aluminum	Copper	Molybdenum	Rhodium	Silver	Tin	Iodine
Chemical sign	Al	Cu	Mo	Rh	Ag	Sn	I
Atomic number	13	29	42	45	47	50	53
K edge energy in keV	1.6	8.98	20	23.22	25.51	29.2	33.16

Material	Barium	Cerium	Neodimium	Europium	Gadolinium	Holmium
Chemical sign	Ba	Ce	Nd	Eu	Gd	Ho
Atomic number	56	58	60	63	64	67
K edge energy in keV	37.45	40.44	43.56	48.5	50.2	55.6

Material	Erbium	Ytterbium	Tantalum	Tungsten	Gold	Bismuth	Uranium
Chemical sign	Er	Yb	Ta	W	Au	Bi	U
Atomic number	68	70	73	74	79	83	92
K edge energy in keV	57.5	61.3	67.41	69.5	80.72	90.53	115.6

Table 1. K edge energies for different materials already used or that can be used in K-edge X-ray imaging.

As shown in Figure 6, at an anode voltage of 28 kV, a Mo anode - Mo filter combination gives a lower mean energy of 17.6 keV better suited for thinner, lower density breasts, while the Rh anode - Rh filter combination has a mean energy of 18.3 keV, which is better for thicker and denser breast imaging. Different Mo and Rh anode and filter combinations are used in some specialized mammography imagers and various anode voltages to fine tune the optimum energy spectrum to obtain maximum contrast at minimum dose for different breast types. Tungsten (W) anodes with higher anode voltages (40kV) and Silver (Ag) filters could also be used. This combination would be especially useful for imaging very large and dense breasts.

Evaluation of different x-ray sources with varying anode voltages is given by Jennings et al. (Jennings, Quinn et al. 1993) and Venkatakrishnan (Venkatakrishnan, Yavuz et al. 1999). Optimization of spectral shape for digital mammography is given by Fahrig and Yaffe (Fahrig and Yaffe 1994). Dose versus image quality was also experimentally studied on a CsI flat panel mammo imaging system using Mo/Mo anode/filter combination. (Huda W Fau - Sajewicz, Sajewicz Am Fau - Ogden et al.) Optimization of the anode-filter combination is provided by Varjonen et al. (Varjonen and Strommer 2008) and a very good Monte Carlo analysis of different combinations is provided by Dance et al. (Dance, Thilander et al. 2000) for both film and digital imaging. Fahrig et al. (Fahrig, Rowlands et al. 1996) investigated the a-Se based digital imagers and found that the optimal x-ray spectra is similar to the indirect (scintillator + photodiode) based imagers.

An X-ray tube at 30 kVp anode-cathode voltage does not provide enough flux for fast three dimensional breast imaging (breast CT). Generally higher tube voltage (60-80kVp) is applied (Boone, Nelson et al. 2001) to keep the imaging time within reasonable limits (breath withholding during the CT scan). However, it is known that the X-ray contrast decreases with increasing X-ray energies. However, in the following we will investigate how we can improve the visualization of tumors in X-ray CT images utilizing K edge filtering.

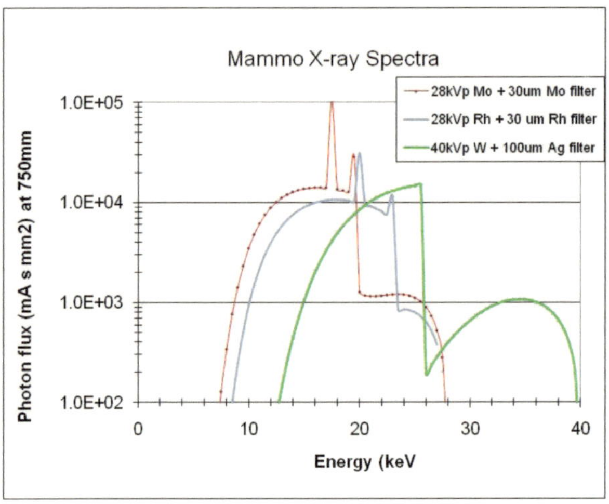

Fig. 6. X-ray applications with K edge filtering.

It is known that iodine has a high Z number which provides reasonable X-ray absorption. It dissolves in water and it has been used for intravenous injection to check blood flow in the body. It is common knowledge that most tumors have generally leaky blood vessels. Blood leaks from the vessels near tumors into the intercellular tissues and it generally takes a longer time to be re-circulated than blood that has not leaked out. So if we inject iodine into the blood stream, this iodine will also leak out in the tumor region and it will stay there for a period of time while the iodine in the rest of the vessels clears up more quickly. The presence of the iodine at the tumor will enhance the contrast of the image for several minutes following the iodine injection.

We know that Iodine has a K edge energy of 33.16 keV. To enhance the contrast of the iodine we have to use K edge filters which have K edges somewhat above the Iodine K edge. These materials are Cerium (Ce) Neodymium (Nd) And Europium (Eu). Figure 7 provides a comparison of the x-ray spectra using these different K edge filters for Iodine contrast enhancement.

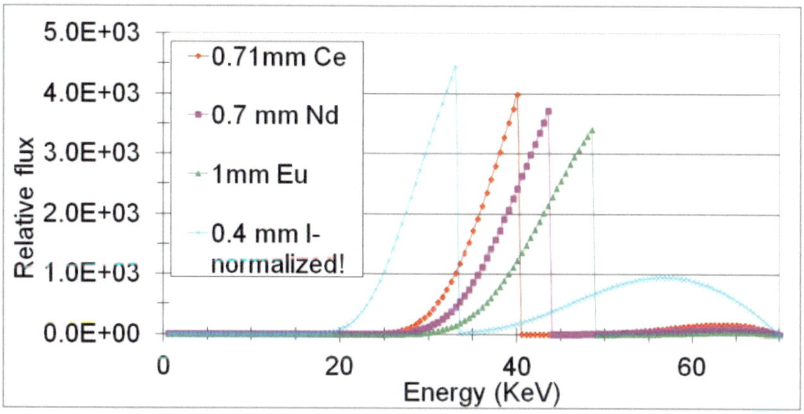

Fig. 7. Iodine (I) as a contrast agent and a few possible K edge filters: Cerium (Ce) Neodymium (ND) and Europium (Eu).

Another contrast material, Gadolinium (Gd) has been extensively used in MRI due to its special magnetic properties. In the bloodstream it behaves similar to the Iodine; it also accumulates in the tumor region when injected in the blood and clears out slower from tumors than it clears from the bloodstream. However, it also has a K edge energy for X-rays at 50.2 keV versus the 33.16 keV K edge of Iodine. This makes Gd a contrast material candidate not so much for X-ray mammography but rather for general radiographic applications. To improve the visibility of Gd absorption, K edge filters with K edge energies slightly over that of the Gd can be used. Possible candidates are Holmium (Ho), Erbium (Er), Ytterbium (Yb) and Tantalum (Ta) or even Tungsten (W).

Figure 8 gives a comparison of the X-ray spectrum of some K edge materials for Gd. It shows the spectra of Gd in red and a few possible K edge filters in other colors. Ta and W spectra have very similar shapes, both showing the W anode K edge spectra, but W has a higher K edge energy than Ta so it cuts off the spectra at higher keV.

An interesting approach for K edge filtering is to use an X-ray tube target material made of K edge filter materials, as was demonstrated by Sato et al (Sato, Tanaka et al. 2004) with Cerium and Samarium anodes (Sato, Tanaka et al. 2007).

A further possibility is to combine dual energy imaging with K edge filters. Taking an image with a filter which has a K edge over the K edge of the contrast agent and one which has a K edge below and then using weighted subtraction can further improve the contrast. This is also seen from Table 4 in section 6.4.2. The Ce filter enhances the contrast while the Iodine filter decreases the Iodine contrast. So further contrast improvement can be obtained by weighted subtraction of the two spectra rather than by just using the Ce filter image alone (see also in Section 7).

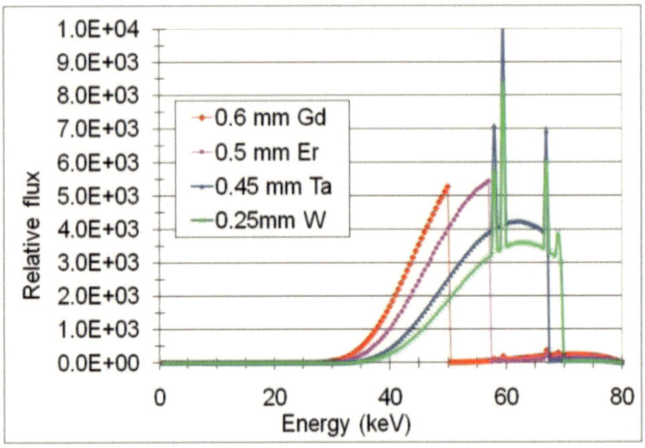

Fig. 8. Gd spectrum is in red. To enhance the contrast, Er, Ta or W can serve as K edge filters, which have higher K edges as Gd.

6.3 Experimental work with K edge filters

This section describes some of the author's own work on different K edge filters used for mammographic CT applications (Zentai 2011).

For the CT tests, so called HU (Hounsfield Unit) Phantoms were prepared. One set was made for HU calibration. This set consisted of small bottles filled with different water and alcohol solutions for densities less than water and also with water and glycerin mixtures for densities higher than water. The bottles were pushed into holes in a large polyethylene cylinder as shown in Figure 9. Polyethylene plugs were used for keeping the bottles in place and also for having the same material densities below and above the bottles. However, small holes were drilled in the center of the plugs for letting the extra air out when pushing the plugs in place. These holes contained air, so HU numbers for the air could also be evaluated by using the air pocket images of these holes. We found that for alcohol-water and glycerin-water solutions the X-ray absorption is proportional to the density. So the numbers written over the bottles of Figure 9 represent the relative densities of the solutions in g/cm^3.

As we know, HU numbers are proportional to the absorption (densities) of these liquids; water has HU=0 and air has HU=-1000. HU from 0 to 2000 represent liquids and solids denser than water. For instance, the density of pure alcohol is 0.782 and the approximate Hounsfield number for alcohol can be calculated (-1000 × 0.782) = -782. Similarly, the density of pure glycerin is 1.14 and the Hounsfield number is then 114. So a set of five different solutions and air were used for calibrating the HU numbers for different X-ray tube voltages and different filters.

To compare the HU numbers of different iodine solutions another fixture was designed as shown in Figure 10. The numbers in the figure give the relative density of the iodine solutions in mg/ml.

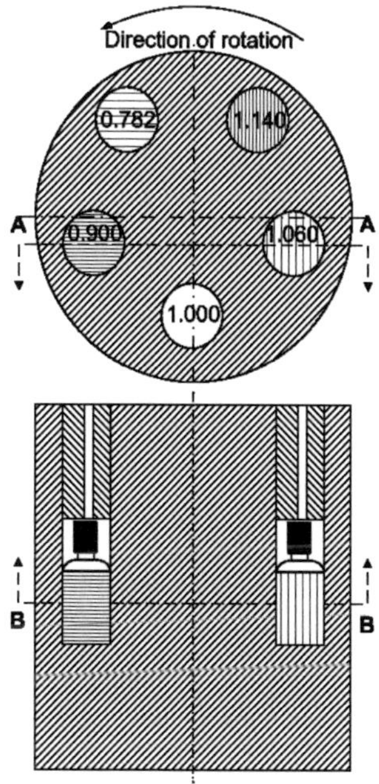

Fig. 9. Hounsfield unit CT phantoms.

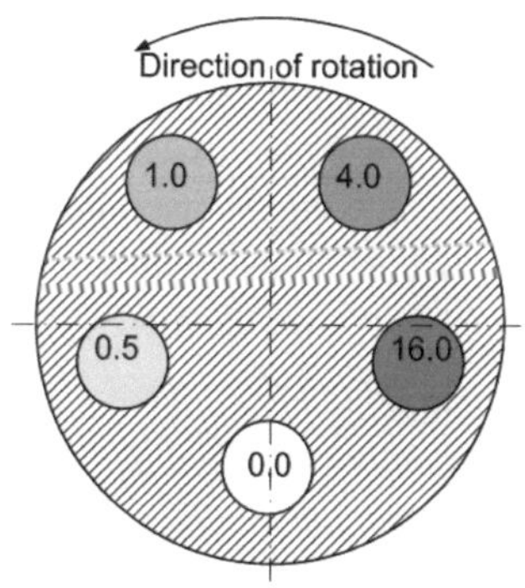

Fig. 10. Iodine solution phantoms.

A rotational table was used to rotate the phantoms during CT image sequences. First it was verified that the center (focal spot) of the X-ray radiation was lined up with the center of the X-ray imager and that the imaginary line between these two points crossed the pivot-line of the rotation. This alignment was done with the help of a so called Isocal phantom. This phantom consists of a graphite cylinder with BBs, which are arranged in a spiral pattern alongside the perimeter. A detailed description of this method and the phantom is given by A. Jeung et al (Jeung, Sloutsky et al. 2005). We also processed a norm factor calibration when we used a cylindrical object of the same size and material as the bulk of the CT phantoms but without any holes in it. This calibration method is described in more details by Matsinos et al (Matsinos 2005).

The rotational table was driven by a stepper motor for precision rotational speed. 625 images were taken during one 360° rotation. The rotational speed and the imaging speed were synchronized. From these values the angles were calculated for each transmission image required for the CT reconstruction. A modified Feldkamp back-projection (Feldkamp, Davis et al. 1984) algorithm was used for cone beam CT reconstruction developed by John Pavkovich at Varian (Pavkovich 1979; Pavkovich).

Imaging was done on a Varian 4030CB CsI/photodiode flat panel imager. The readout ASICs of the imager were set to dynamic gain mode. In this mode the readout ASICs can automatically switch from a high to a low gain mode during the integration time when the signal level exceeds a given limit. This mode provides about 16.5 bit resolution even when the A/D converter has only a 14 bit range. A detailed description of the functions of this readout ASIC is given in (Roos, Colbeth et al. 2004). Imager calibrations were also performed to assure areas of the image where the gain is in transition still appear smooth and continuous.

Different filters were used to evaluate the effect of filtering on the S/N (Signal to Noise) value of the reconstructed CT images and also for the contrast ratio in comparison to CT images without any beam filtering. Lists of the filters and their thicknesses and the corresponding K edges are given in Table 2.

Filter parameters	Iodine (I)	Cerium (Ce)	Neodymium (Nd)	Europium (Eu)	Aluminum (Al)	Copper (Cu)
Effective thickness	0.4 mm	0.71 mm	0.7 mm	1.0 mm	2.24 mm	0.5 mm
K edge (in KeV)	33.16	40.44	43.56	48.50	1.56	8.98

Table 2. Filters applied during the experiments and their consecutive K edge energies.

The entrance doses for each imaging case were measured with a Radcal dose meter, which was placed in the center of the rotational table, where the geometrical center of the object was during the imaging data collection using the exact same conditions.

It is clear that Al and Cu have K edges at very low energies and in this experiment these materials were used as beam hardening filters, filtering out the low energy X-rays. Cerium, Europium and Neodymium all have K edges slightly over the K edge of iodine so they could provide narrow bandwidth filtering for iodine imaging. For comparison we also used a 0.4 mm equivalent thickness iodine solution as a filter. For the K edge filter and no filter experiments we used 60 and 70 kVp X-ray tube anode voltage and 100 kVp for the Cu and Al filters for higher X-ray flux.

6.4 Measurements, results and discussions

6.4.1 Calculation and measurement of X-ray spectra

Spectra of some K edge materials with the given thicknesses were calculated. The calculation was based on the Report 78 Spectrum Processor Program IPEM 1997 (Cranley, Gilmore et al. 1997). The original program contained only absorption spectra of a few materials so additional absorption spectra were obtained from the NIST XCOM website (NIST 2009). Some calculated spectra are given in Figure 11, Figure 12, and in Figure 13.

Figure 11 shows that the CsI scintillator used in the 4030CB flat panel detector has some filtering effects because of the K edge of Iodine contained in the CsI.

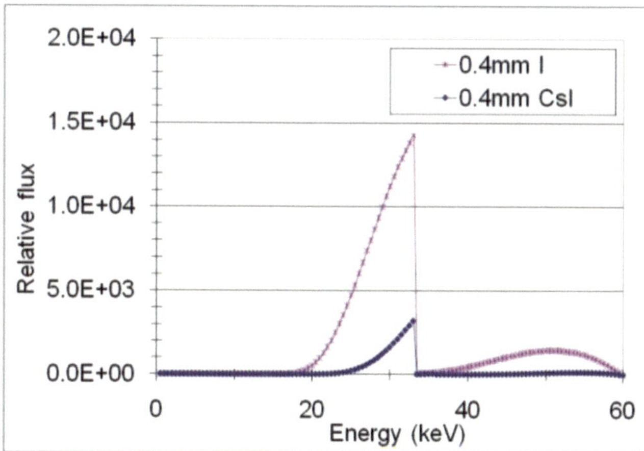

Fig. 11. Calculated 60kVp X-ray spectra with 0.4mm Iodine and 0.4 mm CsI filter.

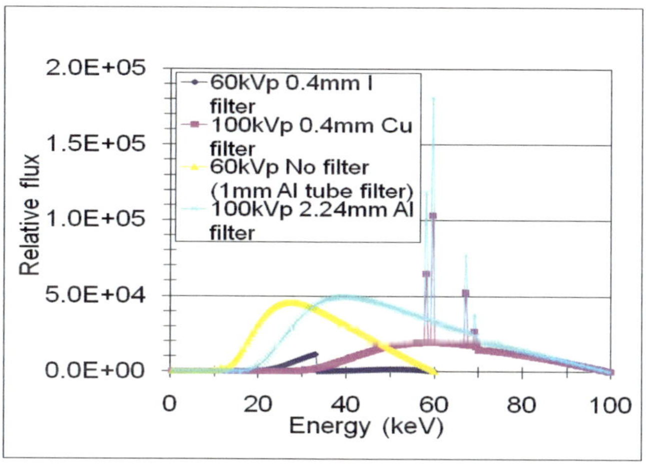

Fig. 12. 60 kVp spectra without any external filter and with 0.4 mm I filter are compared with 100 kVp spectra of 2.24 mm Al and 0.4 mm Cu filters.

From Figure 12 it is clear that while Al effects only the low energy X-rays, copper shifts the mean energy to higher values and K edge filters (Figure 13) significantly decrease the total flux having only single transmission peaks about the K edge energy.

The calculated and measured spectra of the K edge filter materials were compared. Figure 14 contrasts measured and calculated spectra of 0.71mm thick Ce filter. Very good agreement is shown in the 20 - 69 keV energy range. The flux drop of the measured spectra over 69 keV is attributed to the so called heel effect, which was simulated by Monte Carlo method and also measured by Bhat et al (Bhat, Pattison et al. 1999). This effect refers to a falloff of intensity in the X-ray radiation when the electron beam from the cathode hits the anode at a small angle. Because of the thick anode material, part of the X-ray generated deeper in the anode is also absorbed in the anode (in our case tungsten). This is practically the same filtering effect which is shown in Figure 5. It is especially significant above the 69.5 keV K edge of the tungsten anode where this absorption sharply increases causing a sharp decrease above this X-ray energy as can be seen in the measured spectra. However, this decrease would not affect the filter materials K edge behavior since those energies are much lower than the tungsten K edge as shown in Figure 13. Furthermore, most of the measurements with K edge filters were taken only at 60 or 70 kVp X-ray energies, the heel effect does not even show up at these low energies (below the tungsten K edge).

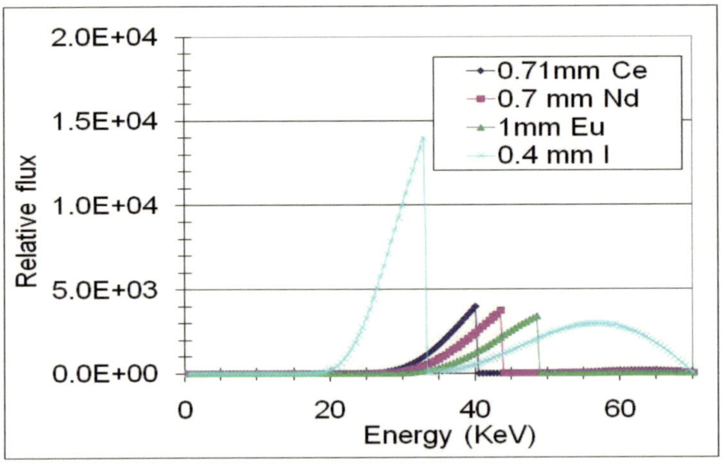

Fig. 13. Simulated spectra for 70 kVp X-ray source and 0.71 mm Ce, 0.7 mm Nd, 1 mm Eu and 0.4 mm I filtering.

Similarly, good agreement between the calculated and measured spectra for the Nd, I and Eu filters was found. Furthermore, our Ce, Nd and Eu spectra calculations and measurements are also very consistent with similar measurements taken by Crotty et al. (Crotty, McKinley et al. 2006).

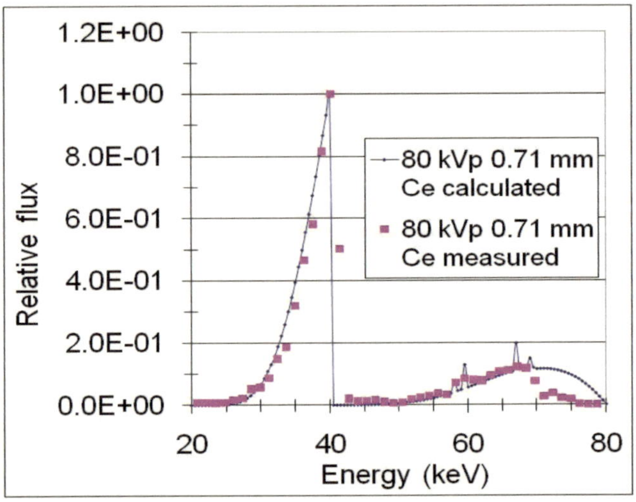

Fig. 14. Comparison of calculated and measured X-ray spectra after 0.71 mm Ce filter. Both the measured and the calculated spectra were normalized for the maximum flux value.

6.4.2 Cone beam measurements

After good agreement between the measured and calculated spectra was demonstrated, CT scans were carried out. It is noted that the K edge filtered X-ray scans require much longer exposure time per frame than scans with the non-filtered or Al and Cu filtered beams in order to get comparable dose results.

CT scans were taken first with the HU phantoms (Figure 9). For each filter and at each kVp, CT reconstructions were carried out and the HU numbers were normalized with the help of the known densities of the HU phantoms. During the normalization an offset and a slope value had to be adjusted at the reconstructed numbers for the best match with the theoretical values.

Next, CT scans were taken of the iodine samples of Figure 10 and the offset and slope calibration numbers from the HU phantom results were applied. A typical CT reconstructed axial view image of the iodine samples with Eu filter is shown in Figure 15. The iodine content increases from top right clockwise.

It is known that HU numbers depend on the energy and spectrum of the X-ray beam and that is why HU calibrations are always performed using the HU phantoms at each X-ray energy and with each filter. Furthermore, some comparisons were made of how much the HU numbers were different if the calibration values from the no filter case were applied instead of applying the calibration values for the proper energy and filter.

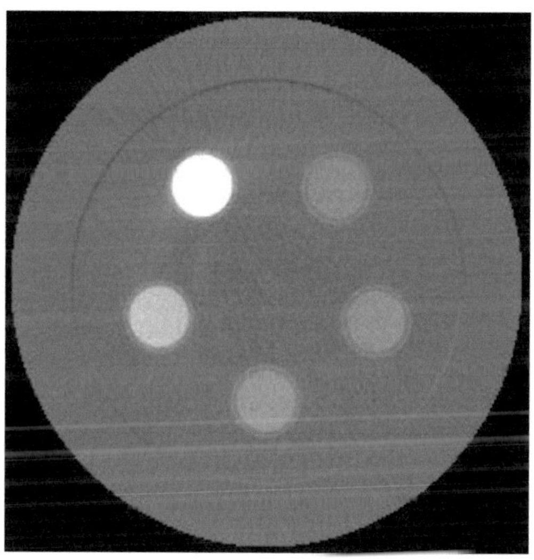

Fig. 15. A CT reconstructed axial image slice of iodine bottles. Image sequence was taken at 2 fr/s with 1.0 mm Eu filter at 70 kVp_20 mA continuous X-ray exposure. From top right to clockwise the iodine content of the bottles is 0, 0.5, 1.0, 4.0 and 16.0 mg/ml.

Using the calibrated offset and gain numbers for the iodine samples, HU numbers were obtained for the same iodine filtering as shown in Figure 10. To double check the numbers the air and water (0.00 mg/ml) values were used, which should be close to the nominal -1000 and 0 HU numbers. In this case the largest error is for the air, where the difference between the nominal and reconstructed values was about 20 HU.

Iodine content in water mg/ml	Nominal (HU) values	Reconstructed (HU) values
Air	-1000	-980.00
0.00	0	20.20
0.50		52.00
1.00		73.76
4.00		219.64
16.00		738.37

Table 3. CT reconstruction (HU) values for iodine samples with iodine filter.

Table 3 shows that the HU number increases with increasing iodine content, as expected. The HU slopes for iodine with different filters are plotted in Figure 16. It is shown that higher HU numbers were obtained (better iodine contrast) with Ce, Nd and Eu filters than without using any filter (No-filter case). The K edges all of these materials are above the K edge of iodine as shown in Figure 13. Furthermore, good HU linearity with iodine content was also observed for all cases.

However, if an Iodine filter is used for the iodine samples, lower contrast is obtained than in the no filter case. It is also noticeable that using higher energy X-rays with Al and Cu filters, which filter out the low energy part of the X-ray spectra, the contrast (HU number) further drops. Table 4 summarizes the HU differences with different filters and X-ray energies.

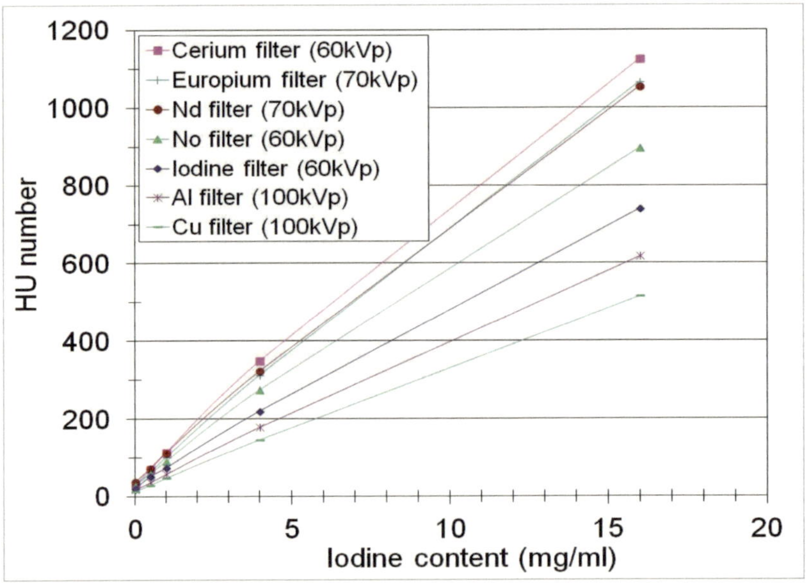

Fig. 16. HU slope with different filters.

It is quite obvious that the Cerium filter at 60kVp energy significantly increased the HU number (increased the contrast) of iodine. It shows a 26% improvement. Eu and Nd filters also improved the contrast by 16 and 17% respectively. The Al and Cu filters made the X-ray beam harder, so the iodine contrast considerably decreased when these filters and higher X-ray energies were used. However, it is interesting to note that the iodine contrast enhancement with K edge filters drastically depends on the X-ray tube voltage. When the X- ray energies were increased from 60 kVp to 70 kVp, the Ce filter contrast enhancement effect had nearly gone and it gave about the same contrast as the no filter case (see Table 4). This means that to obtain the maximum HU (contrast) improvement with iodine, the right X-ray tube voltage has to be set for each filter material. Furthermore, the material of the imaged object also has an effect on beam hardening, which needs to be considered in the optimization process.

Filter	HU(16 mg/ml)-HU(0 mg/ml)	[HU(16)-HU(0)] filter / [HU(16)-HU(0)] nofilter
No filter (60kVp)	866	1.00
Cu filter (100kVp)	501	0.58
Al filter (100kVp)	599	0.69
I filter (60kVp)	718	0.83
Ce filter (60kVp)	1093	1.26
Ce filter (70kVp)	874	1.01
Eu filter (70kVp))	1007	1.16
Nd filter (70kVp)	1015	1.17

Table 4. HU number difference comparison between the 16 mg/ml iodine and 0 mg/ml (pure water) solutions and the relative HU change for different filters and X-ray energies.

After the iodine contrast improvement, S/N (Signal-to-Noise) ratio was optimized. Dose per frame was varied to find the highest S/N. Generally the X-ray flux, after the filters were applied, was an order of magnitude lower than the flux in the no filter case or when the Al or Cu filters were used. To compensate for this effect the exposure time was increased by decreasing the framerate. However, the maximum exposure time per frame was also limited by the heat load limit of the X-ray tube because 625 frames had to be taken for CT reconstruction. Finally, the dose per frame numbers for the filter cases versus the no filter case was still about 2-3 times lower.

The S/N ratios were measured at all sample positions and also inside the bulk polyethylene far from the samples. Finally these numbers were averaged for a given measurement to find the $(S/N)_{filter}$. It is known that for the ideal case, when the electronics noise is negligible, the signal to noise (S/N) value is proportional to the square root of the number of incoming photons (flux). For equivalent image quality the S/N values have to be the same and so we calculated the filtered dose values corresponding to equivalent S/N (Zentai 2011).

$$\frac{\text{Dose}_{\text{equivalent}}}{\text{Dose}_{\text{filter}}} \approx \frac{\left(\frac{S}{N}\right)^2_{\text{nofilter})}}{\left(\frac{S}{N}\right)^2_{\text{filter}}} \quad (9)$$

Where $Dose_{equivalent}$ is the dose for the filter, which gives the same S/N ratio as the no filter case, and $Dose_{filter}$ is the dose measured when a given filter was applied. $(S/N)_{nofilter}$ is the signal to noise ratio for the no filter case while $(S/N)_{filter}$ is for the filtered case. The dose per frame difference during the measurement was only 2-3 times lower for the filtered cases so we thought that the above approximation would not introduce significant error. This approximation was double checked with measurements and S/N evaluation at two different dose-rates and for 8 times dose difference the error using the above approximation was less than 10%.

The equivalent dose from equation (9):

$$\mathrm{Dose}_{\mathrm{equivalent}} \approx \frac{\left(\frac{S}{N}\right)^2_{\mathrm{nofilter)}}}{\left(\frac{S}{N}\right)^2_{\mathrm{filter}}} \times \mathrm{Dose}_{\mathrm{filter}} \qquad (1)$$

After calculating the equivalent doses for each filter, these dose values were divided by the no filter case dose and dose equivalent S/N dose ratios were obtained. Both the equivalent doses and dose ratios are reported in Table 5. These numbers tell how much absolute and relative dose is needed when using these filters to get the same S/N value as the no filter case.

Table 5 tells that practically all of the filter materials used in these experiments provide the same S/N ratio at lower dose as the no filter case. From the dose point of view a Cu filter gives nearly the same very low dose as a Eu filter. However, it is important not just to get lower dose but at the same time to provide better contrast resolution and therefore higher HU numbers for iodine as explained previously.

Filter	Measured Dose uR/fr	S/N Average @ Measured Dose	S/N Equivalent Dose (uR/fr)	Dose ratio
No filter (60kVp)	1111	94.0	1111	1.00
Cu filter (100kVp)	569	114.3	385	0.35
Al filter (100kVp)	858	121.3	516	0.46
I filter (60kVp)	598	92.8	614	0.55
Ce filter (60kVp)	404	80.3	830	0.50
Ce filter (70kVp)	598	87.9	685	0.62
Eu filter (70kVp))	648	121.4	389	0.35
Nd filter (70kVp)	627	98.5	571	0.51

Table 5. Equivalent dose and dose rates.

6.4.3 Some other applications of K edge filters

In addition to mammography, Iodine and K edge filters are used for other medical x-ray imaging applications, such as lung tumor imaging and, frequently, angiography. (Nyman U Fau - Elmstahl, Elmstahl B Fau - Leander et al.), (Sato, Tanaka et al. 2004; Sato, Tanaka et al. 2007), (Sato, Hayasi et al. 2006).

A further enhancement of K edge filters involves using these filers in combination with counting mode energy resolution detectors mostly in CT applications (Alvarez and Macovski 1976; Roessl, Brendel et al. 2008; Schlomka and et al. 2008; Watanabe, Sato et al. 2008).

It is interesting to note that K edge imaging is also used in NDT (non Destructive Testing) applications by Jensen et al (Technology ; Jensen, Aljundi et al. 1997), when they measure the total uranium content in reactor fuel plates using the K edge technique. A further interesting application of K edge imaging is in the analysis of paintings where researchers verify authenticity and hunt for paintings that have been painted over (Dik 2004).

7. Conclusion

This chapter presented different methods used in mammography to improve the contrast between adipose and glandular tissues but especially to find cancerous cells and regions.

First of all the right energy range has to be determined for minimum patient dose with maximum contrast. Dual energy imaging, which uses two images taken at different energies, further enhances the contrast between different tissues and especially when contrast material is used.

Monochromatic X-ray beams are ideal for getting high quality images with optimal dose level and avoiding beam hardening artifacts. Moreover, monochromatic imaging can provide phase contrast images with excellent soft tissue contrast. The major drawbacks are that the synchrotrons, which can provide monochromatic beams with enough flux for medical imaging, are very large and expensive sources of X-rays.

Quasi monochromatic X-rays can be obtained by diffraction of X-rays emitted by an X-ray tube onto a mosaic crystal. The output beam has a limited bandwidth, low output flux, and has a fan beam shape. This limits its application only for scanning type imagers.

Another method of generating quasi monochromatic beams uses K edge filters. These filter materials have K edge electrons with bonding energies in the diagnostic X-ray energy range. The material can absorb an X-ray photon, whose energy is equivalent to or slightly higher than the K edge energy, by releasing an electron. The material's X-ray absorption level dramatically increases at or above this energy. As a result, x-rays higher than the K edge energy are suddenly cut off. Using these materials as X-ray filters, a narrow x-ray transmission energy range below the K edge energy can be obtained. One advantage of the K edge filters is that they provide cone beam shaped X-ray radiation rather than fan beam shaped radiation.

Iodine and Gadolinium are contrast agents injected into the blood flow They absorb the x-rays better than body tissues providing an x-ray shadow. They accumulate in the cancerous cells and remain there longer than they remain in the blood stream. This enhanced x-ray absorption provides extra contrast for better visibility of tumors. Using K edge filters X-ray image contrast of the I or Gd absorption can be further increased. I and Gd are frequently used as contrast agents for CT imaging. The experimental part of this paper describes evaluation of a few K edge filter materials using Iodine contrast material. These filters were compared to the non filtered case and also to Al and Cu filters, which provided only X-ray beam hardening. CT scans were performed and the HU numbers were calculated for iodine contrast agents. It was found that the beam hardening Al and Cu filters and even the iodine filter decreased the iodine HU number, but the K edge filters, which have K edge energy slightly above the K edge of iodine, increased the HU number (increased iodine contrast). This increase can be as high as 26% for Ce filter at 60 kVp. However, it is seen that using an Iodine filter for an Iodine contrast agent decreases the HU number to the no-filter case. That creates an option to further enhance the contrast by subtracting the Iodine filtered image from the Ce filtered one. This would provide an additional ~17% contrast enhancement of iodine. A drawback of this method is that we need two images (practically dual energy imaging), which increases the dose to the patient and increases noise.

We also found that the increase of HU number is linearly proportional with the iodine content in water.

Furthermore, the doses required for S/N number equivalent to the no filter case are lower for each filter material. However, we need not just lower dose but want to increase the iodine contrast (higher HU number for iodine). From this point of view Eu is a much better choice than Cu even if their dose improvement is nearly the same. The dose improvement is nearly 3 times for both filters but Cu decreased the HU number (the iodine visibility) nearly to half of the no filter case. So both the HU increase and the dose improvement have to be considered in parallel. From these considerations Ce, Eu and Nd are all promising candidates for iodine contrast imaging enhancement. Moreover, the HU contrast enhancement effect depends strongly on the X-ray tube voltage as seen in Table 4 for Ce and also on the object material, which contains the iodine, so careful optimization is required for getting the maximum HU improvement with a significantly decreased dose to the patient.

Mc. Kinley et al investigated the effect of K edge filtering on breast CT and found dose reduction possibility up to 6 times while keeping the same contrast ratio (McKinley Iii, Tornai et al. 2007).

Watanabe et al (Watanabe, Sato et al. 2008) and Roessl et al (Roessl, Brendel et al. 2008) also investigated how K edge imaging improves the signal to noise ratio but they used a photon counting CT method. S/N ratio improvement was demonstrated by using the K edge technique but the photon counting method is much more expensive and a slower process than multislice or cone beam CT with K edge filter. These drawbacks come from the high price of the large area pixellated energy resolution detectors and the counting speed is very limited.

Finally, it is very important that for HU calibration we have to use the same kVp setting and filter that we use for scanning the CT object otherwise huge reconstruction errors could be introduced (Zentai 2011).

We need to add that we used heavy K edge filtering of 200th value layer K edge filters for Ce, Eu and Nd. These thick filters significantly decreased the X-ray intensity even around the K edge. From our measurements and calculations we concluded that thinner filters may provide the same advantages that these thick filters without the large flux reduction. This could ease the tube flux requirement and so decrease the maximum heat load and/or increase the CT scanning speed.

8. References

Alvarez, R.E. and Macovski, A. (1976) *Energy-selective reconstructions in X-ray computerized tomography.* Physics in Medicine and Biology 21, 733-44.

Arvanitis, C.D., Royle, G. et al. (2007) *Dual energy contrast enhanced breast imaging optimization using contrast to noise ratio.* In, Medical Imaging 2007: Physics of Medical Imaging, SPIE, San Diego, CA, USA, Vol. 6510, pp. 65102Y-10.

Baldelli, P. and et al. (2005) *A prototype of a quasi-monochromatic system for mammography applications.* Physics in Medicine and Biology 50, 2225.

Baldelli, P., Taibi, A., Tuffanelli, A. et al. (2003) *Quasi-monochromatic x-rays for diagnostic radiology.* Physics in Medicine and Biology 48, 3653-3665.

Bhat, M., Pattison, J., et al. (1999) Off-axis x-ray spectra: *A comparison of Monte Carlo simulated and computed x-ray spectra with measured spectra.* Medical Physics 26, 303-309.

Boone, J.M., Nelson, T.R., et al. (2001) *Dedicated Breast CT: Radiation Dose and Image Quality Evaluation.* Radiology 221, 657-667.

Boone, J.M., Shaber, G.S., et al. (1990) *Dual-energy mammography: a detector analysis.* Medical Physics 17, 665-75.

Carton, A.-K., Lindman, K., et al. (2007) *Dual-energy subtraction for contrast-enhanced digital breast tomosynthesis.* In, Medical Imaging 2007: Physics of Medical Imaging, SPIE, San Diego, CA, USA, Vol. 6510, pp. 651007-12.

Chen, B., Jing, Z., et al. (2006) *Dual-energy contrast-enhanced digital mammography (DE-CEDM): optimization on digital subtraction with practical x-ray low/high-energy spectra.* In, Medical Imaging 2006: Physics of Medical Imaging, SPIE, San Diego, CA, USA, Vol. 6142, pp. 61422N-10.

Coello, C.S., Dinten, J.-M., et al. (2007) *Dual-energy technique for digital flat-panel detectors without x-ray tube voltage switching.* In, Medical Imaging 2007: Physics of Medical Imaging, SPIE, San Diego, CA, USA, Vol. 6510, pp. 651005 10.

Cranley, K., Gilmore, B.J., et al. (1997) *Catalogue of Diagnostic X-ray Spectra and Other Data.* The Institute of Physics and Engineering in Medicine, UK.

Crotty, D.J., McKinley, et al. (2006) *Experimental spectral measurements of heavy K-edge filtered beams for x-ray computed mammotomography.* In, Medical Imaging 2006: Physics of Medical Imaging, SPIE, San Diego, CA, USA, Vol. 6142, pp. 61421V-11.

Dance, D., Thilander, A., et al. (2000) *Influence of anode/filter material and tube potential on contrast, signal-to-noise ratio and average absorbed dose in mammography: a Monte Carlo study.* Br J Radiol 73, 1056-1067.

Dik, J. (2004) Using XRF and *Dual Energy K-edge Absorption imaging in the study of paintings.* In http://neutra.web.psi.ch/cost-g8/presentations/dik.pdf

Donath, T., Pfeiffer, F., et al. (2008) *Phase-contrast imaging and tomography at 60 keV using a conventional x-ray tube.* In, Developments in X-Ray Tomography VI, SPIE, San Diego, CA, USA, Vol. 7078, pp. 707817 8.

Ersahin, A., Molloi, S.Y. et al. (1994) *Scatter and veiling glare corrections for quantitative digital subtraction angiography.* SPIEVol. 2163, pp. 172-183.

Fahrig, R., Rowlands, J.A. et al. (1996) *X-ray imaging with amorphous selenium: optimal spectra for digital mammography.* Med Phys 23, 557-67.

Fahrig, R. and Yaffe, M.J. (1994) *Optimization of spectral shape in digital mammography: Dependence on anode material, breast thickness, and lesion* journal article. AAPMVol. 21, pp. 1473-1481.

Feldkamp, L.A., Davis, L.C. et al. (1984) *Practical cone-beam algorithm.* J. Opt. Soc. Am. A 1, 612-619.

Fiedler, S., Elleaume, H., et al. (2000) *Dual-energy coronary angiography in pigs using a Gd contrast agent.* In, Medical Imaging 2000: Physics of Medical Imaging, SPIE, San Diego, CA, USA, Vol. 3977, pp. 96-103.

Fiedler, S. and et al. (2004) *Imaging lobular breast carcinoma: comparison of synchrotron radiation DEI-CT technique with clinical CT, mammography and histology.* Physics in Medicine and Biology 49, 175.

Gambaccini, M., Fantini, A., et al. (2001a) *Development of a quasi-monochromatic CT system for breast cancer study with combined emission-transmission tomography.* Nuclear Science, IEEE Transactions on 48, 703-706.

Gambaccini, M., Tuffanelli, A., et al. (2001b) *Spatial resolution measurements in quasimonochromatic x rays with mosaic crystals for mammography application.* Medical Physics 28, 412-8.

GE GE Lunar DPX *Bravo Bone Densitometer.* In. http://www.mechealthcareonline.com/p-127-ge-lunar-dpx-bravo-bone-densitometer.aspx

Hologic *Hologic Bone Densitometry.* In. http://www.hologic.com/en/skeletal/osteoporosis-assessment/discovery/

Huda W Fau - Sajewicz, A.M., et al. *Experimental investigation of the dose and image quality characteristics of a digital mammography imaging system.* Medical Physics (2003), Vol.30 (3) 442-448

Jennings, R.J., Quinn, et al. (1993) *Evaluation of x-ray sources for mammography.* SPIE Vol. 1896, pp. 259-268.

Jensen, T., Aljundi, T., et al. (1997) X-ray, *K-Edge Measurement of Uranium Concentration in Reactor Fuel Plates.* In. http://www.osti.gov/bridge/servlets/purl/671994-VS0FZp/webviewable/671994.pdf

Jeung, A., Sloutsky, A., et al. (2005) WE-C-T-617-10: *Geometry Calibration of An On-Board KV Imaging System.* Medical Physics 32, 2129-2130.

Johns, P.C., Drost, D.J., et al. (1983) *Dual Energy Mammographic Imaging.* In Fullerton, G.D. (ed.), SPIE Application of Optical Instrumentation in Medicine SPIE, Vol. 0419, pp. 201-208.

Johns, P.C. and Yaffe, M.J. (1985) *Theoretical optimization of dual-energy x-ray imaging with application to mammography.* Medical Physics 12, 289-96.

Kappadath, S.C., Shaw, C.C., et al. (2004) *Dual-energy digital mammography for calcification imaging: theory and implementation.* In, Medical Imaging 2004: Physics of Medical Imaging, SPIE, San Diego, CA, USA, Vol. 5368, pp. 751-760.

Kashani, H., Varon, C.A., et al. (2010) *Diagnostic Performance of a Prototype Dual-Energy Chest Imaging System: ROC Analysis.* Academic radiology 17, 298-308.

Matsinos, E. *(2005) Current status of the CBCT project at Varian Medical Systems.* In, Medical Imaging 2005: Physics of Medical Imaging, SPIE, San Diego, CA, USA, Vol. 5745, pp. 340-351.

McKinley Iii, R.L., Tornai, et al. (2007) *A contrast-detail comparison of computed mammotomography and digital mammography.* In, Medical Imaging 2007: Physics of Medical Imaging, SPIE, San Diego, CA, USA, Vol. 6510, pp. 65101D-10.

NIST (2009) *Photon Absorption data for elements compounds and mixtures in the 1 keV-100GeV range.* In. http://physics.nist.gov/PhysRefData/Xcom/html/xcom1.html

Nyman U Fau - Elmstahl, B., et al. *Are gadolinium-based contrast media really safer than iodinated media for digital subtraction angiography in patients with azotemia?* Radiology 2002 Vol. 232 (2) pp. 311-318.

Pavkovich, J. (1979a) *Tomographic apparatus and method for reconstructing planar slices from non-absorbed and non-scattered radiation.* In, US Patent, Varian Associates, Inc., US Patent # 4149247.

Pavkovich, J.M. (1979b) *Apparatus and method for reconstructing data.* In, US Patent, Varian Associates, Inc., US Patent # 4149248.

Puong, S., Bouchevreau, X., et al. (2007a) *Dual-energy contrast enhanced digital mammography using a new approach for breast tissue canceling.* In, Medical Imaging 2007: Physics of Medical Imaging, SPIE, San Diego, CA, USA, Vol. 6510, pp. 65102H-12.

Puong, S., Patoureaux, F., et al. (2007b) *Dual-energy contrast enhanced digital breast tomosynthesis: concept, method, and evaluation on phantoms.* In, Medical Imaging 2007: Physics of Medical Imaging, SPIE, San Diego, CA, USA, Vol. 6510, pp. 65100U-12.

Roessl, E., Brendel, B., et al. (2008) *Sensitivity of photon-counting K-edge imaging: Dependence on atomic number and object size.* In, Nuclear Science Symposium Conference Record, 2008. NSS '08. IEEE, pp. 4016-4021.

Roos, P.G., Colbeth, R.E., et al. (2004) *Multiple-gain-ranging readout method to extend the dynamic range of amorphous silicon flat-panel imagers.* In, Medical Imaging 2004: Physics of Medical Imaging, SPIE, San Diego, CA, USA, Vol. 5368, pp. 139-149.

Rutherford, R.A., Pullan, B.R. et al. (1976) *X-ray energies for effective atomic number determination.* Neuroradiology 11, 23-8.

Sato, E., Hayasi, Y., et al. (2006) *K-edge angiography utilizing a tungsten plasma X-ray generator in conjunction with gadolinium-based contrast media.* Radiation Physics and Chemistry 75, 1841-1849.

Sato, E., Tanaka, E., et al. (2004) *Demonstration of enhanced K-edge angiography using a cerium target x-ray generator.* Medical Physics 31, 3017-3021.

Sato, E., Tanaka, E., et al... (2007) *Demonstration of Enhanced K-edge Angiography Utilizing a Samarium X-ray Generator.* In, World Congress on Medical Physics and Biomedical Engineering 2006, Springer, Vol. 14 (10), pp. 1359-1362.

Saunders, R., Samei, E., et al. (2008) *Optimization of dual energy contrast enhanced breast tomosynthesis for improved mammographic lesion detection and diagnosis.* In, Medical Imaging 2008: Physics of Medical Imaging, SPIE, San Diego, CA, USA, Vol. 6913, pp. 69130Y-11.

Shimura, K., Nakajima, N., et al. (1993) *Basic investigation of dual-energy x-ray absorptiometry for bone densitometry using computed radiography.* SPIE Vol. 1896, pp. 121-129.

Sukovic, P. and Clinthorne, N.H. (1999) *Basis material decomposition using triple-energy X-ray computed tomography.* In, IEEE 16th Instrumentation and Measurement Technology Conference 1999, IEEE, Venice, Italy, Vol. 3, pp. 1615-18.

Sutton, D. (2009) *Spectral Impact on Dose and Image Quality in Conventional Radiography. In. Technology, I. Portable X-Ray, K-Edge Heavy Metal Detector.* In. www.dundee.ac.uk/medphys/documents/SPIMAPCT.pdf

Varjonen, M. and Strommer, P. (2008) *Optimizing the anode-filter combination in the sense of image quality and average glandular dose in digital mammography.* In, Medical Imaging 2008: Physics of Medical Imaging, SPIE, San Diego, CA, USA, Vol. 6913, pp. 69134K-8.

Venkatakrishnan, V., Yavuz, M., et al. (1999) *Experimental and theoretical spectral optimization for digital mammography.* SPIEVol. 3659, pp. 142-149.

Walter, D.J., Wu, X., et al. (2004) *Dual kVp material decomposition using flat-panel detectors.* In, Medical Imaging 2004: Physics of Medical Imaging, SPIE, San Diego, CA, USA, Vol. 5368, pp. 29-39.

Watanabe, M., Sato, E., et al. (2008) *Energy-discriminating K-edge x-ray computed tomography system.* In, SPIE Penetrating Radiation Systems and Applications IX, SPIE, San Diego, California, Vol. 7080, pp. 70800B-1-5.

Zentai, G. (2011) *Signal-to-Noise and Contrast Ratio Enhancements by Quasi-Monochromatic Imaging.* IEEE Transactions on Instrumentation and Measurement Vol. 60, 908-915.

7

Standards for Electrical Impedance Mammography

Marina Korotkova and Alexander Karpov
Clinical Hospital #9, Yaroslavl
Russia

1. Introduction

1.1 Imaging technique, employing feeble alternating current

Currently, a variety of electrical impedance diagnostic systems is used both in academic studies and in clinical practice. A significant part of such systems employs electrodes which reside in a single array and two-dimensional mathematical conductivity reconstruction algorithms in the array of the electrodes. Electrical impedance mammograph belongs to the class of 3D tomography systems. Thus, all the measurements are made on the surface of the object under investigation. The change of surface potential difference (compared with the homogeneous case), as a rule, is caused by the presence of a local heterogeneous area in the object. It is mainly concentrated in the area which is a projection of the local heterogeneous area on the surface of the object. Therefore, the main objective of electrical impedance mammography is to visualize the reconstructed three-dimensional electrical conductivity distribution of the object basing on the results of electrical measurements on its surface. For this purpose various modifications of mathematical method of "back projection" are employed. Mathematical methods provide also cross-sectional slices of conductivity.

The usage of alternating current for this purpose is justified from several positions. Extreme complication of electrical conductivity measuring in biological systems at direct (i.e. unidirectional) current is conditioned by high degree of polarization of cellular membranes. Moreover, the flow of direct current through biological tissues is accompanied by irreversible chemical reactions at the electrodes, through which the object is connected with the external part of the circuit. Therefore, only alternating electric current of sufficiently high frequency is employed in medical diagnostics.

1.2 Tissue-specific peculiarities of electrical conductivity

In biological tissue, electric current affects the components and structures that have a net electric charge and / or an electric dipole moment. This influence is carried out in an environment characterized by the presence of numerous interface regions. An example of such interface regions are cell membranes. In the space, surrounding cell membranes from both sides, the changes are carried by electric charges, mainly in the form of ions and the sources of dipole moment in the form of polar water molecules and mobile polar macromolecules. Moreover, the polarization ability of the cell membrane itself due to protein and lipid structures determines its exceptional electrical properties. Thus, the electrical properties of biological tissue as a colloid-disperse system in an alternating electric field are determined by the concentration and «the behaviour» of chemical compounds in it.

2. Indications for application

- Evaluation of palpable lesions of the mammary gland.
- Evaluation of the impalpable changes which do not manifest clinically.
- Formation of groups of people with heightened risk of breast cancer development, using the percentile curves of the age-related electrical conductivity.
- Screening for oncopathology.
- Additional examination of the dense tissue of the mammary gland.
- Examination in the age group under 50, including adolescents.
- Examination of pregnant and lactating women.
- Monitoring during hormonal contraception and hormone replacement therapy.
- Monitoring after pharmacotherapy or operative therapy.
- Examination of the women after cosmetic surgery.

3. Technical requirements and safety assurances for doctors and patients

- Parameters of current employed: alternating current, frequency - 50 кHz, current intensity - 0.5 mA.
- The abovementioned characteristics are allowed for medical use and are safe both for a doctor and a patient; also they are significantly lower than «threshold values», i.e. do not induce pain or other sensations.
- Patient's name/code, examination date, probing current characteristics and initial adjustments shall be displayed on the screen.
- Examination results digital recording.
- Penetration depth ≥ 4.0 cm.

4. Examination quality criteria

For high-quality diagnostic and continuity of work it is necessary that electrical impedance mammograms met specific quality criteria.

- Appropriate visualization of mammary gland tissue: the nipple shall be in the centre of the image.
- If the mammary gland is not completely covered by the panel or if there are palpable lesions out of the electrodes panel area, the examination shall be carried out by segments, clockwise (upper - external - lower - internal segment of the mammary gland).
- Proper designation: patient data, indication of the side and the date of the examination, physiological period, other features, for example, skin changes.
- Sufficient compression: optimal number of good contacts. It is necessary to achieve the maximum possible number of good contacts, however, excessive compression of the breast shall be avoided.

- The absence of motion distortions and artifacts.
- The absence of skin folds.
- The images acquired using improper examination techniques are not accepted for interpretation.

5. Types of mammary gland structure from the perspective of electrical impedance mammography

Electrical conductivity index (IC), calculated during the electrical impedance examination, is a quantitative value, which characterizes the status of the breast. The results of 1,632 electrical impedance mammograph examinations, obtained from healthy women from different age groups, were analyzed. The women were selected for the examination according to the following criteria: absence of complaints on the mammary glands, a normal menstrual cycle, uncomplicated perimenopausal period, absence of chronic somatic and gynaecological diseases and absence of hormonal contraceptives taking or hormone replacement therapy. The women were distributed by age in years as follows: 20-30 (380 women), 31-40 (428), 41-50 (449) and 51-60 (375). All the examinations described in the chapter were carried out with the help of the electroimpedance computer mammograph "MEIK" v.5.6 (0.5 mA, 50 kHz), developed and manufactured by PKF "SIM-Technika", Russia.

Fluctuations of electrical conductivity index in 1,632 studies were as follows: lower limit - 0.01 conventional units, upper limit - 0.68 conventional units. In order to identify the structure of electrical impedance index distribution there were elaborated 8 ranges of criteria at a step of 0.09 and the quantity of studies was calculated in each range (Table 1).

Electrical conductivity index	Number of studies
0.00 - 0.09	67
0.10 - 0.19	279
0.20 - 0.29	471
0.30 - 0.39	435
0.40 - 0.49	299
0.50 - 0.59	75
0.60 - 0.69	6
Total	1632

Table 1. Arrangement of electrical conductivity index frequencies.

Fig. 1 shows the frequency histogram of electrical conductivity index data. Mean electrical conductivity index constituted 0.29, median value - 0.29 and mode - 0.26.

Taking into consideration a bell-shaped curve, close mean, median and mode values one can speak about standard (Gauss) distribution of the quantitative value, in this case, of electrical conductivity index. Typically, mean value and standard deviation are used to describe standard distribution. More detailed data can be obtained using 3th, 10th, 25th, 40th, 75th, 90th and 97th percentiles (Figure 2). In this case, the information on the shape of criterion distribution graph is not required.

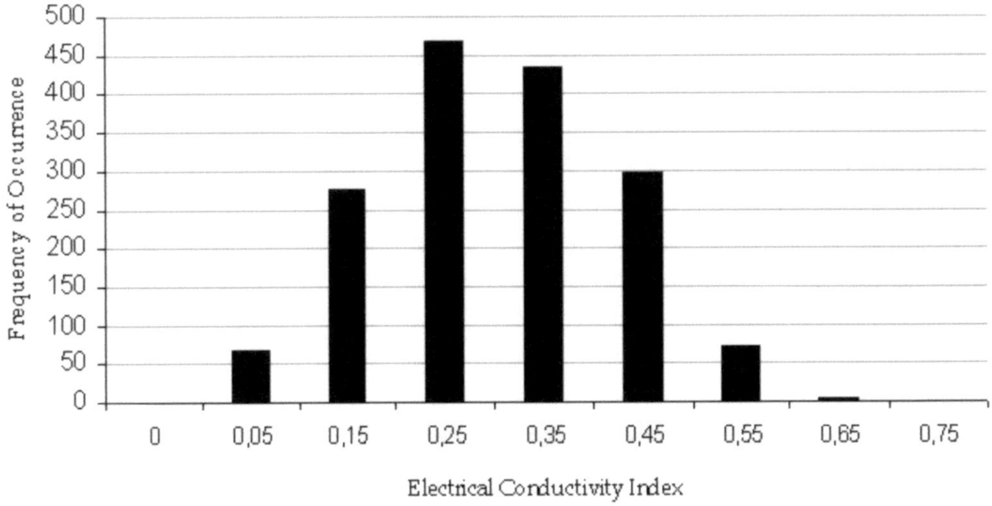

Fig. 1. Frequency histogram of electrical conductivity index data.

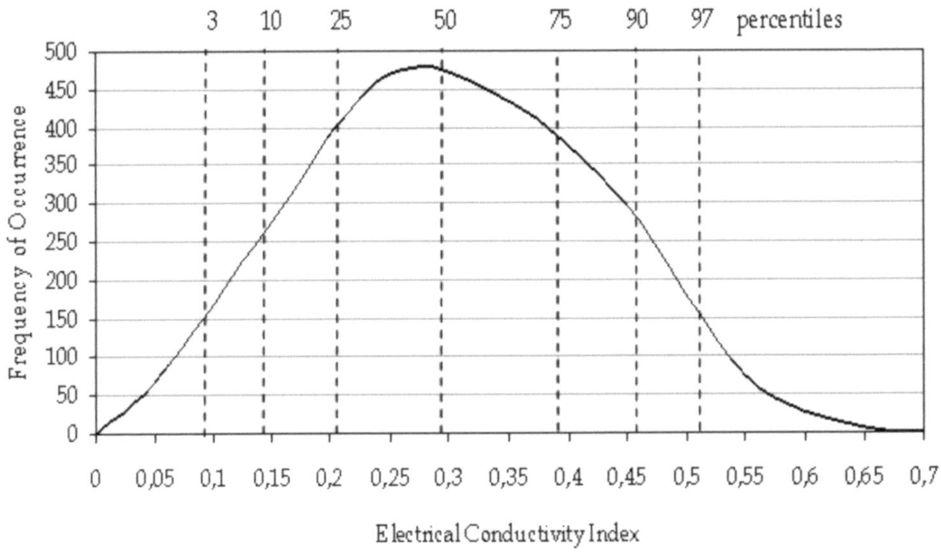

Fig. 2. Frequency histogram of electrical conductivity index data and percentile ranges.

The following pattern was identified after the age-related characteristics of women belonging to the percentile ranges were analyzed. Women aged from 20 to 30, whose data fell to the ranges less than 3rd percentile (IC<0.09) and from 3rd to 10th percentile (IC=0.1-1.4) constituted more than 50%. Women aged from 50 to 60, whose data fell to the ranges higher than 97th percentile (IC>0.53) and from 90th to 97th percentile (IC=0.47-0.52) constituted more than 50%. Age of the women whose data ranged between 25th and 75th percentiles (IC=0.21-0.39) distributed in a uniform manner, the percentage of each age-group constituted from 20 to 30% without any prevalence (Figure 3).

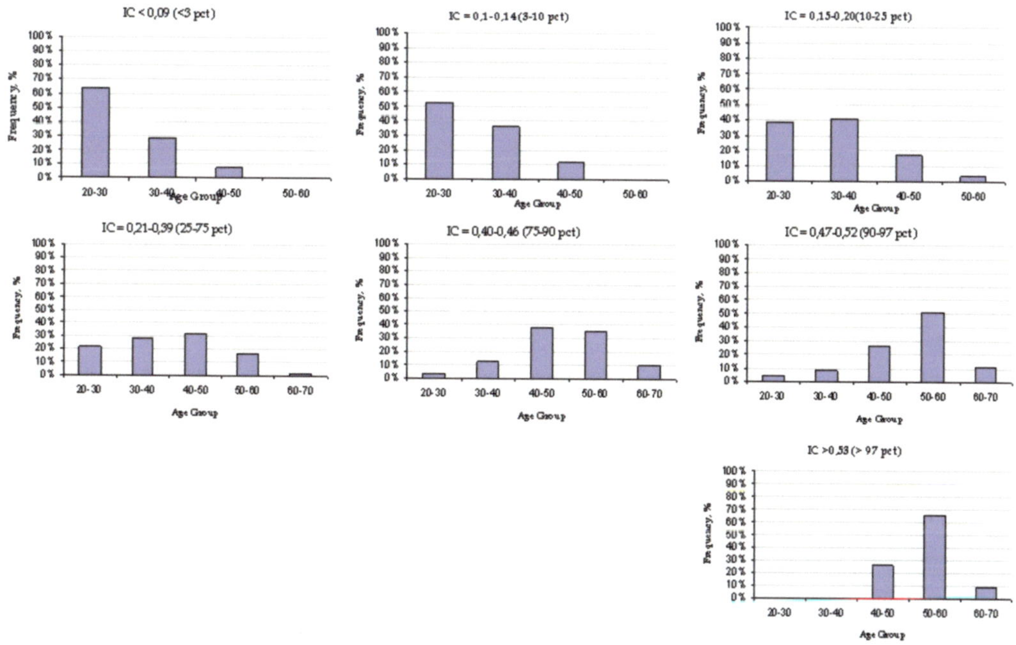

Fig. 3. Age-related characteristics of percentile ranges.

The low electrical conductivity index of the mammary glands typical for women aged from 20 to 30 are conditioned by the peculiarities of breast's anatomy. This group of women is characterized by the prevalence of ductal and acinar epithelium over connective tissue in the mammary gland structure. The phenomenon of low conductivity can be explained by the presence of a large number of membranes of epithelium cells in the mamma. It is known that cell membranes possess capacitance and act as a strong barrier for electrical current. Therefore, a large amount of lactiferous ducts and lobules in the mamma (implying the presence of a large number of cell membranes) conditions low electrical conductivity. The predominance of women in this age group is observed in two percentile ranges - less than 3rd percentile and from 3rd to 10th percentile. Therefore, the status of mammary glands possessing electrical conductivity index lower than 0.14 cu, should be regarded as ductal and acinar type of the breast structure (Fig. 4).

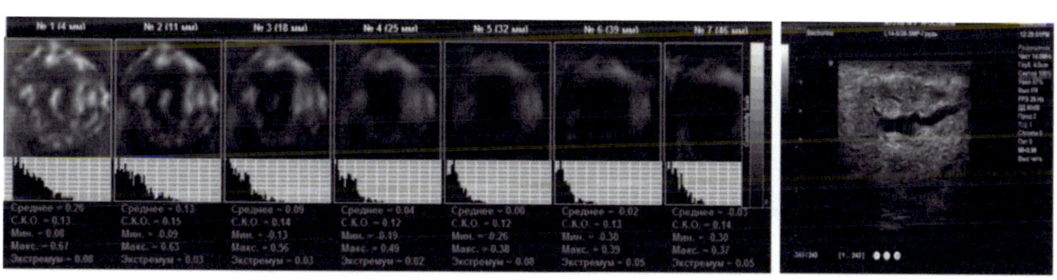

Fig. 4. EIM. Seven scan planes. A 21 years-old patient. Acinar/ductal type of mammary gland structure. Low values of electrical conductivity index (less than 10 pct). On the right - ultrasound image.

"Loss" of acinar/ductal epithelium in women aged from 50 to 60 is the reason for high electrical conductivity index of the mammary glands. When progressive decrease of estradiol secretion occurs, terminal-duct secretory epithelium is substituted by connective tissue with a varied correlation of tissue elements. Intercellular substance includes the ground substance, which contains a large amount of mucopolysaccharides. Loose connective tissue, filling the space between bodies, blood vessels, nerves, muscles and other structures of the body, creates the internal environment, through which the delivery of nutrients to cells and the removal of the waste products of their metabolism are carried out. The major mucopolysaccharide of the ground substance of connective tissue is hyaluronic acid, which carries a large number of negative charges. Its ability to bind and retain water dipoles determines the electrical properties of amorphous substance of connective tissue, making it a good conductor. Therefore, the predominance of connective tissue in the breast should expect high electrical conductivity. The predominance of women in this age group is observed in two percentile ranges - more than 97th percentile and from 90th to 97th percentile. Therefore, the status of mammary glands possessing electrical conductivity index higher than 0.47 cu, should be regarded as amorphous type of the mammary gland structure (Fig. 5).

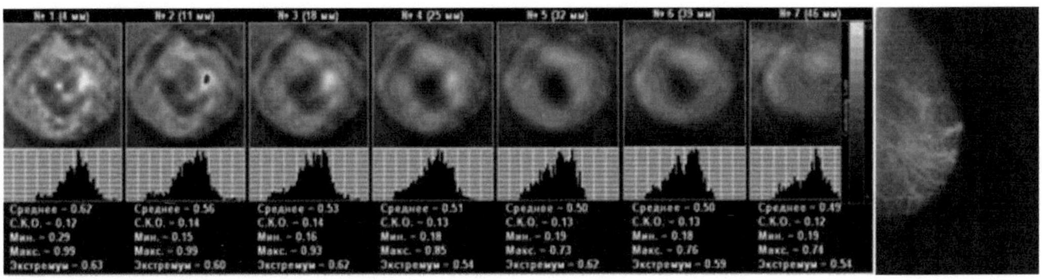

Fig. 5. EIM. Seven scan planes. A 52 years-old patient. Amorphous type of mammary gland structure. High values of mean electrical conductivity index – (> 90 pct). On the right - X-ray mammogram.

Different combinations of acinar/ductal components and connective tissue with adipocytes are the reasons for electrical conductivity index variations from 0.21-0.39 in women of all age groups. Therefore, the status of mammary glands possessing electrical conductivity index within the range from 0.21 to 0.39 cu, should be regarded as a mixed type of the mammary gland structure. Different combinations of the structures that determine the conductivity of tissues, define the wide range of the values of electrical conductivity index (Fig. 6).

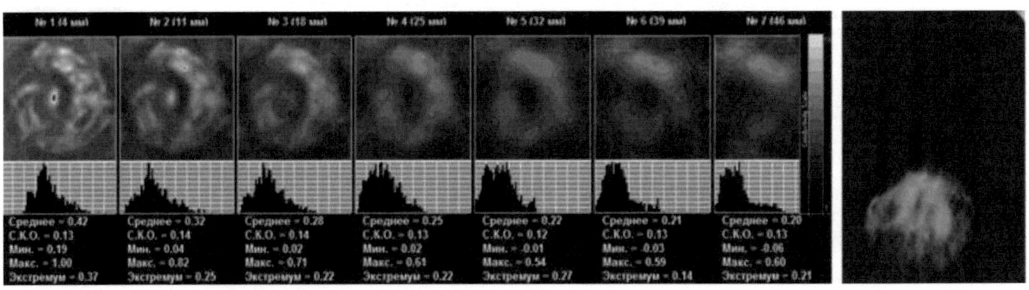

Fig. 6. EIM. Seven scan planes. Age 39 years. Mixed type of mammary gland structure. Mean electrical conductivity index – 25-75 pct. On the right - X-ray mammogram.

Within the ranges from 10th to 25th percentile and from 75 to 90th percentile the data of two age groups of women prevail. Therefore, the status of mammary glands possessing electrical conductivity index within these ranges, should be regarded as a mixed type of the mammary gland structure with prevalence of acinar/ductal or amorphous component respectively.

Below the summary table of structure estimates for the breast in terms of electrical impedance mammography is provided (Table 2).

	Formulation	Electrical conductivity	Percentiles
Type Ia	Amorphous type of mammary gland structure.	above 0.47	>90‰
Type Ib	Mixed type of mammary gland structure with amorphous component predominance.	0,40 – 0,46	75-90‰
Type II	Mixed type of mammary gland structure.	0,21 – 0,39	25-75‰
Type III	Mixed type of mammary gland structure with acinar/ductal component predominance. High density of ductal component.	0,14 – 0,20	10-25‰
Type IV	Acinar/ductal type of mammary gland structure. Extremely high density of acinar/ductal component	below 0.14	<10‰

Table 2. Types of mammary gland structure from the perspective of electrical impedance mammography.

Thus the estimation of mammary gland structure from the perspective of electrical impedance mammography using electrical conductivity index is possible. It is known that the structure of the mammary gland determines their density. Thus, the defined ranges of electric conductivity correspond to different types of mammary gland "density". Low values of electric conductivity correspond to "dense" breasts of the so-called combined ductal/lobular type. High values of electrical conductivity index are characteristics of the amorphous type of breasts, consisting mainly of fat and connective tissue. A distinctive feature of this method for evaluating structure of the breast is the expression of its anatomical and histological structure in numerical terms. Estimation of the density of mammary glands from the perspective of electrical impedance mammography using electrical conductivity index in *ACR* terms is provided below (Table 3).

	EIM classification	*ACR* classification
Type Ia	Amorphous type of mammary gland structure. IC >90‰.	Predominantly fat. Under 25% of tissue is represented by parenchyma
Type Ib	Mixed type of mammary gland structure with amorphous component predominance. IC=75-90‰.	
Type II	Mixed type of mammary gland structure. IC=25-75‰.	Fat with some fibroglandular tissue. 25-50% of tissue is represented by parenchyma
Type III	Mixed type of mammary gland structure with acinar/ductal component predominance. High density of acinar/ductal component. IC=10-25‰.	Heterogeneously dense. 50-75% of tissue is represented by parenchyma
Type IV	Acinar/ductal type of mammary gland structure. Extremely high density of acinar/ductal component. IC < 10‰.	Extremely dense. 75-100% of parenchyma tissue.

Table 3. Mammary gland structure from the perspective of electrical impedance mammography execution and breast density types according to the classification of the American College of Radiology (ACR).

6. System for description of mammary glands images

6.1 Terminology

- Electrical conductivity scale - electrical conductivity index values from 0 to 1.00, or in gray-scale - changes from black to white, respectively.
- Hyperimpedance structure, lesion - electrical conductivity is lower than electrical conductivity of the surrounding tissue of the breast and corresponds to IC < 0.20.
- Isoimpedance structure, lesion - electrical conductivity is approximately equal to the electrical conductivity of the surrounding tissue of the breast and corresponds to IC = 0.3-0.5.
- Hypoimpedance structure, lesion - electrical conductivity is higher than the electrical conductivity of the surrounding tissue of the breast and corresponds to IC = 0.6-0.8.
- Animpedance structure, lesion - electrical conductivity is considerably higher than the electrical conductivity of the surrounding tissue of the breast and corresponds to IC > 0.90.

6.2 Normal signs in the electrical impedance mammogram

6.2.1 The septa

The septa (layers) consisting of delicate fibrillary tissue are going deep into the mass of the mammary gland from connective tissue capsule that surrounds it. The septa, radiating from the centre, which form the connective tissue stroma of the mammary gland are characterized by a hyperimpedance structure (Fig. 7).

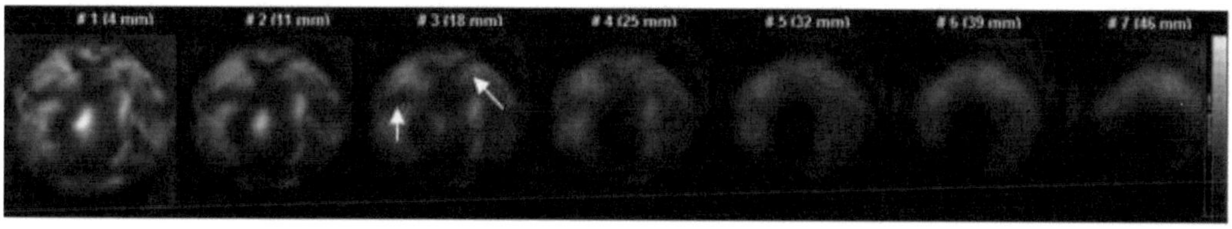

Fig. 7. EIM. Seven scan planes. Connective tissue septa, radiating from the areola (indicated with arrows).

6.2.2 The parenchyma

One distinguishes the parenchyma, which consists of alveolar-tubular glands, and the connective tissue stroma, which is represented by a small amount of cells, delicate fibres and ground intercellular substance. The parenchyma is characterized by an isoimpedance structure and is located between the septa. (Fig. 8).

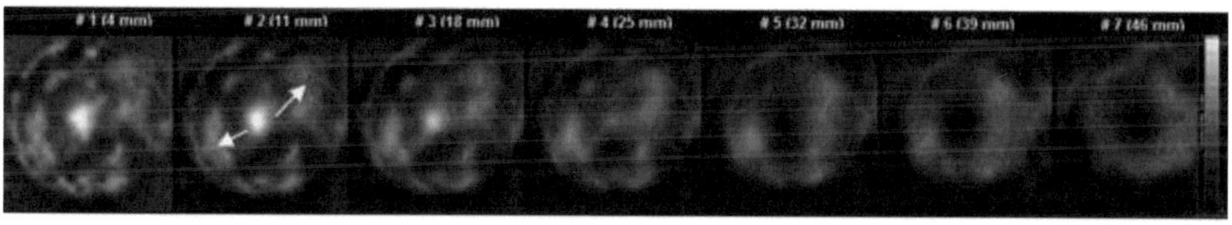

Fig. 8. EIM. Seven scan planes. Parenchyma as isoimpedance areas located between the connective tissue septa (indicated with arrows).

6.2.3 The lactiferous sinus zone

Before reaching the nipple milk ducts gain in breadth and create a lactiferous sinus (sinus lactiferi) which accumulates secreta as well as the milk. There are about 15-25 sini in the retromammilary area. The lactiferous sinus zone is visualized as a vast hypoimpedance area located in the centre of the mammogram (fig. 9).

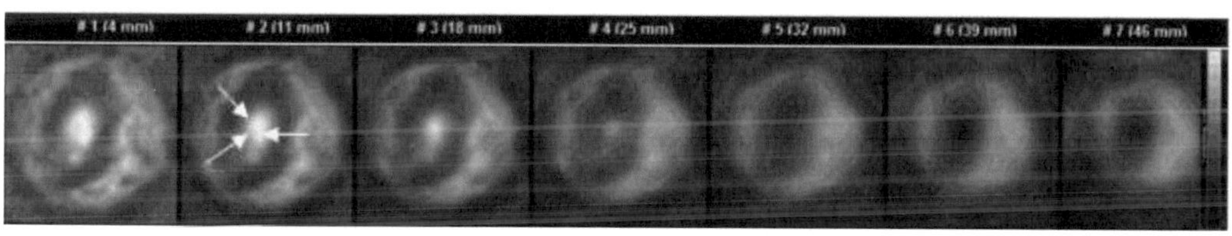

Fig. 9. EIM. Seven scan planes. A hypoimpedance area in the centre of the mammogram corresponds to the location of the lactiferous sinus zone (indicated with arrows).

6.2.4 The nipple

The nipple consists of the excretory ducts of the breast lobes, surrounded by fibrous tissue and a large number of sebaceous glands. High electrical impedance of the nipple is determined by the absence of the excretory ducts of perspiratory glands in it. In the electrical impedance tomogram the nipple is visualized in the centre as a circular or linear hyperimpedance area, located closely to the lactiferous sinus zone (fig. 10).

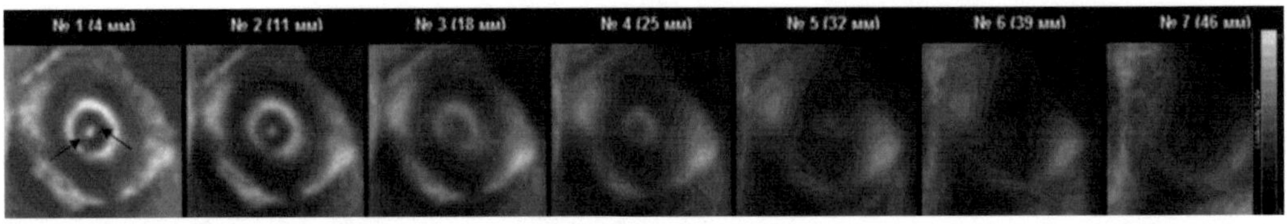

Fig. 10. EIM. Seven scan planes. The nipple is visualized in the centre as a rounded hyperimpedance area (indicated with arrows). In the centre of the nipple there are excretory ducts which are characterized by hypoimpedance. Around the nipple there is the hypoimpedance area of the lactiferous sinus zone.

6.2.5 The areola

In the dermis of areola there are circular smooth muscle fibres, numerous sebaceous glands and a large number of pigment cells. Large sebaceous glands located on the periphery of the areola cause the formation of protrusions (Montgomery's tubercles). High electrical impedance of the areola, as well as that of the nipple, is determined by the absence of the excretory ducts of perspiratory glands in it. In the electrical impedance mammogram the areola is visualized as a circular hyperimpedance formation surrounding the lactiferous sinus zone (fig. 11).

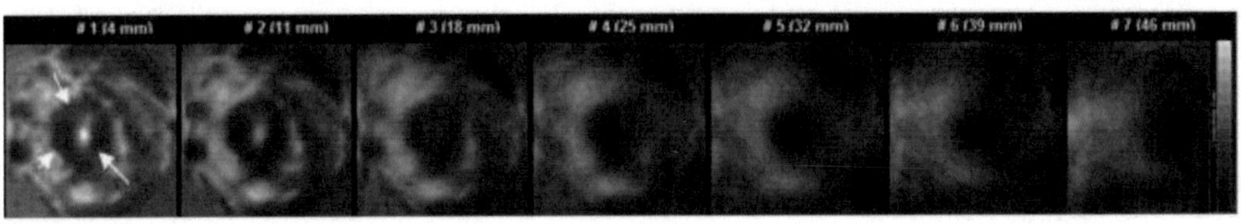

Fig. 11. EIM. Seven scan planes. A hyperimpedance area in the centre of the mammogram corresponds to the location of the areola (indicated with arrows).

6.3 Volumetric lesion

Volumetric lesion - a dimensional lesion, detected in several scan planes. The analysis of images includes assessment of the shape, contour, internal electrical structure and changes of the surrounding tissues.

6.3.1 Assessment of volumetric lesion shape in accordance with the terms of BI-RADS ACR

a. Round - a lesion of a spherical, circular or spherical shape (Fig. 12). The size is determined by lesion's diameter. Typical example - a cyst.

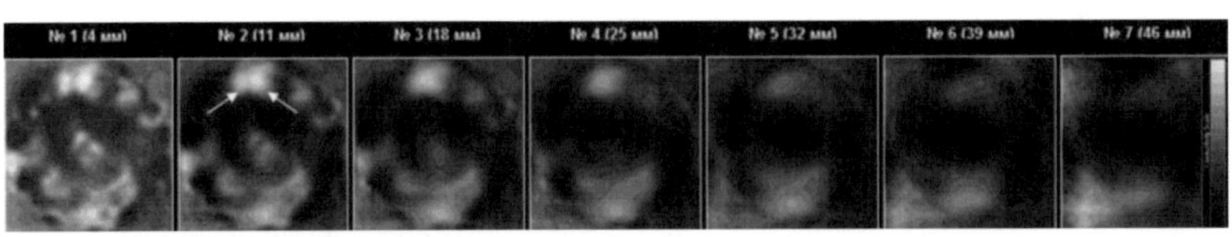

Fig. 12. EIM. Seven scan planes. In the upper segment there can be visualized two lesions of rounded shape (indicated with arrows).

b. Oval – an ellipsoid or obovoid lesion (Fig. 13). The size is determined by longitudinal and lateral axes. Typical example – fibroadenoma, cancer.

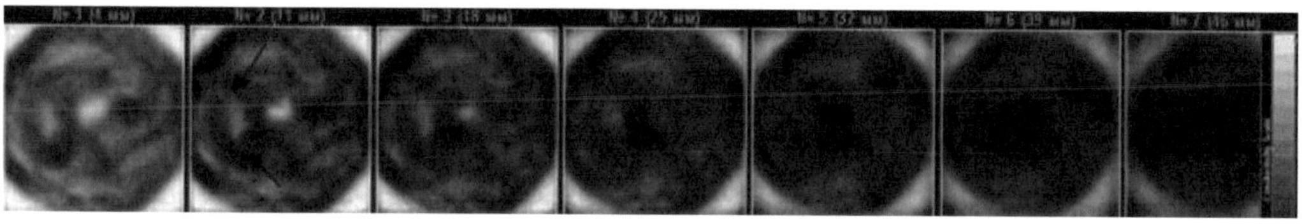

Fig. 13. EIM. Seven scan planes. The obovoid lesion is visualized at 9 on the clock dial (indicated with arrows).

c. Lobular – a lesion with the undulated contour (Fig. 14). The size is determined by longitudinal and lateral axes. Typical example – fibroadenoma.

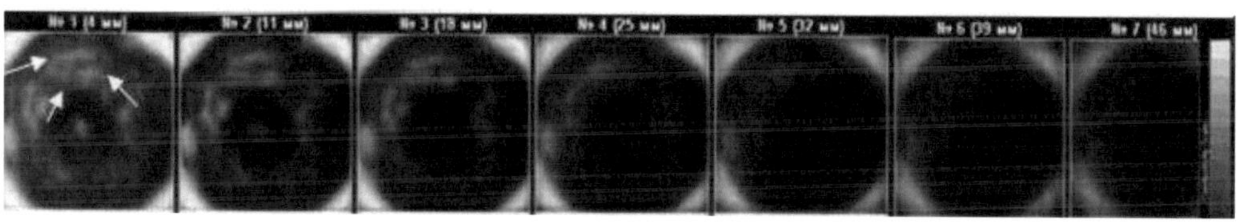

Fig. 14. EIM. Seven scan planes. In the upper segment at 12 on the clock dial, there can be observed two round hypoimpedance lesions.

d. Irregular - the shape of a lesion cannot be characterized and does not correspond to round, oval or lobular (Fig. 15). Typical example – breast cancer.

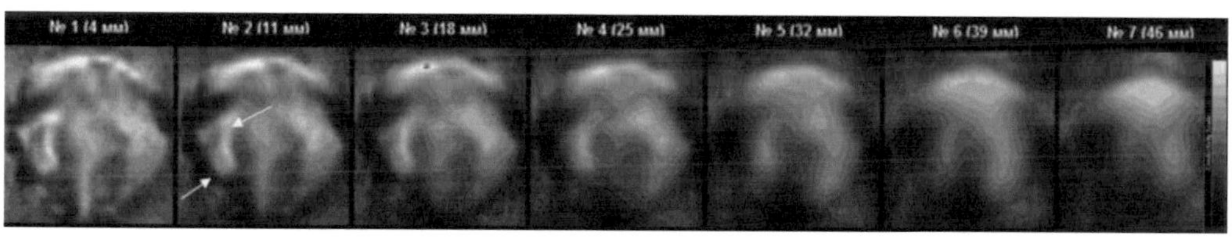

Fig. 15. EIM. Seven scan planes. In the upper segment there can be visualized a lesion with a lobed contour (indicated with arrows).

6.3.2 Assessment of volumetric lesion contours in accordance with the terms of BI-RADS ACR

a. Sharp (well defined or distinct) – the contours of a lesion are clearly observable. Abrupt junction of the lesion and surrounding tissues (Fig. 16).

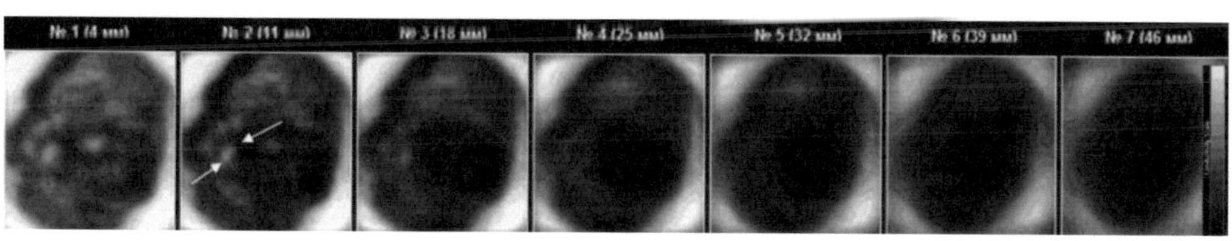

Fig. 16. EIM. Seven scan planes. The lesion with a sharp distinct contour is visualized at 9 on the clock dial (indicated with arrows).

b. Vague, indistinct (poorly observable) – the contours of a lesion are uneasy to define. The transition between the lesion and surrounding tissues is gradual and indistinct (Fig. 17). Typical example of an invasive ductal carcinoma.

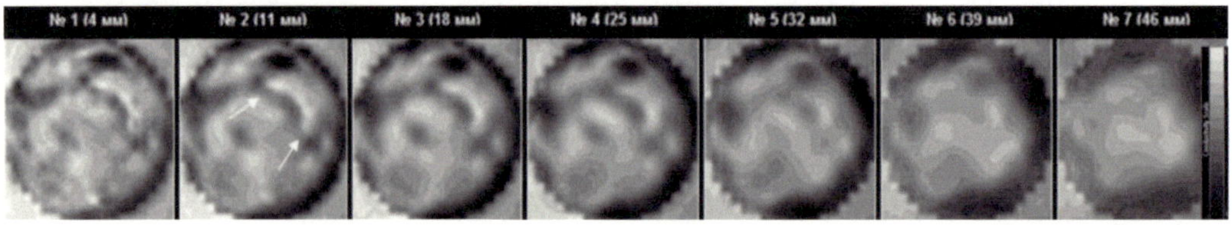

Fig. 17. EIM. Seven scan planes. The irregular-shaped lesion with indistinct contours is visualized at 12-3 on the clock dial (indicated with arrows).

c. Infiltrated - the contours of a lesion are clearly distinguishable and are characterized by hyperimpedance (Fig. 18). Typical example – breast cancer.

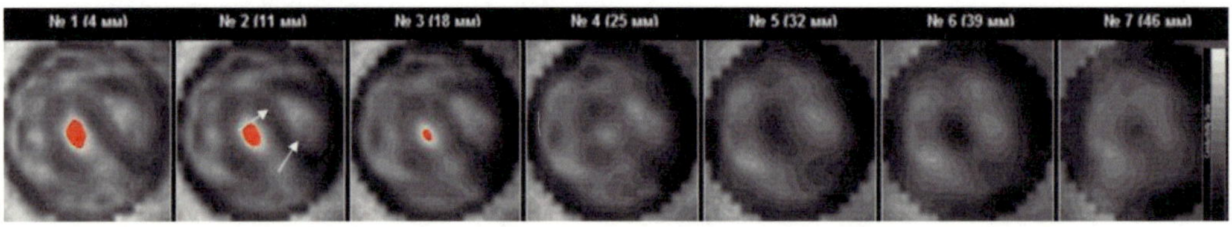

Fig. 18. EIM. Seven scan planes. The obovoid lesion with hyperimpedance contours is visualized at 3 on the clock dial (indicated with arrows).

6.3.3 Assessment of the internal electrical structure of a volumetric lesion

Taken separately, the internal electrical structure of the lesion is not the criterion for judging on its possible malignancy. However, it is an important characteristic, especially in combination with other evaluation criteria. The increase of electrical conductivity is correlated with an increase of the probability of malignancy.

a. Hyperimpedance - electrical conductivity of the lesion is lower than electrical conductivity than that of the surrounding tissue of the breast (Fig. 19). Typical example – mastitis in the stage of infiltration.

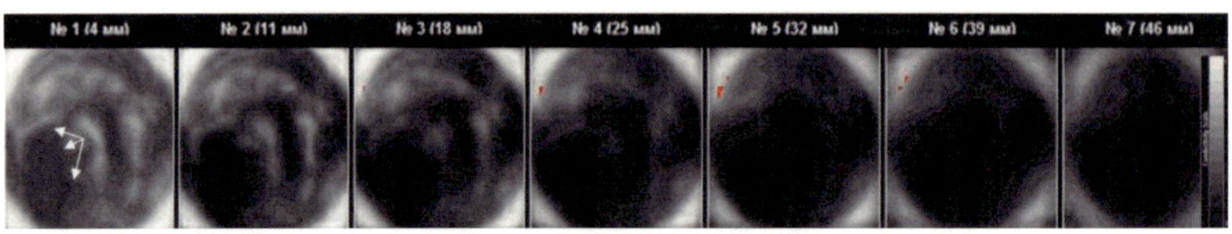

Fig. 19. EIM. Seven scan planes. The obovoid lesion with hyperimpedance structure is visualized at 8 on the clock dial (indicated with arrows).

b. Isoimpedance - electrical conductivity of the lesion corresponds to that of the surrounding tissue of the breast (Fig. 20). Typical examples – fibroadenoma, cancer.

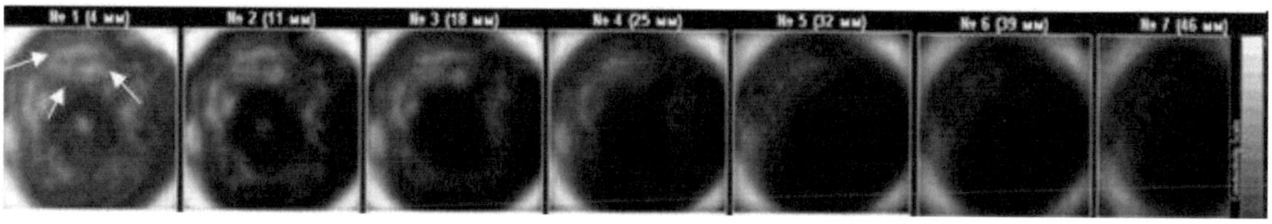

Fig. 20. EIM. Seven scan planes. The lesion with isoimpedance structure is visualized at 12 on the clock dial (indicated with arrows).

c. Hypoimpedance - electrical conductivity of the lesion is higher than that of the surrounding tissue of the breast (Fig. 21). Typical example - a cyst.

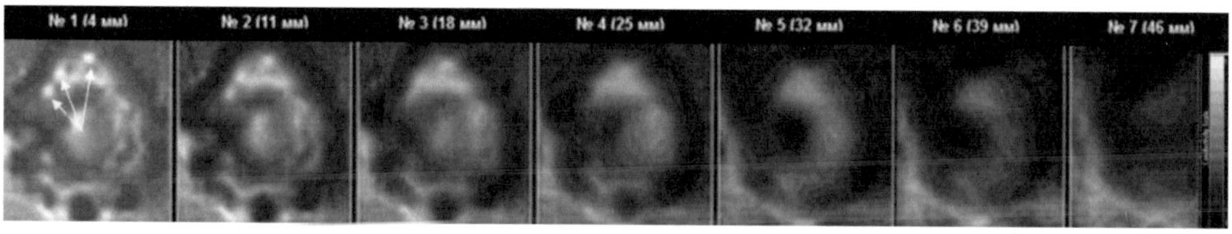

Fig. 21. EIM. Seven scan planes. In the upper segment there can be visualized three hypoimpedance lesions of rounded shape (indicated with arrows).

d. Animpedance - electrical conductivity of the lesion is considerably higher than that of the surrounding tissue of the breast (Fig. 22). Typical example - breast cancer.

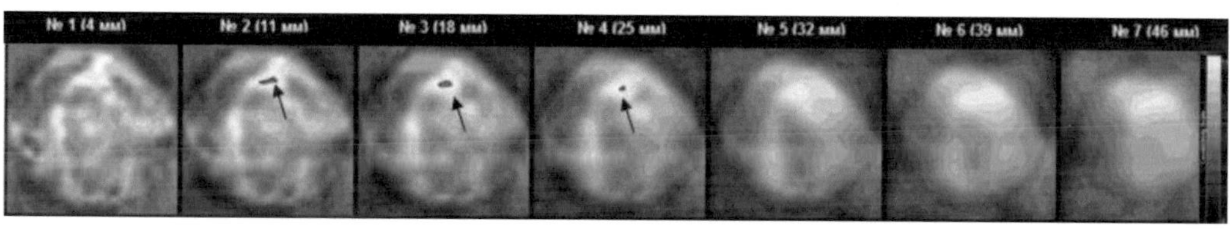

Fig. 22. EIM. Seven scan planes. In the upper segment, at 12 on the clock dial there is an irregular-shaped lesion with animpedance structure (highlighted in red and indicated with arrows).

6.4 Assessment of volumetric lesion influence on the surrounding tissue in accordance with the terms of BI-RADS ACR

a. Skin thickening - a significant one-sided hyperimpedance change of the contour around the mammary gland (Fig. 23). Typical example - mastitis-like carcinoma.

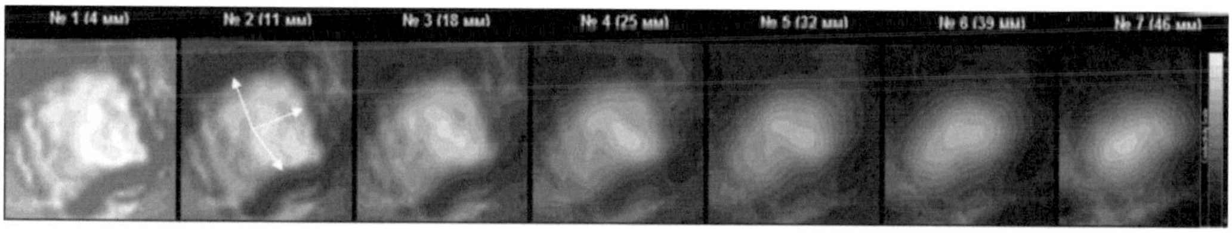

Fig. 23. EIM. Seven scan planes. A pronounced hyperimpedance change of the contour around the mammary gland (indicated with arrows).

b. Skin extrusion or retraction - a local change of mammary gland contour: In case of the retraction - into the mamma, in case of extrusion - entoectad (Fig. 24, 25). Typical example - breast cancer, mastitis.

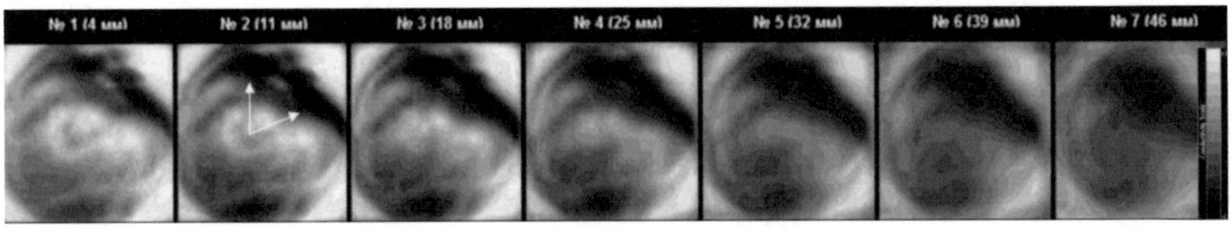

Fig. 24. EIM. Seven scan planes. In the upper segment, a change of the contour (retraction) of the mammary gland (indicated with arrows)

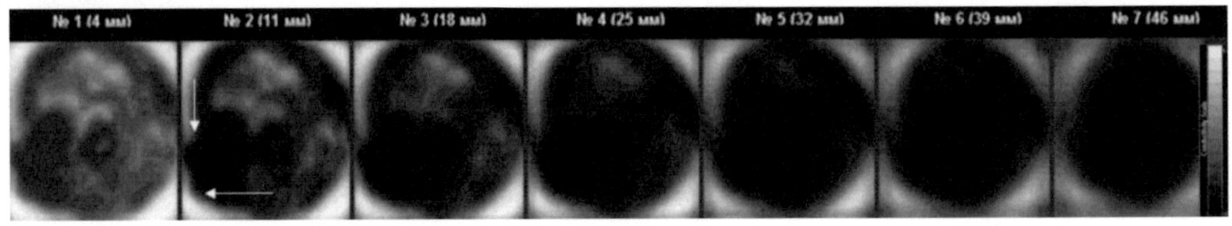

Fig. 25. EIM. Seven scan planes. At 7 on the clock dial, a change of the contour (extrusion) of the mammary gland (indicated with arrows).

c. Skin or nipple infiltration - a local hyperimpedance change of the contour of a mammary gland or of a nipple (Fig. 26, 27). Typical example - breast cancer, Paget's cancer.

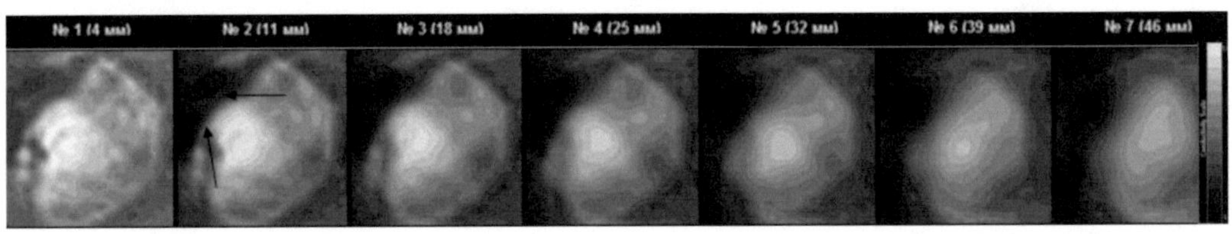

Fig. 26 EIM. Seven scan planes. A unilateral local hyperimpedance change of the mammary gland contour (indicated with arrows).

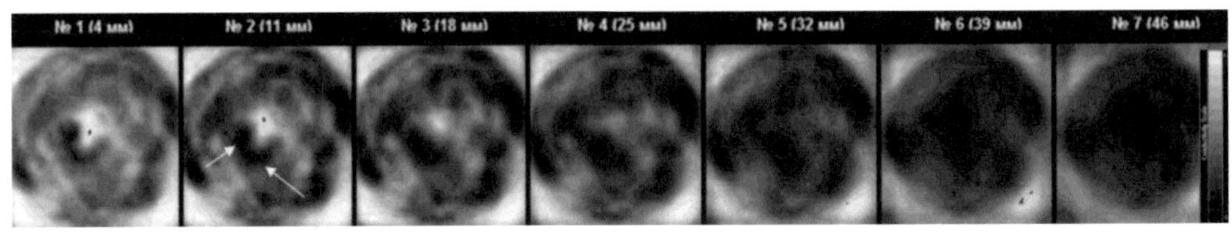

Fig. 27. EIM. Seven scan planes. A unilateral hyperimpedance change of the nipple contour (indicated with arrows).

d. Alterations of the breast anatomy - focal disruption of the normal mammographic scheme. Alteration of the age-related electrical impedance structure (Fig. 28, 29). Typical example - mastitis, breast cancer.

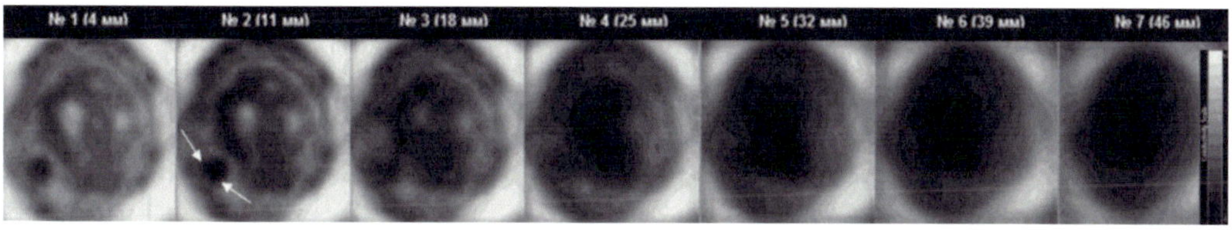

Fig. 28. EIM. Seven scan planes. Alteration of the normal mammographic scheme represented by a hyperimpedance lesion at 7 on the clock dial (indicated with arrows).

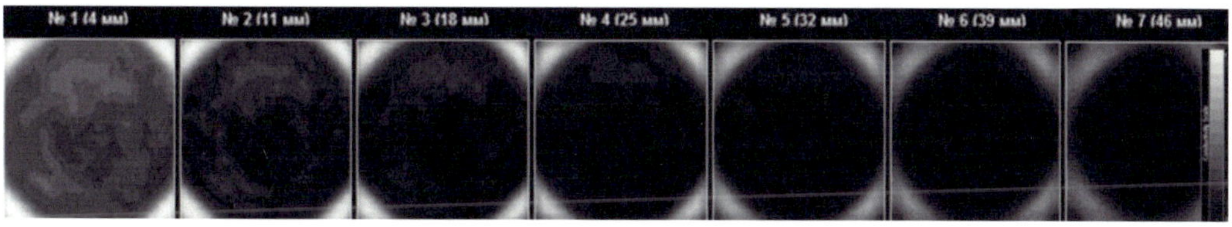

Fig. 29. EIM. Seven scan planes. Total alteration of the age-related electrical impedance structure.

6.5 Lactiferous sinus zone assessment

The visualization of lactiferous sinus zone depends on the age and physiological period of a patient. In women of elder age during the postmenopause the lactiferous sinus zone is hardly visualized. An extensive round hypo- or animpedance area in the centre of the mammogram is typical for the lactation period (Fig. 30). When pathology, there can be observed deformation and fragmentation of the lactiferous sinus zone (Fig. 31).

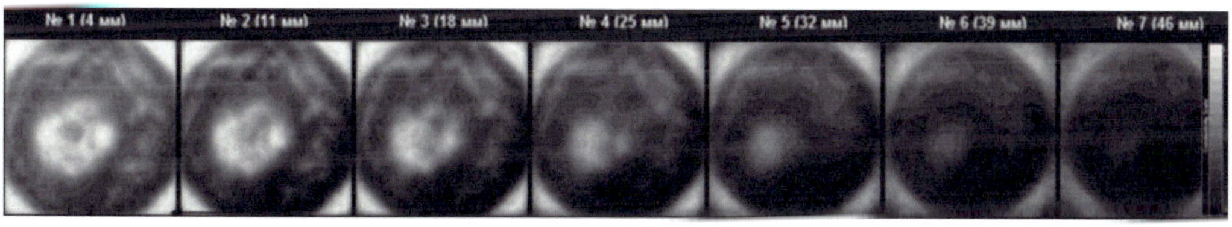

Fig. 30. EIM. Seven scan planes. There is a vast undistorted hypoimpedance area in the centre of the mammogram, which corresponds to the location of the lactiferous sinus zone.

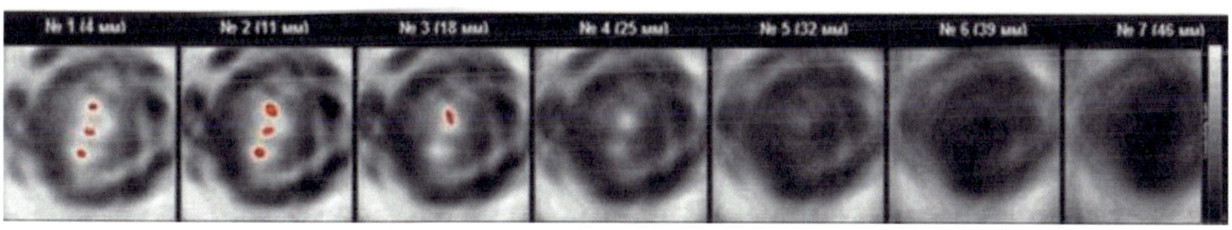

Fig. 31. EIM. Seven scan planes. There is a divided hypoimpedance area in the centre of the mammogram, which corresponds to the location of the lactiferous sinus zone. It is highlighted in red.

6.6 Age-related and comparative electrical conductivity

6.6.1 Age-related conductivity

Age-related conductivity is the alteration of electrical conductivity of the breast with respect to age-related percentile curve of electrical conductivity (Fig. 32). The so-called percentile method as an approach to brief description of distributions is wide-spread in medical and biological research. This method does not require the data on distribution structure, i.e. it is non-parametric. The assessment of the average electrical conductivity in healthy women of different ages allowed creating the percentile curves of age-related electrical conductivity.

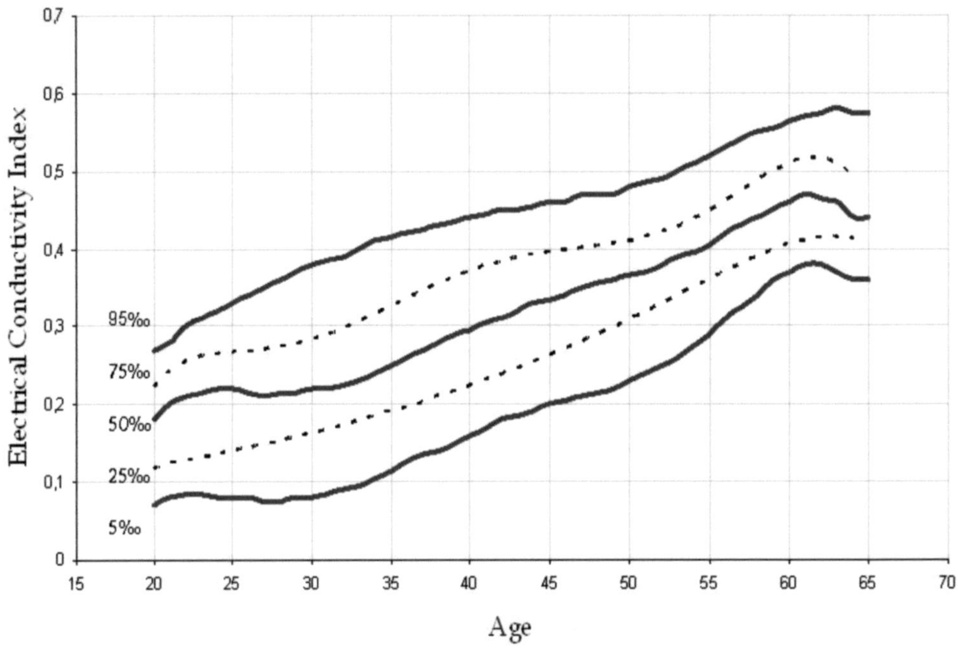

Fig. 32. Percentile curves of age-related electrical conductivity.

According to these curves each age group corresponds to a certain range of electrical conductivity. In accordance with the proposed assessment rules, the values which are less than 5th percentile shall be considered as pronouncedly low, from 5 to 25 percentiles - as low, from 25 to 75 percentiles - as medium, from 75 to 95 percentiles - as heightened and above 95 percentile – as pronouncedly heightened (Fig. 32). Formation of groups of people with heightened risk of breast cancer development can be performed using the percentile curves of the age-related electrical conductivity.

6.6.2 Comparative conductivity

Comparative conductivity is the alteration of electrical conductivity of one breast with respect to the other (Fig. 33). The histograms of the electrical conductivity distribution variance percent is chosen with the help of the Kolmogorov-Smirnov nonparametric test (more than 40%) and is highly informative (j>3.0 according to Kullback). Typical example – breast cancer, mastitis.

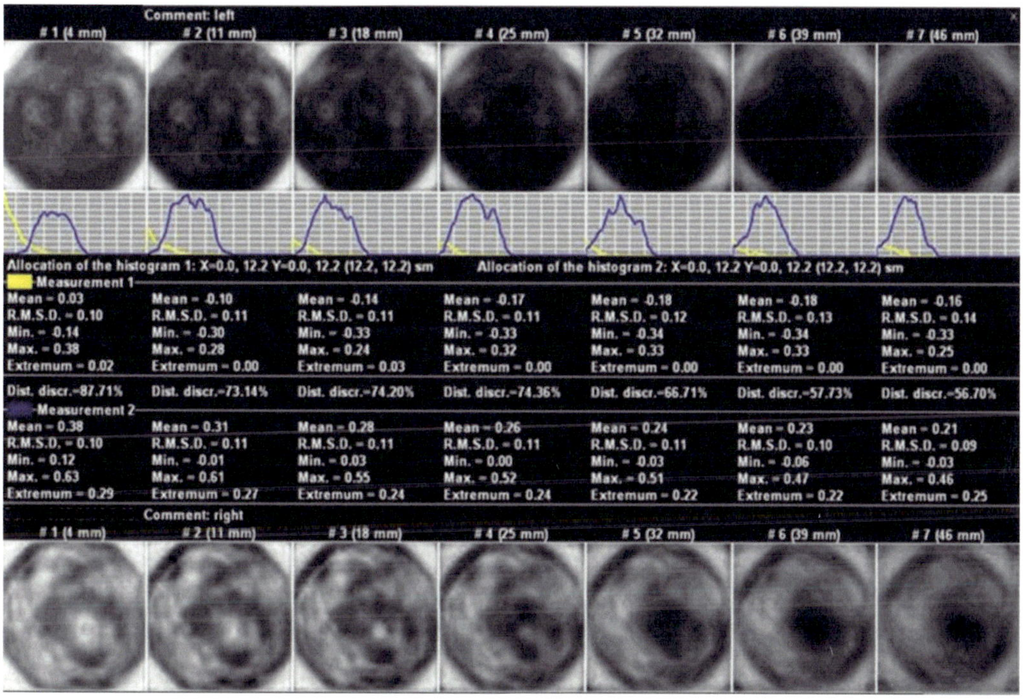

Fig. 33. Upper row - EIM. Seven scan planes. Breast cancer. Bottom row - EIM. Seven scan planes. Healthy gland. The second row shows the divergence between the histograms of electrical conductivity distribution of the affected and healthy gland.

7. Diagnostic criteria for electrical impedance mammography

In order to sort out the diagnostic criteria the diagnostic chart was created, in which each criterion was measured in points (Table 4).

Using the numerical score for evaluation of volumetric and non-volumetric lesions within the mammary gland in electrical impedance mammography allowed comparing this information to BI-RADS ACR categories (See Table 5).

The above description of the system of images and diagnostic criteria for electrical impedance mammography provides diagnostics of various breast diseases, including neoplastic, inflammatory, dishormonal and other disorders. However, we believe the detection of breast cancer at early stages to be the high-priority of the method. The basic features of electrical impedance mammography in early diagnostics of breast cancer are the following.

8. Early diagnostics of breast cancer

If the method of diagnostics under examination permits to acquire a numerical result, the so-called "breaking point" (the value exceeding of which is considered as a sufficient cause for qualitative assessment) should be determined. In this case the estimation of diagnostic

Diagnostic criteria	Electrical impedance mammography points
Shape	
round, oval	1
lobular, irregular	2
Contour	
sharp	1
hyperimpedance, indistinct	2
Surrounding tissues	
preserved	0
structure alteration/displacement	1
thickening/extrusion/retraction	2
Internal electrical structure	
hyperimpedance (IC <0.2)	0
iso- and hypoimpedance (IC = 0.3-0.8)	1
animpedance (IC > 0.90)	2
Comparative electrical conductivity	
divergence between the histograms < 30%	0
divergence between the histograms 30-40 %	1
divergence between the histograms > 40%	2

Table 4. Diagnostic criteria for differentiating volumetric lesions in electrical impedance mammography.

EIM	ACR
Common scale	*BI-RADS categories*
no score	BI-RADS 0 poor image
0-1	BI-RADS 1 lesion is not defined
2-3	BI-RADS 2 benign tumours - routine mammography
4	BI-RADS 3 probably benign findings
5-7	BI-RADS 4 suspicious abnormality - biopsy
8-10	BI-RADS 5 highly suggestive of malignancy - treatment/biopsy

Table 5. EIM numerical score allows for standardizing the description of volumetric lesions and for the usage of patient monitoring algorithm, developed by the American College of Radiology in electrical impedance mammography.

technique efficiency may be limited to sensitivity and specificity assessment. The diagnostic criterion when screening for early stages of breast cancer is the following: high electrical conductivity areas (above 0.95 cu) outside the lactiferous sinus zone - the so-called animpedance areas, which differ markedly from electrical conductivity of healthy mamma's areas (Fig. 34).

It seems that membrane permeability increase is necessary in both directions to support vital activity of dedifferentiated cells during the intraductal stage of oncologic process. The membrane permeability of cancer cells during intraductal and early extraductal stage increases both for chemical compounds and electric charges. This process results in increase of electrical conductivity.

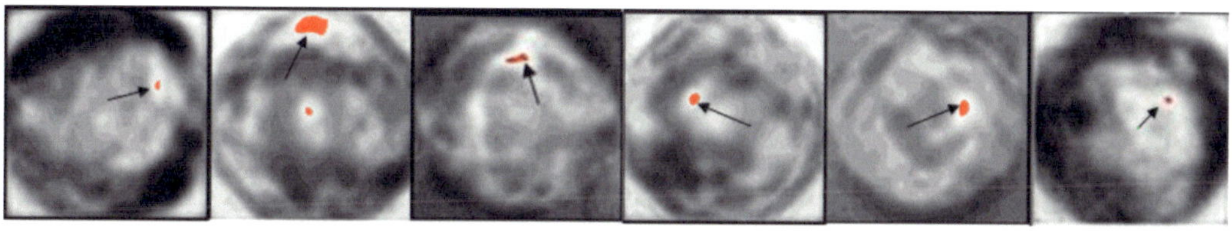

Fig. 34. High electrical conductivity area (above 0.95 cu) outside the lactiferous sinus zone, which is highlighted with red (indicated with arrows).

The example of electrical impedance diagnostic. Figure 35 represents the electrical impedance mammogram of a patient. There can be distinguished a focal lesion, in the form of animpedance area, highlighted with red, with electrical conductivity index over 0.95 conditional units. This is the criterion for early diagnostics of breast cancer. Roentgenogram and US image of the same mammary gland are represented below (Fig. 36).

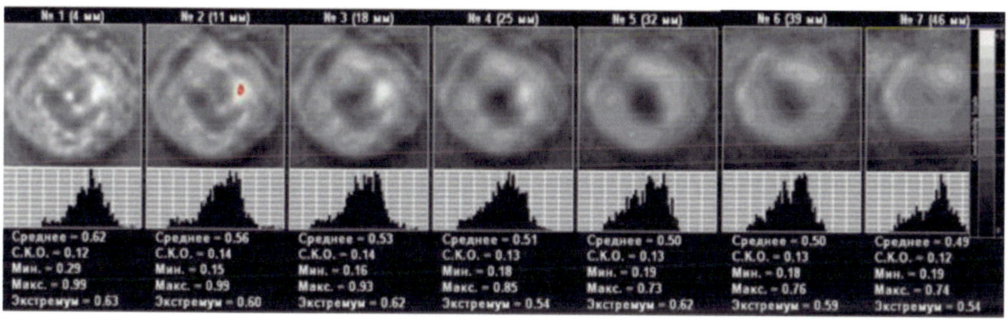

Fig. 35. EIM. Amorphous type of mammary gland structure. In the outer segment of the left mammary gland, at 3 o'clock position there is observed an animpedance area, which is highlighted with red in the second scan plane, less than 10 mm in size.

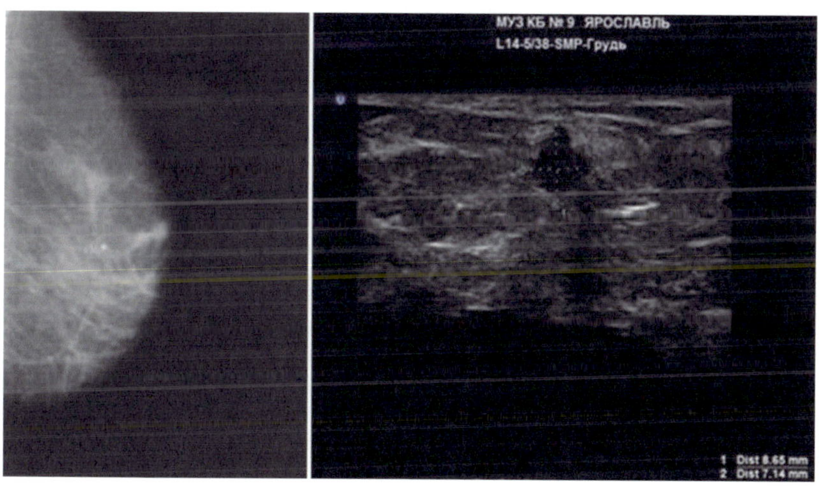

Fig. 36. Roentgenogram (left): fibro-fatty involution. In upper-outer segment there is observed a lesion up to 1 cm in size with a radiant contour. Ultrasound (right): The structure of parenchyma with adipose lobules and connective tissue layers. An inhomogeneous 8x7 mm lesion of irregular shape is located at 28 mm distance from the nipple and at 12 mm depth.

With such a breaking point the sensitivity and specificity of electrical impedance mammography are quite high: sensitivity is 84-93%, specificity - 87-99% (according to the data given by different authors).

Impedance mammography is in the beginning of its development. The authors sincerely hope that their modest paper will help to arouse interest of a wide range of medical researchers.

9. Acknowledgement

The authors would like to express their gratitude to radiologists A. Bulatov and A. Frizyuk, oncologists N. Sotskova and S. Korotkov as well as to all the staff of PKF "SIM-technika" for their help in conducting clinical trials.

10. References

Glants S. Medical and Biological Statistics. McGraw-Hill, 1994

Gubler E. Quantitative methods for analysis and identification of pathology. Leningrad, 1978

Karpov A.; Korotkova M., Mumtazuddin Ahmed M., Myachin M., Tsofin Yu. Seminar on electrical impedance potential mammography. Yaroslavl, 2011, Biomedical Engineering, v24/is4-6, 1996

Cherepenin V.; Karpov A., Korjenevsky A., Kornienko V., Mazaletskaya A., Mazurov D. A 3D electrical impedance tomography (EIT) system for breast cancer detection. *Physiological Measurement.* 2001, 22, 9-18.

Dunaeva O.; Gerasimov D., Karpov A., Machin M., Tchayev A., Tsofin Yu., Tsyplyonkov V. Using Backprojection Algorithm for 3D Image Reconstruction in EIT. *World Congress on Medical Physics and Biomedical Engineering*, Munich, Germany, 2009, Electrical Impedance Tomography. IOP, 2005

Karpov A.; Korjenevsky A., Mazurov D., Mazaletskaya A. 3D Electrical Impedance Scanning of Breast Cancer. *World Congress on Medical Physics and Biomedical Engineering, Chicago*, 2000, p.62

Korotkova M.; Karpov A. Procedure for assessment of the mammary gland electrical impedance images. *XIII international conference on electrical bio-impedance.* Graz, Austria, 2007.

Mumtazuddin Ahmed M. Histology functional and Clinical. HEC Islamabad, 2009

8

The Role of Molecular Imaging Technologies in Breast Cancer Diagnosis and Management

Anne Rosenberg, Douglas Arthur Kieper, Mark B. Williams, Nathalie Johnson and Leora Lanzkowsky
Jefferson University, Hampton University, University of Virginia, Legacy Good Samaritan, Nevada Imaging Center
USA

1. Introduction

Anatomic breast imaging techniques such as mammography and ultrasound are very useful in the detection of breast cancer, but can have limited sensitivity and positive predictive value, particularly in patients with dense breasts (Kolb et al., 2002). These limitations have provided the impetus for adjunctive technologies such as nuclear medicine and PET based diagnostic imaging procedures. The nuclear medicine based technique is referred to as Breast-Specific Gamma Imaging (BSGI) or molecular breast imaging (MBI) while the positron-emission tomography (PET) based technique is referred to as Positron Emission Mammography (PEM). Both have demonstrated good results in clinical studies and are increasingly being adopted into clinical practice. Although these imaging techniques have similarities, they are different in several aspects. This chapter is designed to provide an overview of these imaging technologies and their potential roles in patient management.

2. Radiotracers

Both BSGI/MBI and PEM are physiologic imaging modalities conducted through the injection of a pharmaceutical, called a tracer, which is tagged with a radioactive isotope and the resulting molecule is called a radiotracer. Each radiotracer is designed to bind to a specific target (organ, tissue, physiologic process, cell receptor or protein) while the isotope tag emits radiation that is detected by cameras placed near the patient. The cameras provide an image of the distribution of the radiotracer tracer and thus measure a specific physiologic process in the area being imaged.

2.1 Isotopes

There are two types of radioactive isotope tags used in medical imaging: single gamma emission isotopes and positron emission isotopes. Single gamma emission isotopes release a gamma ray from the nucleus. There are a variety of single gamma isotopes used in nuclear medicine. The most common isotopes used in diagnostic imaging are referred to as low-energy isotopes with gamma-ray energies ranging from 80 – 200 kiloelectron volts (keV). The gamma ray is a photon with sufficient energy to exit the body and be captured by specially designed detectors called gamma cameras. Positron emission isotopes emit a positron, an antimatter particle with the same mass as an electron, but with a positive charge. This positron travels a short distance from the nucleus prior to colliding with an electron. Since the positron is a particle traveling through the tissue until this collision, the patient radiation dose associated with positron emission isotope studies is generally higher than that from single gamma emission isotope examinations. This collision results in annihilation of both particles converting the mass of the two particles into energy and producing a pair of 511 kiloelectron volt (keV) gamma rays traveling approximately 180° from each other. In positron emission tomography imaging (PET) these gamma rays exit the body and are captured by a pair of opposed gamma cameras.

The units for measuring the activity of radiotracer delivered to the patient are the Becquerel and the Curie. The Becquerel (symbol Bq) is the SI-derived unit of radioactivity. One Bq is defined as: one decay (emission) per second. The curie (symbol Ci) is a unit of radioactivity, defined as 3.7×10^{10} decays per second. In breast imaging, the megabecquerel (MBq) and millicurie (mCi) are the most common units used; one millicurie equals 37 Megabecquerel. These units only describe the number of decays per second for a given sample and are not to be confused with the units used to describe the radiation dose they deliver to a patient. A more detailed discussion of radiation dose is provided in Section 4.

2.1.1 Pharmaceuticals for BSGI/MBI

BSGI/MBI is a single photon imaging technique that has been conducted using a variety of imaging agents, but the most common is ^{99m}Tc-hexakis-2-methoxyisobutylisonitrile also referred to as ^{99m}Tc-Sestamibi or MIBI. MIBI is a 140 KeV gamma ray emitting isotope in a lipophilic cation molecule. It was originally cleared by the US FDA for use as a cardiac perfusion agent; breast imaging was subsequently added subsequently breast imaging was added as an indication following additional clinical studies to determine its efficacy in this application. It is injected intravenously and is retained in cells likely by electronegative cellular and mitochondrial membrane potentials (Piwnica-Worms et al., 1990). Studies show that its accumulation is roughly proportional to blood flow, desmoplastic activity and cellular proliferation and therefore it accumulates preferentially in breast cancers compared with surrounding tissues (Cutrone et al., 1998). It is a lipophilic substrate for the P-glycoprotein (Pgp), a cellular efflux pump for various compounds (Ballinger et al., 1995). Therefore, Sestamibi exhibits rapid tumor wash-in (within about 2 minutes) followed by a slow tumor washout (over the course of several hours) (Sciuto et al., 2002). Based on these factors, imaging can begin within minutes after injection and can continue for up to about 90 minutes post injection, providing ample time for all required views to be conducted before the washout cycle negatively impacts lesion-to-background tracer concentration ratio. In addition, since the level of Pgp expression correlates with tumor response to cytotoxic chemotherapy, a comparison of immediate and delayed images (4 hours post injection) may be used to quantify the radiotracer washout as a measure of Pgp expression and the probability of multi-drug resistance.

There are no known contraindications for use. Reactions to Sestamibi are generally minor according to the Cardiolite drug data sheet. In the analysis of potential reactions, 3068 patients (77% men, 22% women, and 0.7% not recorded) were documented from the cardiac clinical trials and 673 were recorded from the breast imaging trials. Of the 673 breast imaging patients, all of whom were women, the most common reported reaction was taste perversion with most of those patients reporting a metallic taste at the time of injection. The other minor reactions are listed in table 1. More serious reactions were reported in less than 0.5% of patients and included: signs and symptoms consistent with seizure occurring shortly after administration of the agent; transient arthritis, angioedema, arrythmia, dizziness, syncope, abdominal pain, vomiting, and severe hypersensitivity characterized by dyspnea, hypotension, bradycardia, asthenia, and vomiting within two hours after a second injection of Technetium Tc99m Sestamibi. However the list of serious reactions is from the total population of patients including men and women undergoing a cardiac stress test.

Body System	**N = 673**
Body as a whole	21 (3.1%)
Headache	11 (1.6%)
Cardiovascular	9 (1.3%)
Angina	0 (0%)
ST segment changes	0 (0%)
Digestive System	8 (1.2)
Nausea	4 (0.6%)
Special Senses	132 (19.6%)
Taste Perversion	129 (19.2%)
Parosmia	8 (1.2%)

Table 1. Reactions to Sestamibi from 673 breast imaging patients.

2.1.2 Pharmaceuticals for PEM

PEM is a positron emission imaging technique conducted with 2-[fluorine-18] fluoro-2-deoxy-D-glucose (FDG), a modified glucose molecule with a positron-emitting isotope. Breast cancers exhibit a greater uptake of FDG than the surrounding breast tissue due to their hyperglycolytic rate. For some malignant lesions, although they possess an elevated GLUT-1 transmembrane transport function, however this does not necessarily result in increased tracer uptake (Smith, 1999). Studies have established that the uptake of FDG is primarily dependent on blood flow, the type of breast malignancy and the microstructure of the lesion (nodular vs. diffuse) (Avril et al., 2001). For example, lobular carcinoma exhibits a roughly 30% lower uptake than ductal carcinoma (Avril et al., 2001). For the PEM procedure, patients must fast 4 – 6 hours prior to the injection of FDG. It is important to note that patients with compromised glucose metabolism should have their glucose level checked prior to the administration of FDG and at least one study reports that altered glucose metabolism can affect the sensitivity of this procedure (Berg et al., 2006). FDG is administered intravenously and imaging is conducted approximately 60-90 minutes post injection in order to allow sufficient time for glucose uptake into the tissue. Patients should be requested to sit quietly in a dark, calm room to avoid manipulating the distribution of FDG. A dual-phase imaging technique may be used to improve specificity of the study (imaging at both 60 and 90 minutes post injection).

The emitted positron has a mean free path of approximately 1 mm in the breast tissue before annihilation with an electron resulting in the emission of two 511 KeV gamma rays. The random nature of the displacement between the positron and gamma ray points of origin has some impact on the lower limit of spatial resolution in studies using positron-emitting isotopes (Turkington, 2001).

2.2 Comparison of BSGI/MBI and PEM Radiotracers

Both Sestamibi and FDG demonstrate increased accumulation in breast cancers, although the mechanism for this accumulation is better understood for FDG. In addition, although the breast tissue typically has a homogeneous uptake of both tracers, they can accumulate in normal glandular tissue resulting in a diffuse heterogeneous uptake pattern, especially in pre-menopausal women who are in the luteal phase of their menstrual cycle (Lin et al., 2007). This is not surprising as it reflects the heterogeneous nature of the breast tissue and the impact of blood hormone levels on the breast parenchyma. This heterogeneity does not generally impact cancer detection, but may complicate interpretation. The intensity of this pattern can be reduced for both tracers by imaging outside of the luteal phase and several studies report that day 2 - 14 of the menstrual cycle is optimal. Neither tracer is linked to nephrogenic systemic fibrosis, a sometimes fatal condition that is associated with gadolinium contrast agents used in breast MRI. MIBI has some minor pharmacologic considerations and rare reactions occurring in less than 0.5%of patients. FDG imaging requires fasting for a minimum of 4 hours prior to injection and as mentioned in the previous section, it is beneficial to check the blood glucose level prior to FDG administration as the tumor uptake of FDG is reduced in hyperglycemic states (Schelbert et al., 1999) and this results in some potential for complications and reduced sensitivity for the procedure in diabetic patients. In comparison, MIBI does not require fasting and imaging can be conducted within minutes of the injection.

Some of the physical and clinical differences between FDG and MIBI imaging are summarized in Tables 2 and 3 respectively.

	Energy of Emission photon	Half Life (minutes)
FDG	511 KeV	110
MIBI	140 KeV	360

Table 2. gamma-ray emission information for radiotracers.

	Pre-study Fasting	Injection to Imaging time	Recommended Pre-procedural testing
FDG	4 - 6 hours	60 – 90 minutes	Blood glucose
MIBI	None	5 minutes	None

Table 3. Radiotracer administration and imaging considerations.

3. Imaging systems

Both the single gamma and positron isotopes described in section 2.1 ultimately emit gamma rays (the positron isotopes through the annihilation and the conversion of the positron) that exit the patient's body and can be detected with external detectors. The goal of these detector systems is to reconstruct the gamma ray emissions into an image that allows the physician to visualize the distribution of the radiotracer in the body. There are two modes of image reconstruction, plannar and tomographic. The planar method results in a single 2-dimensional image per acquisition, similar to the mammogram. Tomographic reconstruction provides a 3-dimensional reconstruction of the breast similar to MRI. The single gamma detector systems used for BSGI/MBI can be planar or tomographic and can be constructed of a single or multiple detectors. The positron imaging systems used for PEM by their design provide tomographic imaging only and since the detection of the pair of gamma rays is required for image reconstruction, positron systems must consist of either a pair of opposed detectors or a ring detector design.

3.1 Gamma-ray imaging basics

The detection of an abnormality in BSGI and PEM imaging is based on the ability of the imaging system to depict the variations of uptake in the tissue. Unlike anatomical imaging where high spatial resolution is needed to visualize the detailed morphology used to provide differential diagnosis, the molecular imaging system must provide sufficient image contrast in order to visualize the variations in radiotracer uptake; the contrast between radiotracer concentration in the tumor and the uptake of the surrounding breast tissue. While this is partially a function of resolution, there are several other factors impacting imaging. This contrast based imaging requires a careful balance between spatial resolution, image noise and photon sensitivity. Generally, as spatial resolution increases, image noise increases and photon sensitivity decreases proportionally to some degree thus if spatial resolution is increased to a level where the detector has poor photon sensitivity and the resulting image noise is too high, the ability of the system to visualize the contrasting tissue uptake is diminished. A detailed discussion of the balance between these factors is beyond the scope of this text, but it is important to realize that in molecular imaging is a contrast based imaging and spatial resolution is not the only parameter affecting the visualization of lesions. For example, it is possible to detect a 1 mm cancer using a system with a 4 mm spatial resolution if the uptake of that lesion is sufficiently enough higher than the background to overcome the partial volume effect. Conversely, a 40 mm cancer could be missed by the same imaging system if the lesion uptake is not sufficiently higher than the surrounding tissue.

As an illustration, nearly all commercially available large field-of-view gamma cameras, typical to the nuclear medicine department, have a variable matrix setting, including 512 x 512, 256 x 256 and 128 x 128. Although the 512 x 512 setting produces the highest spatial resolution, nearly all nuclear medicine studies are conducted on the 256 x 256 or 128 x 128 settings because the resulting image noise at the 512 x 512 setting diminishes image quality for the majority of studies.

System photon sensitivity is another important parameter in BSGI/MBI and PEM imaging. As photon sensitivity increases, the amount of radiotracer, the length of time the image is acquired, or some combination of both parameters can be decreased. For Example: a given detector system is providing good clinical images using a dose of 300 MBq and an acquisition time of 10 minutes. If the photon sensitivity of this system can be increased 50% the clinician would have three possible options. First, they could reduce the patient's radiation exposure by reducing the amount of radiotracer delivered to the patient by 50%, to

150 MBq and maintain the same imaging time, 10 minutes. Second, they could reduce the imaging time by 50% to 5 minutes using a 300 MBq dose. Or third, they could reduce both the time and the dose by roughly 25% resulting in a dose of 225 MBq and an imaging time of 7.5 minutes. It is important to remember that in molecular imaging techniques such as BSGI/MBI and PEM, the imaging time and the dose delivered can be manipulated, but reducing both to any large degree is not possible unless significant improvements in photon sensitivity are obtained.

3.1.1 BSGI/MBI Imaging

BSGI/MBI imaging is conducted with a single-head or dual-head detector system (see Figure 1). Only one detector equipped with a collimator is required for image reconstruction. Generally, gentle breast compression (normally less than 12 lbs or 53 newtons) is used to provide breast immobilization. This compression is noticeably lower than that used in mammography for two reasons. First, the typical imaging time for a single BSGI/MBI image is significantly longer than that needed for a mammographic projection, 5 - 10 minutes, thus lower pressures are better tolerated by patients and second, the 140keV gamma ray emitted in BSGI/MBI has sufficiently higher tissue penetration than the 8 - 35 keV x-ray used in mammography therefore these images benefit less from higher compression. As shown in figure 1, in the single-head design a paddle is used to provide compression and in the dual-head system, the breast is compressed between the detectors. The compression paddle used in the single head system can be exchanged for a fenestrated paddle to allow biopsy. Biopsy is currently not available on the dual-head design.

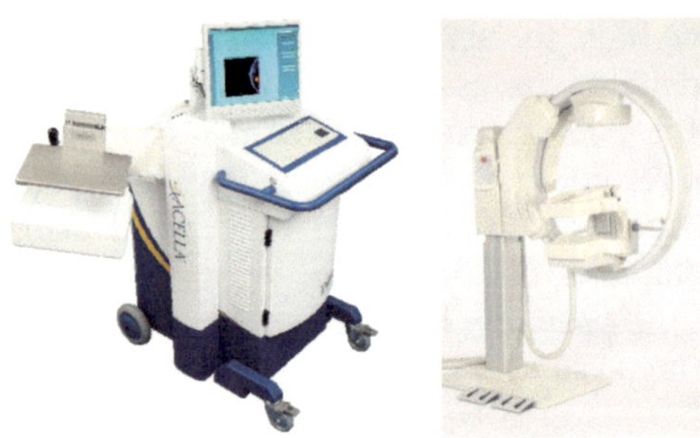

Fig. 1. A single and dual head imaging system for BSGI/MBI.

3.1.2 BSGI/MBI detectors

As mentioned in the previous section, there is generally an inverse relationship between photon sensitivity and spatial resolution however both are important to imaging. These parameters are determined by several aspects of the detector design, especially that of the collimator. The most commercially available systems have an extrinsic spatial resolution of between 1.9 and 3.3 mm at the surface of the detector however it is important to note that the spatial resolution of planar, single gamma imaging systems decreases with increasing source-to-collimator distance, thus the spatial resolution of a lesion near the detector is better than that of one deep in the breast tissue, relative to the detector face. For example, if the breast is being imaged in the cranio-caudal position (detector inferior to the breast tissue), lesions in the inferior portion of the breast tissue will be somewhat more visible than those in the superior portion of the breast. This resolution loss is, at least in part, the driving logic behind the dual-head opposed detector design. In theory, if the breast is imaged using a dual-head system in the cranio-caudal position, the upper detector would maximize visualization of the superior portion of the breast while the lower detector optimizes visualization of inferior lesions.

Although there is a theoretical benefit to the dual-head design, it is interesting to note that clinical data from the dual-head and single-head systems shows similar performance in terms of lesion sensitivity (see section 5 below). This is likely due to the two-view imaging protocol adopted from mammography that is standard in BSGI/MBI protocols. Just as in mammography, the optimal coverage of breast tissue is obtained by acquiring an MLO and CC image of each breast and additional images are obtained as needed. Since all patients have a minimum of two views obtained, the likelihood of a lesion being deep to both projections is quite small. In addition, similar to mammography, when a lesion is seen in only one image, additional images are obtained in order to determine the location of the lesion in the breast tissue. As long as this two-view protocol remains the standard, it is unlikely that the dual-head system will result in significant improvements in the sensitivity of the detection of breast malignancies. However, provided the two detector images are fused properly, it may be possible to reduce either the injected dose or the acquisition time to facilitate low-dose imaging or higher throughput on the imaging system.

Single photon emission computed tomography (SPECT) is a recent development in BSGI/MBI. Currently these devices are only available in the research setting (Williams et al., 2010). Additional research is needed to determine if dual-head image combination techniques or the implementation of SPECT imaging will provide a clear benefit to BSGI/MBI in terms of breast cancer detection. Such studies are underway, but the data is not yet available for analysis.

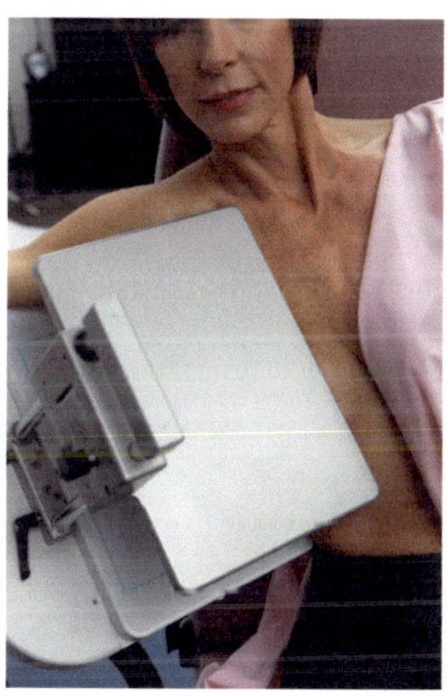

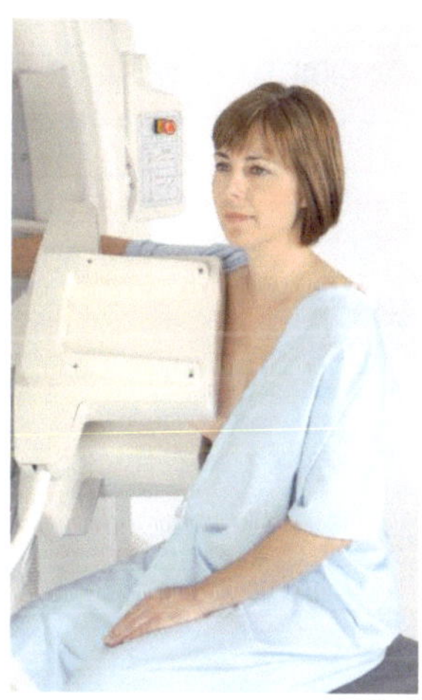

Fig. 2. Left and Center - a single-head BSGI/MBI system with a compression paddle used for positioning. The left image illustrates the cranio-caudal (CC) position and the center image illustrates the medial lateral oblique position (MLO). The right image illustrates the MLO position with the dual-head system where the compression paddle is replaced by a second detector.

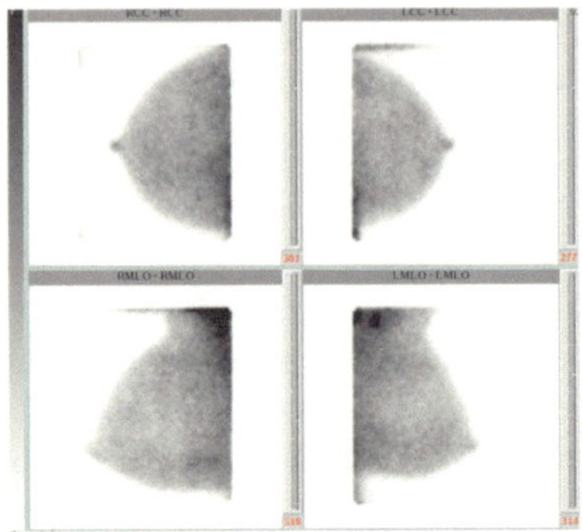

Fig. 3. A typical 4-view BSGI study.

3.1.3 Detectors for PEM

PEM imaging is conducted with either a dual head or ring style gamma-ray detector. Both systems are designed to detect the coincident gamma rays which, are traveling approximately 180° from each other after the annihilation reaction (see figure 4). Unlike BSGI imaging devices, PEM devices do not use a collimator to help determine the location of each event. In PEM imaging, since there are two gamma-rays traveling 180° apart, the event location is calculated as a line of response between the location that each gamma-ray strikes the pair of opposed detectors. One advantage to PEM is that it does not have the same loss of resolution with distance that BSGI/MBI systems experience. As mentioned in the previous section, the mean free path of the ^{18}F positron within the breast tissue is approximately 1 mm and commercially available PEM systems report an in-plane spatial resolution of about 2 mm. One limitation of the dual-head PEM detector design is that, due to the limited angle of acquisition, it has limited resolution in the Z-axis (depth). Ring detectors do not suffer from this limitation as they provide a 360° acquisition for reconstruction however there is currently no biopsy capability on the ring detector systems. A needle biopsy localization device was recently introduced for the opposed dual-head detector system.

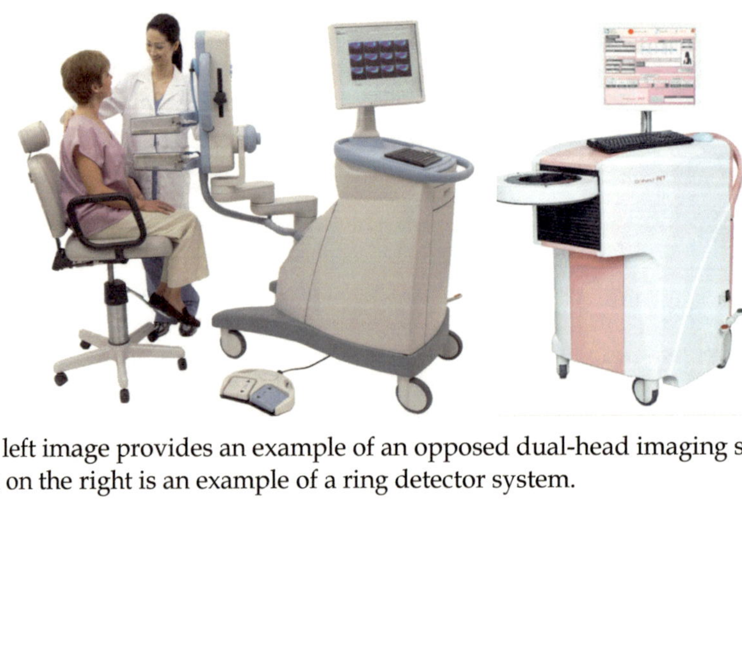

Fig. 4. The left image provides an example of an opposed dual-head imaging system while the system on the right is an example of a ring detector system.

One limitation to PEM image reconstruction is that the detector photon sensitivity is not linear across the field-of-view with lower sensitivity along the detector edges. This causes a higher level of noise to be present in the breast images, along the chest wall. Figure 5 provides a schematic representation of factors affecting the photon sensitivity in a PEM detector. The maximum angle of reconstruction (MAR) is a setting used in PEM software and it is defined as the maximum angle away from the detector normals (90° from the detector face) for which coincident gamma ray detections are included in tomographic image reconstruction. Larger MAR values yield greater overall photon sensitivity but with potential loss in spatial resolution due to the depth-of-interaction (DOI) blur. The blue lines in Figure 1 show the angular range over which gamma rays emitted from two points in the breast are accepted. Figure 1A shows a point near the nipple, and Figure 1B shows one near the chest. For events that occur in the center of the field-of-view (FOV), all of the events within the MAR are captured by the detector system. However a significant fraction of events occurring near the FOV edges go uncounted for because one of the paired gamma rays traveling outside the edges of the detector is not detected. As a recent study found, this loss of photon sensitivity along the edges limits the ability of the PEM system to detect lesions located near the chest wall (Rosen et al, 2005).

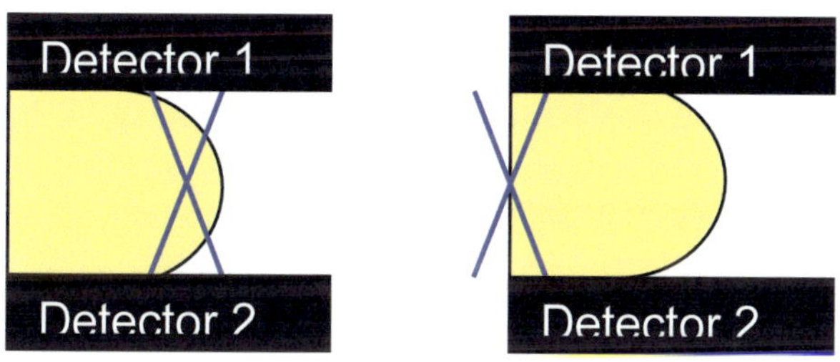

Fig. 5. A and B: a schematic example of the maximum angle of reconstruction near the center of the detector field-of-view and then near the chest wall respectively.

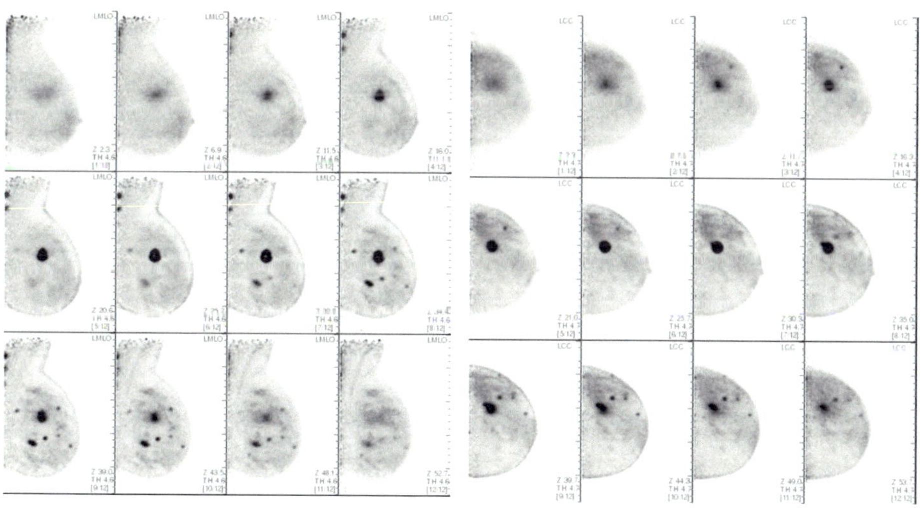

Fig. 6. a typical PEM study with multiple slice reconstruction for each projection.

PEM detectors are tomographic imaging devices, an example image from the opposed detector system is provided in Figure 6. Note the noise level along the chest wall and the Z-resolution affect is expressed as a blurry, low intensity focus in the reconstruction planes outside of the plane the lesion is located in. In this particular case, it is most noticeable in the MLO projection images. There is noticeable residual blur in the area of the largest lesion in all of the projections, including those outside of the lesion.

4. Radiation dose

As with all nuclear medicine procedures, the detector systems do not emit radiation. The radiation dose delivered to the patient in these procedures comes from the radiotracer and is dependent on both the activity of the radiotracer injected and the biologic distribution of the tracer in the organs.

4.1 BSGI/MBI radiation dose

Sestamibi (MIBI) was cleared by the US FDA in 1991 for cardiac perfusion studies. In 1997, breast imaging was added as an indication to the drug package insert following a clinical trial conducted with standard gamma cameras equipped with high-resolution collimators. According to the drug package insert, the patient whole-body radiation dose is 4.8 milligray at 1110 megabecquerels (0.5 rads at 30 millicuries), see Table 4. According to the Dosage and Administration section of the drug package insert, breast imaging is to be conducted using a dose of 740 - 1110 MBq (20 - 30 mCi).

At the time of the US FDA approval, the breast imaging studies were being acquired with standard, large field-of-view gamma cameras, typical to a nuclear medicine department and the dose required for imaging was determined largely by the low photon sensitivity of these imaging systems when equipped with high-resolution collimators (Khalkhali et al., 2004) Since that time, several breast optimized gamma camera systems have been developed with significantly higher photon sensitivity and several studies indicate that it is possible to lower the injected dose of MIBI required for breast imaging with these systems.

A recent clinical trial was conducted to examine breast tissue uptake as a function of injected dose. The results of this analysis indicate that breast tissue uptake of MIBI appears to be linear relative to the injected dose thus implying there is no physiologic limitation to using lower doses (Böhm-Vélez et al., 2011). According to additional studies, conducted by the Mayo Clinic, the new, breast optimized detector systems provide a photon sensitivity roughly 3 times higher than that of the older imaging systems (Hruska et al., 2008).

From the available data, it is evident that these new detector technologies can reduce the dose required to conduct breast imaging with MIBI. Reducing the dose MIBI from 740 - 1110 MBq (20 - 30 mCI) to 259 - 370 MBq (7 - 10 mCi) reduces patient radiation exposure by nearly a factor of 3. The radiation exposure from a 259 MBq injection of MIBI is approximately 2 millisieverts (mSv) and is approximately equivalent to the radiation dose diagnostic breast patients receive from the combination of screening and diagnostic mammograms (Hendrick, 2010; Valinten, 2007).

Estimated Radiation Absorbed Dose				
	STRESS			
	2.0 hour void		4.8 hour void	
Organ	rads/ 30 mCi	mGy/ 1110 MBq	rads/ 30 mCi	mGy/ 1110 MBq
Breasts	0.2	2.0	0.2	1.8
Gallbladder Wall	2.8	28.9	2.8	27.8
Small Intestine	2.4	24.4	2.4	24.4
Upper Large Intestine Wall	4.5	44.4	4.5	44.4
Lower Large Intestine Wall	3.3	32.2	3.3	32.2
Stomach Wall	0.6	5.3	0.5	5.2
Heart Wall	0.5	5.6	0.5	5.3
Kidneys	1.7	16.7	1.7	16.7
Liver	0.4	4.2	0.4	4.1
Lungs	0.3	2.6	0.2	2.4
Bone Surfaces	0.6	6.2	0.6	6.0
Thyroid	0.3	2.7	0.2	2.4
Ovaries	1.2	12.2	1.3	13.3
Testes	0.3	3.1	0.3	3.4
Red Marrow	0.5	4.6	0.5	4.4
Urinary Bladder Wall	1.5	15.5	3.0	30.0
Total Body	0.4	4.2	0.4	4.2

Table 4. Radiation dosimetry of Sestamibi.

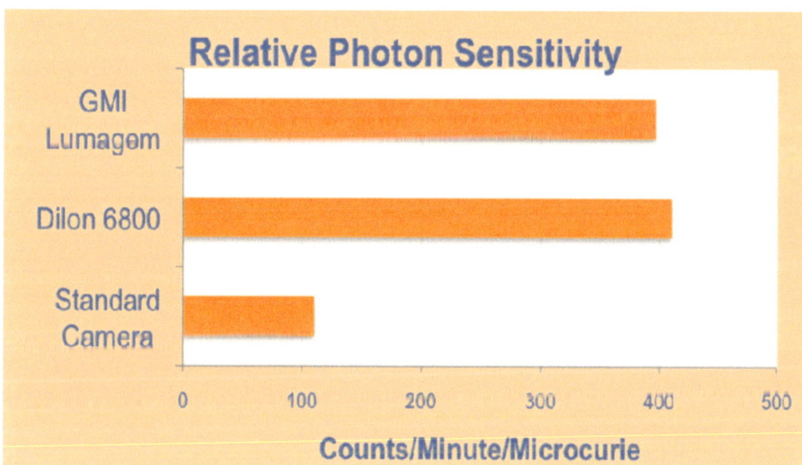

Graph 1. The relative photon sensitivity of commercially available, breast-optimized imaging systems compared to that of the standard gamma camera.

4.2 PEM radiation dose

F-18 fluorodeoxy-D-glucose (FDG) was cleared by the US FDA in 2000 for a variety of uses including tumor localization. The total body radiation dose in FDG PET is 39 mrads per mCi injected activity (Table 5). According to the clinical literature, the typical FDG dose used for imaging with the standard whole body PET detectors ranges between is approximately 370 - 740 MBq (10 - 20 mCi).

TABLE 5. RADIATION DOSE FOR INTRAVENOUS 2FDG(F-18) TO VARIOUS ORGANS

Target organ	Activity per organ (μCi/organ*)	From target organ (mrad/mCi)	From total body (mrad/mCi)	From bladder (mrad/mCi)	Total dose to target organ (mrad/mCi)
Kidneys	8	46.5	37.0	1.18	85
Lungs	25	40.9	35.1	1.52	78
Liver	30	37.2	37.1	0.887	75
Spleen	12	120.	37.1	0.718	160
Red marrow	15†	12.3	35.1	3.84	51
Ovaries	0.1	13.7	37.0	1.90	53
Testes	0.3†	13.5	38.8	15.6	68
Bladder‡	—	—	—	—	440
Brain‡	—	—	—	—	80
Heart	36	134	24.1	—	160
Total body	700	—	33.3	5.9	39

* Based on 1 mCi injection for percent injected activity from Table 1.
† Estimate based on relative weight: 1.5% of dose to red marrow and 0.03% of dose to testes.
‡ The radiation dose to the brain and to the bladder wall for 2-hr void time were evaluated in humans. See Tables 2 and 4.

Table 5. Radiation dose for FDG based on 1 mCi injection.

The dose of FDG used for PEM studies has generally followed the guidelines established with the lager systems, typically using approximately 444 MBq (12 mCi) (Berg et al, 2006). However, more recent studies have demonstrated that doses of 111 - 185 MBq (3 - 5 mCi) are possible with the breast-optimized imaging systems (MacDonald et al, 2010). The resulting radiation dose to the patient is 1.9 - 3.1 mSv using a low dose protocol, nearly identical to that of low dose BSGI/MBI (O'Connor et al., 2010).

5. Clinical evidence

There is a substantial history of clinical literature on imaging breast cancers with nuclear medicine techniques. One of the first reports of breast imaging using MIBI was provided by Campeau and his colleagues in 1992 while the first report of breast cancer imaging using FDG was reported by Wahl the previous year (Campeau et al., 1992; Wahl et al,. 1991) Since that time, hundreds of articles have been published on breast imaging using these radiotracers. However until recently, these imaging studies were conducted with large gamma cameras typical in the nuclear medicine department. The development of breast-optimized detector systems used in BSGI/MBI and PEM is more recent and the primary advantage of these systems is that they provide higher sensitivity for the detection of breast lesions than their predecessors.

5.1 Clinical evidence for BSGI/MBI

There have been several clinical studies evaluating BSGI/MBI in breast cancer detection. In 2008, the group from George Washington Medical University provided an overview of their experience using BSGI/MBI in 146 patients who participated in an IRB approved trial (Brem et al., 2008). Table 6 provides the reported sensitivity of BSGI for various subgroups from that analysis.

Overall	96%
Invasive Cancers	97%
Sub-centimeter lesions	89%
Lobular Carcinoma	93%
DCIS	94%

Table 6. The sensitivity of BSGI in various subgroups.

Other, larger studies have provided evidence of high sensitivity and specificity for BSGI. The first of these larger studies was an analysis performed by Weigert and her associates in more than 500 women who had a BSGI scan performed as part of their routine diagnostic imaging following conventional imaging (Weigert et al., 2007). It is interesting to note that over half of the patients in this study had indeterminate findings following mammography and ultrasound. Two years later, Bertrand presented the results from a retrospective, multicenter study reporting that BSGI provided a higher sensitivity than diagnostic mammography in detection of breast cancer, especially in the high-risk and dense breast populations (Bertrand et al., 2009) Last, in 2011, Lee et al reported that BSGI had a higher sensitivity than mammography and higher specificity than ultrasound in their series of 622 patients who had all three imaging modalities performed as part of their diagnostic examination (Lee et al., 2011). In addition, this work found that there was no change in the sensitivity of BSGI between normally dense and heterogeneously or very dense breast tissue.

	Bertrand, 2009	**Lee, 2011**	**Weigert, 2007**
Total Patients	1,042	662	512
Sensitivity (%)	91	95	89
Specificity (%)	77	88	90
NPV (%)	96	97	98

Table 7. The clinical performance of BSGI from several studies.

5.2 Clinical evidence for PEM

One of the earliest published studies on PEM containing a group of 77 patients examined the effectiveness of PEM in the detection of breast carcinoma (Berg et al., 2006). Table 8 provides the sensitivity of PEM as determined by this work. As expected, the sensitivity for lobular carcinoma was somewhat lower potentially due to the reduced glucose metabolism compared to ductal carcinoma.

	Sensitivity
Overall	90%
DCIS	91%
ILC	75%
Sub-centimeter	63%

Table 8. Sensitivity of PEM by sub-group.

The overall sensitivity and specificity for PEM is very good, especially for DCIS. Table 9 lists for each of the four PEM studies cited, the total number enrolled, the sensitivity, specificity, and negative predictive value.

	Berg, 2006	Tafra, 2005	Schilling, 2011
Total Patients	77	44	182
Sensitivity (%)	90	89	85
Specificity (%)	86	NR	74
NPV (%)	88	NR	NR

Table 9. Clinical results of PEM imaging. NR = not reported.

In clinical studies of BSGI/MBI and PEM, both of these metabolic imaging modalities provide improved sensitivity and specificity for the diagnosis of breast cancer compared to mammography alone. The sensitivity and specificity of BSGI and PEM are generally comparable with both modalities demonstrating the capability to visualize lesions as small as 1 - 2 mm. Both PEM and BSGI/MBI systems have biopsy guidance capabilities.

6. Clinical considerations

Both BSGI and PEM provide valuable clinical information in the detection and treatment of breast carcinoma. Like all imaging studies, each has distinct advantages and limitations. From the clinical data, it is evident that the performance of these modalities is quite comparable.

The biggest differences between the procedures are logistical. First, in most areas, MIBI is more readily available and significantly less expensive than FDG. In addition, the shorter half-life of FDG puts tighter constraints on the clinical schedule. For example, if a patient arrives 1 hour late for a FDG injection, the dose has lost 32% of the intended activity where as a MIBI dose has lost 9%. Also, the use of FDG requires four hours of patient fasting prior to injection and MIBI does not have this constraint. FDG also requires a 1-hour post-injection delay for imaging where as MIBI imaging can begin immediately post injection. Based on the injection-to-imaging time considerations, total time required for a MIBI study is approximately 45 minutes compared to approximately 2 hours for an FDG study.

7. Clinical indications

Several indications for these technologies have been proposed in the medical literature. Generally speaking, BSGI/MBI has been examined as a diagnostic adjunct to mammography and ultrasound when these imaging modalities are inconclusive or discordant with other imaging studies and/or clinical signs and symptoms and there is a remaining diagnostic concern. In addition, there is good data to suggest that it is also useful in pre-operative treatment planning for patients with known malignancy and in monitoring the response of the breast lesion(s) to neoadjuvant chemotherapy, see section 5.1. The majority of studies on PEM have examined its use as in preoperative treatment planning for patients with know malignancy and in monitoring the response of breast tumor(s) to neoadjuvant chemotherapy.

In June of 2009, an interdisciplinary committee established by the American College of Surgeons published a report to provide guidance on the use of imaging techniques in breast patients (Silverstein et al., 2009). This panel grouped BSGI/MBI and PEM together as molecular imaging techniques and issued the following recommendation:

- "The available information suggests that they (BSGI/MBI and PEM) may have equivalent sensitivity and improved specificity when compared with breast MRI. It is recommended that these adjunctive tools be used only after high-quality standard imaging is performed; their results should not prevent performing a biopsy recommended after conventional imaging. Either breast-specific gamma imaging or positron emission mammography may be used as an alternative to breast MRI when MRI is not available or is contraindicated in a particular patient. Both tools may be valuable in pre-operative surgical staging. Breast-specific gamma imaging may also be useful as an additional problem-solving tool in some situations."

7.1 Recognized BSGI/MBI indications

In June 2009, the Society of Nuclear Medicine released the Procedural Guidelines for Breast Scintigraphy with Breast-Specific Gamma Cameras that included several proposed several indications for BSGI/MBI (Goldsmith et al., 2009). The indications are quite specific and echoed those set forth by the American College of Surgeons. The indications can be grouped into 4 primary categories.

1. As a diagnostic adjunct for patients with indeterminate findings on conventional imaging (mammography, ultrasound and/or MRI) and remaining diagnostic concerns such as palpable mass, nipple discharge, pain, etc.
2. Preoperative treatment planning in patients with a known cancer diagnosis to determine the extent of the primary lesion and to detect additional foci of disease.
3. As an alterative to breast MRI for patients whom MRI is indicated, but not possible; ferromagnetic implants, compromised renal function, etc.
4. Monitoring tumor response to chemotherapy.

7.2 Recognized PEM indications

There are no additional published guidelines for PEM other than those of the American College of Surgeons that essentially provided three indications:

1. Pre-operative treatment planning in patients with a known cancer diagnosis to determine extent of the primary lesion and to detect additional foci of disease.
2. To monitor the response of breast tumor(s) to neoadjuvant chemotherapy.
3. As an alternative to breast MRI in patients for whom MRI is indicated, but not possible; ferromagnetic implants, compromised renal function, etc.

8. Conclusion

BSGI/MBI and PEM are adjunctive molecular breast imaging technologies which are becoming more common in the breast center and they provide very similar performance in terms of sensitivity and specificity. The radiation dose associated with these imaging techniques is similar to that patients receive from other diagnostic imaging procedures such as CT, PET and nuclear medicine thus their use is currently limited to the diagnostic patient population. However, several studies are underway to reduce the radiation dose to the level of screening mammography which will likely increase their utility to breast cancer screening in the asymptomatic population. The BSGI/MBI procedure is a useful problem-solving tool for patients with dense or complex breast tissue and an unresolved diagnostic concern following anatomical imaging procedures such as mammography and ultrasound. Both BSGI/MBI and PEM are useful in breast cancer patients to detect the extent of disease (additional occult multifocal or muticentric disease) and to monitor tumor response to neoadjuvant chemotherapy. PEM has the advantage of tomographic reconstruction and uniform spatial resolution with increasing tumor depth. In addition, for the breast cancer patient undergoing a PET/CT scan for staging, it is possible to conduct the PEM study following the PET/CT without an additional administration of FDG. The advantages for BSGI/MBI are superior photon sensitivity along the chest wall, fewer patient restrictions and the wider availability of MIBI (see the considerations section above).

9. References

Avril, N., Menzel, M., Dose, J., Schelling, M., et al. (2001). Glucose Metabolism of Breast Cancer Assessed by 18F-FDG PET: Histologic and Immunohistochemical Tissue Analysis. *Journal of Nuclear Medicine,* Vol.42, No.1, (January 2001), *pp.*9–16, ISSN 0161-5505

Ballinger, J.R., Hua, H.A., Berry, B.W., Firby, P. & Boxen, I. (1995). 99Tcm-Sestamibi as an agent for imaging P-glycoprotein-mediated multi-drug resistance: in vitro and in vivo studies in a rat breast tumour cell line and its doxorubicin-resistant variant. *Nuclear Medicine Communications.* Vol.16, No.4, (April 1995), pp. 253–257, ISSN 0143-3636

Berg, W.A., Weinberg, I.N., Narayanan, D., Lobrano, M.E., Ross, E., Amodei, L., Tafra, L., Adler, L.P., Uddo, J., Stein, W. & Levine, E.A. (2006). High-resolution fluorodeoxyglucose positron emission tomography with compression ("positron emission mammography") is highly accurate in depicting primary breast cancer. *Breast Journal.* Vol.12, No.4, (July 2006), pp. 309-323, ISSN 1524-4741

Bertrand. M., Lanzkowsky, L., Stern, L. & Weigert, J. (2009). Results of a Multi-Center Patient Registry to Determine the Clinical Impact of Breast-Specific Gamma Imaging: A Molecular Breast Imaging Technique. *Radiologic Society of North America Annual Meeting.* Chicago, Illinois, USA, November 29 - December 4, 2009.

Böhm-Vélez, M., Kieper, D.A., Williams, M.B., Chang, T.S., Ward, B.H. & Straka, M.R. (2011) A Clinical Evaluation of Breast Tissue Uptake of Tc99m-Sestamibi as a Function of Injected Dose. *Breast Cancer Imaging: State of the Art 2011 – Poster Abstracts, Journal of Nuclear Medicine,* Vol.52, No.4, (April 2011) pp. 660-675. ISSN 0161-5505, Washington D.C. USA, April 21-22, 2011.

Brem, R., Floerke, A., Rapelyea, J., Teal, C., Kelly, T. & Mathur, V. (2008). Breast Specific Gamma Imaging as an Adjunct Imaging Modality for the Diagnosis of Breast Cancer. *Radiology.* Vol.247, No.3 (June 2008), pp. 651-57, ISSN 0033-8419

Campeau, R..J, Kronemer, K.A. & Sutherland, C.M. Concordant uptake of Tc-99m sestamibi and T1201 in unsuspected breast tumor. (1992). *Clinical Nuclear Medicine,* Vol.17, pp. 936-937

Cutrone, J.A., Yospur, L.S., Khalkhali, I., Tolmos, J., Devito, A. & Diggles, L. (1998). Immunohistologic assessment of technetium-99m-MIBI uptake in benign and malignant breast lesions. *Journal of Nuclear Medicine.* Vol.39, No.3, (March 1998), pp. 449-453, ISSN 0161-5505

Goldsmith, S., et al. (2010). SNM Practice Guideline for Breast Scintigraphy with Breast-Specific λ-Cameras 1.0. Available from http://interactive.snm.org/docs/BreastScintigraphyGuideline_V1.0.pdf

Hendrick, E. (2010) Radiation doses and cancer risks from breast imaging studies. *Radiology.* Vol.257, No.1, (October 2010), pp. 246-53, ISSN 0033-8419

Hruska, C.B., Phillips, P.W., Whaley, D.H., Rhodes, D.J. & O'Connor, M.K. (2008) Molecular Breast Imaging: Use of a Dual-Head Dedicated Gamma Camera to Detect Small Breast Tumors. *American Journal of Roentgenology,* Vol.191 No.6, (December 2008) ISSN 1546-3141

Khalkhali, I., et al. (2004). Society of Nuclear Medicine Procedure Guideline for Breast Scintigraphy 2.0. Available from http://interactive.snm.org/docs/Breast_v2.0.pdf. (June 2004)

Kolb, T.M., Lichy, J. & Newhouse, J.H. (2002) Comparison of the performance of screening mammography, physical examination, and breast US and evaluation of factors that influence them: an analysis of 27,825 patient evaluations. *Radiology,* Vol.225, No.1, pp. 165–175. ISSN 0033-8419

Lee, A., Lee, J., Chang, J., Lim, W., Kim, B., Lee, B. & Moon, B. (2011). The efficacy of Breast-Specific Gamma Imaging with 99mTc-Sestamibi in the diagnosis of breast cancer according to breast density for Korean women. *Yellow Sea International Medical Biennial symposium,* Kintex, Korea, January 22, 2011

Lin, C., Ding, H., et al. (2007) Correlation Between the Intensity of Breast FDG Uptake and Menstrual Cycle. *Academic Radiology,* Vol.14, No.8, (August 2007), pp. 940–944, ISSN 1076 6332

MacDonald, L., Luo, W., Lu, X., Wang, C. & Rogers, J. (2010) Low Dose Lesion Contrast on the PEM Flex Solo II. *Medical Physics, Proceedings of the Fifty-second Annual Meeting of the American Association of Physicist in Medicine,* Vol.37, No.6, (July 2010) Philadelphia Pennsylvania, USA, July 18-22, 2010. ISSN 0094-2405

O'Connor, M., Li, H., Rhodes, D.H., Hruska, C.B., Clancy, C.B., Vetter, R.J. (2010). Comparison of radiation exposure and associated radiation-induced cancer risks from mammography and molecular imaging of the breast. *Medical Physics.* Vol.37, No.12, (December 2010), pp. 6187-1689, ISSN 0094-2405

Piwnica-Worms, D., Kronauge, J.F. & Chiu, M.L. (1990). Uptake and retention of hexakis (2-methoxyisobutyl isonitrile) technetium in cultured chick myocardial cells. Mitochondrial and plasma membrane potential dependence. *Circulation,* Vol.82, No.5, (November 1990), 1826–1838. ISSN 0009-7322

Rosen, E., Turkington, T., Soo, M.S., Baker, J.A. & Coleman, R.E. (2005). Detection of Primary Breast Carcinoma with a Dedicated, Large Field-of-View FDG PET Mammography Device: Initial Experience. *Radiology,* Vol.234, No.2, (February 2005), pp. 527–534. ISSN 0033-8419

Schelbert, H., et al. Society of Nuclear Medicine Procedure Guideline for Tumor Imaging Using F-18 FDG. Available from http://interactive.snm.org/docs/pg_ch28_0403.pdf. 1999.

Schilling, K., Narayanan, D., Kalinyak, J., The, J., et al. (2011). Positron emission mammography in breast cancer presurgical planning: comparisons with magnetic resonance imaging. *European Journal of Nuclear Medicine and Molecular Imaging.* Vol.38, No.1, (January 2011), pp. 23-36, ISSN 1619-7089

Sciuto, R., Pasqualoni, R., Bergomi, S., et al. (2002) Prognostic Value of 99mTc-Sestamibi Washout in Predicting Response of Locally Advanced Breast Cancer to Neoadjuvant Chemotherapy. *Journal of Nuclear Medicine,* Vol.43, No.6, (June 2002), pp. 745-751, ISSN 0161-5505

Tafra, L., Cheng, Z., Uddo, J., et al. (2005). Pilot Clinical Trial of 18F-fluorodeoxyglucose Positron-Emission Mammography in the Surgical Management of Breast Cancer. *American Journal of Surgery,* Vol.190, No.4, (October 2005), pp. ISSN 628-632. 0002-9610

Turkington, T. (2001). Introduction to PET Instrumentation. *Journal of Nuclear Medicine Technology,* Vol.29, No.1, (March 2001), pp. 1-8, ISSN 0091-4916

Silverstein, M., et al. (2009). Image-Detected Breast Cancer: State-of-the-Art Diagnosis and Treatment. *Journal of the American College of Surgeons.* Vol.209, No.4, (October 2009), ISSN 1072-7515

Smith, T.A. (1999). Facilitative glucose transporter expression in human cancer tissue. *British Journal of Biomedical Science.* Vol.56, No.4, (April 1999), pp. 285-292, ISSN 0967-4845

Wahl, R.L., Cody, R.L., Hutchins, G.D. & Mudgett E.E. (1991). Primary and metastatic breast carcinoma: initial clinical evaluation with PET with the radiolabeled glucose analogue 2-[F-18]-fluoro-2-deoxy-D-glucose. *Radiology,* Vol.179, No.3, (June 1991), pp. 765-770. ISSN 0033-8419

Weigert, J. (2007). Breast Specific Gamma Imaging (High Resolution Molecular Imaging of the Breast): A Useful Adjunct to Breast Imaging. *Radiologic Society of North America Annual Meeting.* Chicago, Illinois, USA, November 25–30, 2007.

Williams, M., Judy, P., Gunn, S., Majewski, S. (2010). Dual-Modality Breast Tomosynthesis. *Radiology,* Vol.255, No.1 (April 2010), pp. 191-198, ISSN 0033-8419

Valinten, J. (2007)The 2007 Recommendations of the International Commission on Radiological Protection. ICRP publication 103. Ann ICRP 2007; Vol.37No.2-4, (March 2007) pp. 1–332. ISSN 0146-6453

Cardiolite Drug Data Sheet. Lantheus Medical Imaging Division. Available from http://www.cardiolite.com/pdfs/Cardiolite%20US%20PI%20513121-0710%207-20-2010.pdf

Part 2

Clinical Implications

9

Suspicious Nipple Discharge Diagnostic Evaluation

Yukiko Tokuda[1] and Yoshinori Kodama[2]
National Hospital Organization Osaka National Hospital
Department of Radiology[1] and Pathology[2]
Japan

1. Introduction

Nipple discharge (ND) is the third most common breast-related complaint after breast pain and breast mass, and accounts for nearly 7% of all breast symptoms (Hussain et al., 2006; Simmons et al., 2003 citing Leis et al., 1998).

The diagnosis of ND begins with its characterization as either a physiological or pathological condition (Simmons et al., 2003). Physiological discharge, often a manifestation of breast manipulation, is usually bilateral, is white or green, and emanates from many ducts (Simmons et al., 2003). Possible causes of persistent physiological discharge include oral contraceptives, antihypertensives, tranquilizers, hypothyroidism, and pituitary adenoma (Simmons et al., 2003). Most NDs are physiological and are not associated with an underlying benign or malignant breast neoplasm (Sickles, 2000). A pathological discharge is generally unilateral, spontaneous, persistent, clear, watery, serous or bloody in appearance, and emanates from a single duct (Morrogh et al., 2007). Most of the common pathological causes of ND are benign (Hou et al., 2001; Hussain et al., 2006), and the most frequently encountered benign causes are intraductal papilloma, followed by ductal ectasia and fibrocystic disease (Hou et al., 2001; Morrogh et al., 2010; Sickles, 2000). The most important cause of pathological discharge is breast cancer. For single duct nipple discharges, the incidence of malignant or high-risk pathology is reported to be as high as 15% (Orel et al., 2000 citing Carty et al., 1994; Fung et al., 1990; Leis et al., 1989; Piccoli et al., 1998; Tabar et al., 1983; Winchester et al., 1996). In some cases, ND is the only sign of carcinoma (Hou et al., 2001). NDs that are bloody or serous in appearance, associated with a mass, and present in an elderly patient are more likely to be caused by malignant tumors (Das et al., 2001; El-Daly & Gudi, 2010; Pritt et al., 2004; Tabar, 1983; Tjalma, 2004 citing Seltzer et al., 1970).

We defined suspicious ND as pathological ND, which is spontaneous, unilateral, and localized to a single duct, combined with at least one of the following characteristic findings associated a high risk of malignant disease: bloody or serous appearance, associated with a mass, and occurrence in elderly patients.

If ND is multi-duct or bilateral, breast imaging is not required. However, single-duct ND is considered an indication for further investigation by mammography (MMG) and/or ultrasonography (US) (EUSOMA, 2010).

---

[1] Current Affiliation: NTT West Osaka Hospital, Japan

In this chapter, we review several methods of diagnostic evaluation including MMG, US, conventional ductography (DG), ND cytology, fine needle aspiration (FNA) and histopathology. We also demonstrate how to use the findings of contrast-enhanced magnetic resonance imaging (CEMRI) studies, including direct and indirect MR ductography (MRDG), to localize the causative lesion and to differentiate malignant lesions from benign ones in cases of suspicious ND.

2. Mammography (MMG)

While MMG is considered the standard initial imaging examination and may reveal microcalcifications and other signs of malignancy, it rarely provides information about the etiology of ND (Rissanen et al., 2007 citing Cabioglu et al., 2003; Dillon et al., 2006; Funovics et al., 2003; Sardanelli et al., 1997; Tabar et al., 1983). In the study by Tabar et al. (1983), only half of the patients who presented with ND and were diagnosed with breast cancer had an abnormal mammogram. In the study by Morrogh et al. (2010), the sensitivity of MMG among all patients with pathological ND was 18%. Conversely, MMG had a high negative predictive value (NPV) and specificity (94%), suggesting that MMG can be used to select patients with physiological ND for whom clinical observation alone may be a reasonable management approach.

3. Ultrasonography (US)

Breast US is a non-invasive diagnostic method that has proven to be useful in the evaluation of patients with ND (Sakorafas, 2001). However, US has limitations with respect to depicting causative lesions of small masses and ductal carcinomas in situ (DCIS), especially those in peripheral regions without ductal dilatation or those in high adipose-containing breasts (Berg & Gilbreath., 2000; Nakahara et al., 2003 citing Chung et al., 1995).

The most common sonographic features are duct dilatation, particularly in cases associated with solid internal echoes and duct wall thickening in generally central and/or subareolar areas (Ballesio et al., 2008). Berg & Gilbreath (2000) reported that US identified 45 of 48 (94%) invasive tumor foci and 7 of 16 (44%) foci of DCIS while only 9 of 64 (14%) malignant foci were detected by US. Rissanen et al. (2007) reported that in 52 patients with unilateral nipple discharge, 80% of papillomatous lesions, 58% of other benign lesions, and 20% of malignant lesions were sonographically positive, and among the 6 cases in which duct dilatation was the only sonographic finding, 3 (50%) were malignant lesions and the other 3 (50%) were papillomas and other benign lesions. In a study of 55 patients with bloody ND, Nakahara et al. (2003) reported that of all findings, only the hypoechoic masses with smooth margins (NPV = 90.9%) and hypoechoic masses with irregular margins (positive predictive value (PPV) = 85.7%) were statistically significant.

In addition to the patient's clinical history and cytological evaluation of the ND, performing a US-guided FNA is fundamental for differentiating between malignant and benign lesions (Ballesio et al, 2008 citing Sardanelli et al., 1997).

4. Nipple discharge (ND) cytology

ND cytology is a simple and noninvasive method that includes simply touching the nipple, obtaining a smear of the fluid, or gently scraping the surface of a lesion. Breast pumping, breast massage, or nipple aspiration may be attempted if the discharge does not occur spontaneously during collection of the samples (Gupta et al., 2004; Krishnamurthy, et al., 2003). Gupta et al. (2004) have suggested that the use of routine ND cytology is limited by the small samples obtained and that ND cytology cannot always distinguish between physiological processes, fibrocystic disease, and papillomas. However, studies based on a large number of cases suggest that ND cytology is a reasonable method for diagnosing malignant and suspicious cases (Das et al., 2001; El-Daly & Gudi, 2010; Gupta et al., 2004; Pritt et al., 2004). Cytological examination of ND is valuable mainly for detecting such cancers. The efficiency of ND cytology remains controversial, as an older study has demonstrated low sensitivity, for detection of malignancy, ranging from 11% to 31.2% (Dinkel et al., 2001). However, studies that are more recent have reported higher sensitivity of ND cytology. For example, Pritt et al. (2004) determined a sensitivity and specificity of 85% and 97%, respectively. Likewise, a sensitivity of 58.3% and 63% and a specificity of 100% and 100% were reported by Lee (2003) and El-Daly & Gudi (2010), respectively. Therefore, ND cytology can be useful in the diagnosis of malignant and suspicious cases.

Foam cells are the predominant cytological feature in tissues being subjected to in inflammatory processes, mastopathy, or fibrocystic disease (Fig. 1a). Its secretion occasionally contains duct epithelial cells (Fig. 1b). Apocrine metaplasia of duct epithelial cells is sometimes seen. In intraductal papillomas, large, cohesive clusters of normal duct cells may be observed (Fig. 2).

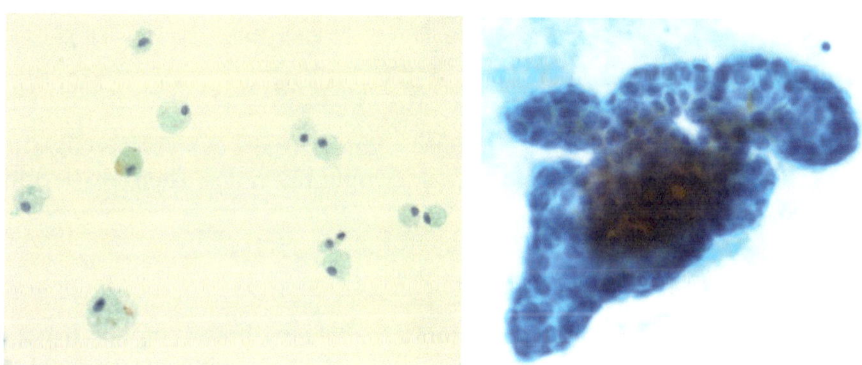

(a) (b)

Fig. 1. Nipple discharge cytology of benign lesions. (a) Several foam cells are observed but no epithelial cells are present. (b) A number of clusters composed of duct cells forming a papillary structure can be seen. (Histological diagnosis, duct papillomatosis)

Clusters of apocrine cells may also be seen. In some cases, papillary structures composed of spherical clusters of large duct cells with atypical features such as cytoplasmic vacuoles, enlarged nuclei, and visible nucleoli may be present. In ductal carcinoma, the clusters composed of atypical cells may be loosely structured and are sometimes thick or spherical. They may also form papillary structures. Necrosis is commonly seen in high-grade lesions (Fig. 3).

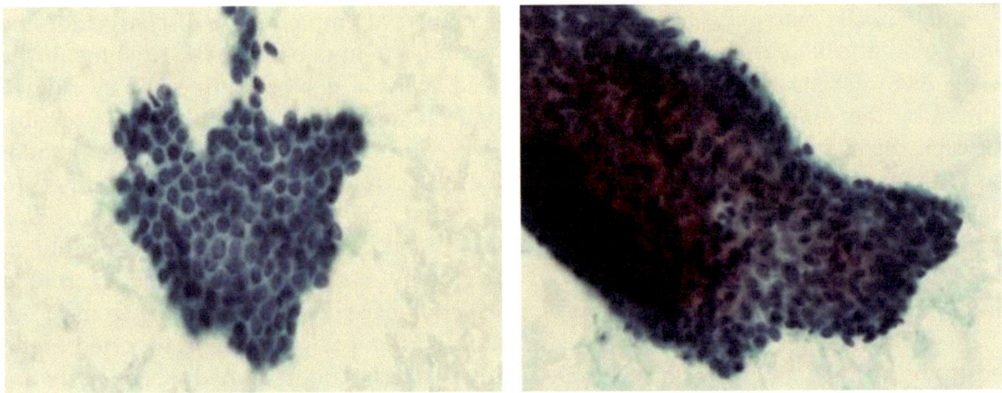

(a) (b)

Fig. 2. ND cytology of intraductal papilloma. (a, b) Cohesive clusters composed of benign duct cells. The histological diagnosis was intraductal papilloma (see Fig. 8)

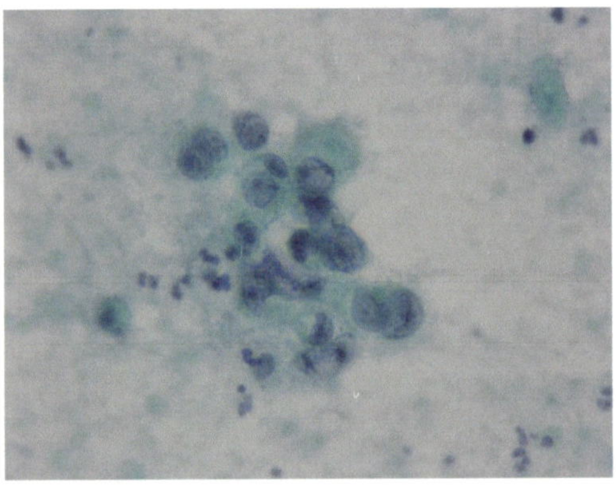

Fig. 3. ND cytology of a malignant lesion. The smear shows clusters of atypical cells with enlarged, irregular-shaped nuclei, and high nuclear cytoplasmic ratios. There are necrotic cells in the background.

5. Fine needle aspiration (FNA)

FNA cytology is now a popular widely used tool for assessing breast tumors. It has been reported that ND cytology is as specific as concomitant FNA cytology but slightly less sensitive for detecting papillomas or malignant lesions (Lee, 2003). However, ND samples are often inadequate. Gupta et al. (2004) showed that 492 of 1948 ND smears (25%) were inadequate for diagnosis. Lee (2003) reported that ND cytology was non-diagnostic in 43 of 82 cases (52%), whereas FNA cytology was non-diagnostic in only 1 of 34 cases (2.9%). Therefore, ND cytology has little complementary diagnostic value. FNA cytology is a sensitive and effective method of diagnosing breast cancer.

6. Ductography (DG, also called Galactography)

DG is a diagnostic modality used for identification of the secreting duct, which is cannulated and injected with a sterile water-soluble contrast material. This is followed by

MMG (Sakorafas, 2001). DG is more sensitive than ND cytology and MMG in detecting intraductal lesions (Rongione et al., 1996; Chung et al., 1995; Orel et al., 2000). It was found that when a standard evaluation was negative for a lesion, the addition of DG localized 19 of 25 (76%) otherwise occult malignant/high-risk lesions and 80 of 88 (91%) benign lesions (Morrogh et al., 2010). The incidence of malignancy, despite negative clinical breast examination and conventional imaging, was found to be as high as 10% (Morrogh et al., 2008). Ductographic findings suggestive of carcinoma include irregular filling defects, ductal irregularities (distortion, displacement, complete obstruction of contrast flow, and non-iatrogenic contrast extravasation), and a deeper position of the lesion (Cardenosa et al., 1994; Ciatto et al., 1998; Tabar et al., 1983). Smooth intraductal filling defects, complete ductal obstruction, ductal expansion with apparent distortion, and irregularity of the ductal wall are more common ductographic features obsreved for solitary papillomas (Cardenosa et al., 1994; Nakahara et al., 2003). Unfortunately, evidence for a predictive role for DG is less convincing because a positive study does not differentiate between malignant and benign causes of discharge and a negative study does not exclude the presence of an underlying carcinoma. The PPV and NPVs of DG have been reported to be 19% and 63%, respectively (sensitivity, 76%; specificity, 11%); these values are consistent with those of other studies and confirm that DG is not effective in distinguishing between malignant and benign causes of nipple discharge (Morrogh et al., 2007). The routine use of DG in cases of suspicious ND remains controversial (Rongione et al., 1996; Chung et al., 1995; Orel et al., 2000).

DG is invasive and time-consuming with potential complications including intense pain, mastitis, lymphatic opacification, and duct perforation (Cardenosa et al., 1994; Lorenzon et al., 2011; Tabar et al., 1983). The rate of incomplete and/or technically inadequate conventional DG has been reported to be as high as 10–15% (Morrogh et al., 2008; Sickles, 2000). All of these technical difficulties may result in the failure to detect and surgically treat the lesion, as most cases of pathological ND have no detectable lump and negative or undefined ultrasonographic findings (Schwab et al., 2008).

7. Contrast-Enhanced Magnetic Resonance Imaging (CEMRI)

Negative or benign findings identified by physical examination, MMG, US, cytological analysis of discharge, and DG are not sufficient to rule out the presence of underlying malignant lesion (Rongione et al., 1996; Tabar et al., 1983), but the physician must still decide whether to manage expectantly or proceed to major duct excision (Morrogh et al., 2010). CEMRI is increasingly being used as a diagnostic modality for breast cancer, with diagnostic sensitivities of 86–100% and 40–100% for invasive and intraductal cancers, respectively (Orel et al., 2001; Tjalma & Verslebers, 2004 citing Esserman et al., 1999; Vichweg et al., 2000).

Preliminary research on the application of CEMRI for evaluation of patients with ND suggests that it is useful for the localization of otherwise occult diseases, identification of both benign and malignant causes of ND, and noninvasiveness relative to DG. However, the available data are limited (Nakahara et al., 2003; Orel et al., 2000; Tjalma & Verslebers, 2004). Therefore, the gold standard diagnostic and therapeutic approach for patients with pathological ND is surgical duct excision (Morrogh et al., 2010 citing Nelson & Hoehn, 2006). However, a frequent criticism of this blind approach is that the pathologists may not always identify a discrete lesion responsible for the discharge. In addition, major duct excision is expected to be undesirable for a woman of childbearing age. Therefore, there is a need to develop more effective tools for localizing the lesions responsible for ND and for distinguishing between malignant and benign causes of ND, the 2 most important roles of imaging (Morrogh et al., 2007; Yau et al., 2011).

7.1 Localization of the disease causing the ND

There is evidence in the literatures that CEMRI offers high diagnostic performance for detecting lesions in patients with suspicious ND, even when no lesions are identified by conventional imaging and when DG is not feasible or inconclusive (Sardanelli et al., 2008 citing Daniel et al., 2003; Hirose et al., 2006; Nakahara et al., 2003; Orel et al., 2000). Lorenzon et al. (2011) found that CEMRI could identify 5/5 cancers (sensitivity = 100%) and 13/14 high-risk lesions (sensitivity = 92.9%) (overall sensitivity, 94.7%; overall specificity, 78.9%). In addition, it was found that 3 of 5 cancers (1 invasive, 1 in situ, 1 contralateral invasive) and 2 of 14 high-risk lesions could be detected only by CEMRI. CEMRI was significantly more sensitive than either MMG or US ($p < 0.0001$ and $p = 0.042$, respectively). Morrogh et al. (2007) reported that the PPV and NPV of CEMRI for detection of the disease causing the ND were 56% and 87%, respectively (sensitivity, 83%; specificity, 62%), and CEMRI performed after negative standard evaluation detected 75% of otherwise occult malignant/high risk lesions. Nakahara et al. (2003) reported that CEMRI identified all malignant lesions (100%) including DCIS. Kramer et al. (Van Goethem et al., 2009 citing Kramer et al., 2000) used CEMRI alone and in combination with MMG and DG to assess 48 women with pathological ND. The sensitivity and specificity values of DG for detection of papillomas were 94% and 79%, respectively, whereas only 1 carcinoma was detected by MMG/DG. CEMRI had a sensitivity of 89% (8/9) for malignant lesions. These authors have concluded that while MMG in combination with DG remains the primary diagnostic tool, the addition of CEMRI can demonstrate the location and distribution of lesions, especially in malignant cases, and therefore recommend performing a CEMRI to detect underlying lesions that may have been misdiagnosed by conventional imaging (Lorenzon et al., 2011; Van Goethem et al., 2009).

7.2 Differentiation of malignant and benign lesions

Predicting whether the causative lesion is malignant or benign is important because it affects the physician's choice of clinical follow-up or surgical treatment.

Nakahara et al. (2003) reported that segmental clumped enhancement (PPV = 100%), a focal mass with a smooth border (NPV = 91.7%), and diffuse or regional stippled enhancement (NPV = 94.1%) were statistically significant features that can be used for differentiating between malignant and benign lesions. Ballesio et al. (2008) reported that 5 papillomatosis lesions appeared as patchy, homogeneously enhanced areas, that among 15 intraductal papillomas, some had an oval appearance with well-defined margins, while other had areas of homogeneous enhancement with a linear shape at the periareolar or subareolar sites, moreover, they reported 2 cases of atypical ductal hyperplasias with diffuse nodular enhancement. One micropapillary DCIS, 1 papillary carcinoma, and 1 invasive ductal carcinoma were visualized as 2 segmental areas of enhancement and 1 mass-like enhancement with poorly defined margins. Morrogh et al. (2007) reported that MRI was use as the first-line test in 32/52 (63%) patients in whom it was performed and yielded a breast imaging reporting and data system (BI-RADS) MRI (American College of Radiology, 2003) ≥

4 diagnosis in 11/32 (34%) patients. Seven of 11 (64%) patients proceeded directly to major duct excision and demonstrated 1 invasive cancer, 2 DCIS, 2 high-risk lesions, and 2 benign lesions. MRI was negative in 21 patients (BI-RADS MRI score, ≤3). Among this group, 4 patients proceeded to major duct excision, yielding 1 invasive cancer and 3 benign lesions. Therefore, an evaluation based using only BI-RADS MRI descriptors has a limited ability to distinguish between malignant and benign lesions.

We analyzed MRI findings in patients with suspicious ND using BI-RADS MRI descriptors and clustered ring enhancement criteria (Tokuda et al., 2009), and compared them with histopathological diagnoses to assess the accuracy of differentiating between malignant and benign lesions. Clustered ring enhancement is characterized by clusters of minute ring enhancements. The clusters include enhanced foci constituting enhanced ring-like patterns, and heterogeneous enhancement of minute internal ring patterns (Tozaki et al., 2006) (Fig. 4). Breast CEMRI was performed on 47 patients to identify lesions causing suspicious ND. The 39 lesions for which histopathological diagnoses were obtained consisted of 17 carcinomas and 22 benign lesions. The types of carcinoma identified included DCIS (n = 10), invasive ductal carcinoma (IDC) with intraductal components (n = 2), and IDC (n = 5). The benign lesions included fibrocystic disease (n = 11), intraductal papillomas (n = 5), duct papillomatosis (n = 2), fibrosis (n = 3), and a fibrous nodule (n = 1). Table 1 shows the frequencies of the BI-RADS MRI descriptors and the presence of clustered ring enhancement for benign and malignant lesions. Among the non-mass-like enhancement patterns, no distribution modifiers such as "linear," "regional," or "multiple regions" were observed, and no internal enhancements such as "reticular" enhancement were detected. Only 2 lesions showing mass enhancement were not diagnosed by histopathology.

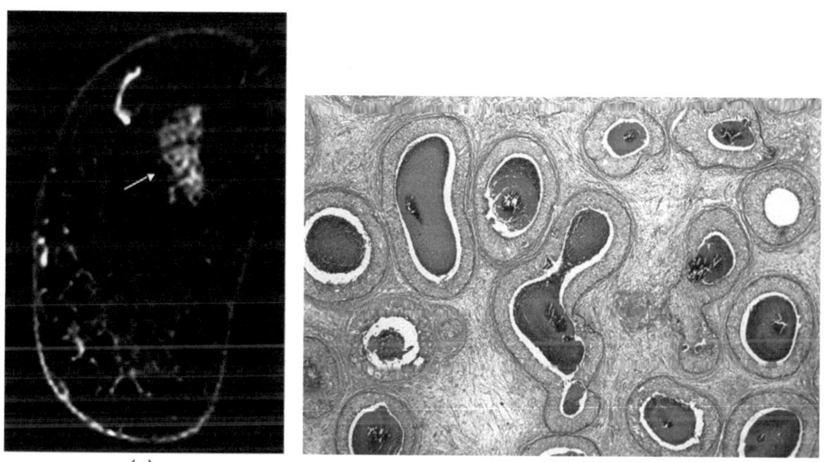

(a) (b)

Fig. 4. Images of the breast of a 54-year-old woman with suspicious microcalcifications observed by mammography. (a) Coronal first contrast-enhanced T1-weighted MR image of the left breast shows regional enhancement in the upper outer quadrant (arrow). The lesion demonstrates heterogeneous enhancement with interior clustered minute ring enhancements (clustered ring enhancement). (b) A photomicrograph of the histopathological specimen shows a ductal carcinoma in situ with intraluminal necrosis and microcalcifications. Clustered ring enhancement corresponds to periductal stroma. However, intraductal cancer cell involvement in the enhancement cannot be ruled out. Reprinted from Tozaki et al. (2006)

Descriptor	Benign (n=22)	Malignant (n=17)	P*
Non-mass-like enhancement			
Distribution modifiers			
Ductal	10 (45)	3 (18)	NS
Focal	1 (5)	1 (6)	NS
Regional	0 (0)	0	NS
Segmental	8 (36)	10 (59)	NS
Diffuse	3 (14)	1 (6)	NS
No enhancement	0	2 (11)	NS
Internal enhancement			
Homogeneous	2 (9)	1 (7)	NS
Heterogeneous	9 (41)	9 (57)	NS
Stippled,punctuate	11 (50)	3 (22)	NS
Clumped	0	2 (14)	NS
Reticular	0	0	NS
Clustered ring enhancement	2	9	0.002

Numbers shown in parentheses indicate percentages.
Masses were not diagnosed by histopathology were excluded from this table.
*Fisher's exact test was used.
NS indicates not significant.

Table 1. Frequency of MRI parameters in cases of suspicious nipple discharge. Reprinted from Tokuda et al. (Tokuda et al., 2009)

The 22 benign and the 17 malignant lesions comprised 15 non-mass-like enhancements and 2 non-enhanced lesions, which had DCIS foci measuring 2 and 2.5 mm in diameter without stromal changes.

The most common findings of the benign lesions were stippled (50%), ductal (45%), and heterogeneous (41%), whereas those of the malignant lesions were segmental (59%) and heterogeneous (57%). Both lesions (2/2) showing clumped internal enhancement were IDCs with an intraductal component. Clustered ring enhancement was observed in 60% (9/15) of the malignant enhancing lesions but in only 9% (2/22) of the benign lesions (p = 0.002). Of the 11 lesions showing clustered ring enhancement, 9 were malignant and 2 were benign. The highest PPVs for carcinoma were associated with the clumped (100% or 2/2), clustered ring enhancement (82% or 9/11), and segmental (56% or 10/18) descriptors.

The specificity of clustered ring enhancement was 90% (20/22). Among the lesions showing clustered ring enhancement, 8 exhibited segmental distribution and 3 ductal enhancement. Both the malignant lesions with clumped enhancement (100% or 2/2) also showed clustered ring enhancement. Although the distribution pattern alone was not useful for differentiating between malignant and benign lesions, the combination of segmental distribution and clustered ring enhancement showed a significant association with breast cancer (p = 0.004). Twelve patients did not undergo a surgical procedure, and no histopathological diagnoses were obtained. We show cases with (Fig. 5) and without (Fig. 6) clustered ring enhancement. Images in Figures 5 and 6 are similar to images in Tokuda et al., (2009) but were obtained using a MRI device with a standard breast-dedicated coil. The most common kinetic pattern observed in the malignant lesions was the plateau pattern (40% or 6/15), and the most common kinetic pattern in the benign lesions was the persistent pattern (55% or 12/22). The washout pattern had the highest PPV for carcinoma, 100% ($p = 0.02$). The highest PPVs for carcinoma were associated with a clumped internal enhancement (100%), clustered ring enhancement (82%), and a washout pattern (100%).

Tozaki et al. (Tozaki et al, 2006) reported that clustered ring enhancement combined with the BI-RADS MRI descriptors appear to be useful in differentiating between benign and malignant lesions. Most of the lesions causing suspicious ND were observed to have non-mass-like enhancement. Many DCISs have been reported to have non-mass-like enhancement and a segmental or ductal distribution and clumped internal enhancement (Liberman et al., 2002; Morakkabati-Spitz et al., 2005). Tozaki et al. (2006) reported that all lesions showing segmental distribution were malignant. In this study, of the lesions showing segmental distribution, 8 were benign and 10 were malignant. In addition, among the lesions showing ductal distribution, 10 and 3 were benign and malignant, respectively, and the difference was insignificant. The PPV of segmental distribution alone was 44%. Morakkabati-Spitz et al. reported that segmental distribution and linear enhancement were the most common features of DCIS on dynamic MRI. In that study, 13 fibrocystic disease lesions showed segmental distribution. The PPV of segmental distribution in our study was similar to that reported by Morakkabati-Spitz et al. (2005), but was markedly lower than that of Tozaki et al. (2006). This may be due to different biases in patient selection for MRI. We analyzed lesions causing suspicious ND, Morakkabati-Spitz et al. (2005) examined lesions showing a segmental distribution and linear enhancement, and Tozaki et al. (2006) evaluated lesions showing non-mass- like enhancement. Similar to the results reported by Tozaki et al. (2006), the most common internal enhancement patterns was a heterogeneous pattern for the malignant lesions (59%) and a stippled/punctuate pattern for the benign lesions (45%); this difference was not significant. In this study, both the clumped internal enhanced lesions (2/2) were found to be malignant. Although the number of cases studied was small, Liberman et al. (2002) reported similar results (Liberman et al., 2002).

All lesions (4/4) showing a washout kinetic pattern were malignant. Ten benign and 6 malignant lesions showed a plateau pattern. Kuhl et al. (Kuhl et al., 1999) pointed out that segmental and ductal enhancements are the imaging hallmarks of DCIS in breast MRI and concluded that the sensitivity of breast MRI for the detection of DCIS can be increased by performing additional morphological analysis of the enhancement pattern. However, in this study, the combination of distribution modifiers and a washout pattern was not significant. The presence of clustered ring enhancement was useful for differentiating between malignant and benign lesions ($p = 0.002$) and had a high PPV (82%) for breast cancer. Although the distribution pattern alone was not useful for differentiating between malignant and benign lesions, the combination of segmental distribution and clustered ring enhancement showed a significant association with breast cancer ($p = 0.004$) and a high PPV (88%). This indicates that clustered ring enhancement is a useful parameter in CEMRI analysis.

We conclude that the most common CEMRI finding in patients with suspicious ND is non-mass-like enhancement. The combination of segmental distribution and clustered ring enhancement showed the highest PPV for malignancy, and MRI can provide clinically useful information for distinguishing between benign and malignant causes of suspicious ND.

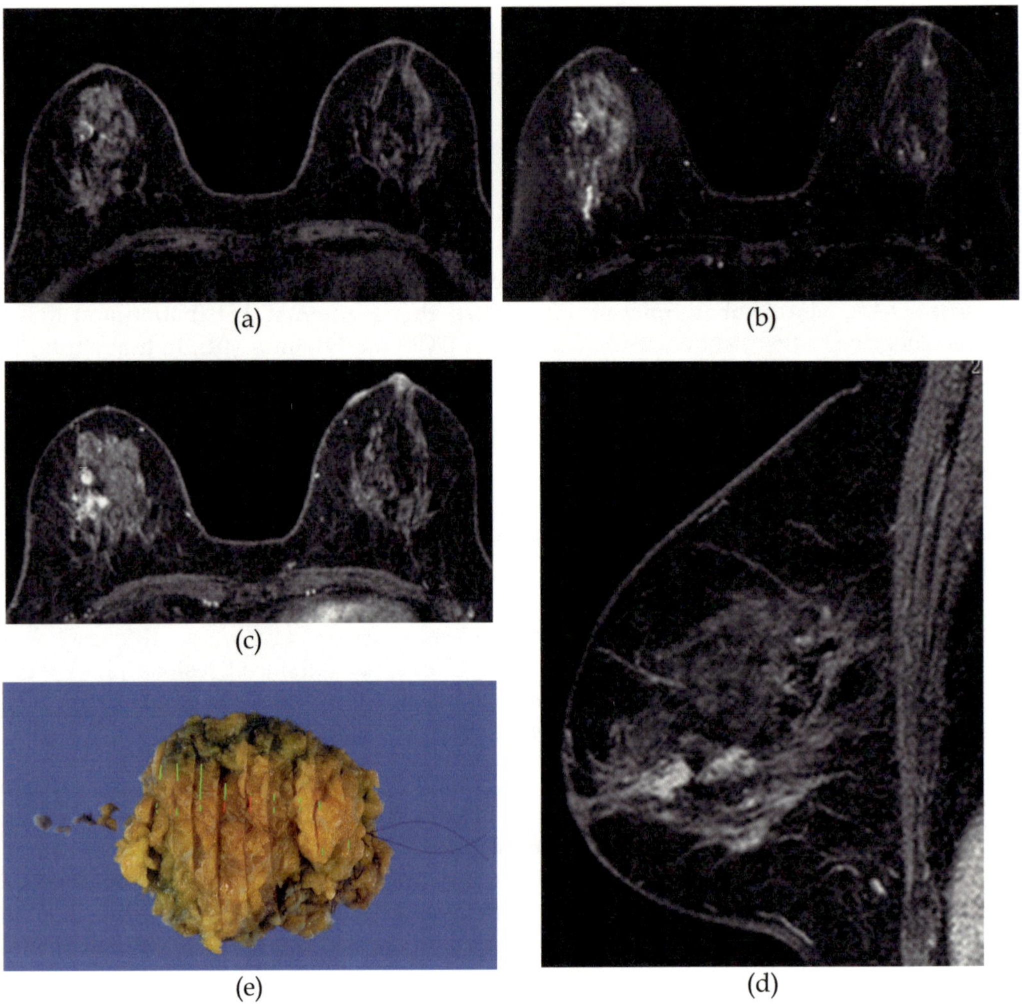

Fig. 5. Images of the breasts of a 70-year-old woman who presented with bloody discharge from the right nipple. (a) Pre-contrast enhanced fat-suppressed T1-weighted image showing intraductal high intensity corresponding to bloody discharge. (b) A fast short-tau inversion-recovery (STIR) image showing peripheral duct ectasia and intraductal fluid accumulation. (c) Dynamic contrast-enhanced early phase image showing clumped enhancement with segmental distribution. (d) Post-contrast-enhanced sagittal image showing heterogeneous tramline-like and clustered ring enhancement. The histopathological diagnosis was invasive ductal carcinoma with predominant intraductal components. (e) Mapping of the lesion (green line area, ductal carcinoma in situ; red line area, invasive ductal carcinoma).

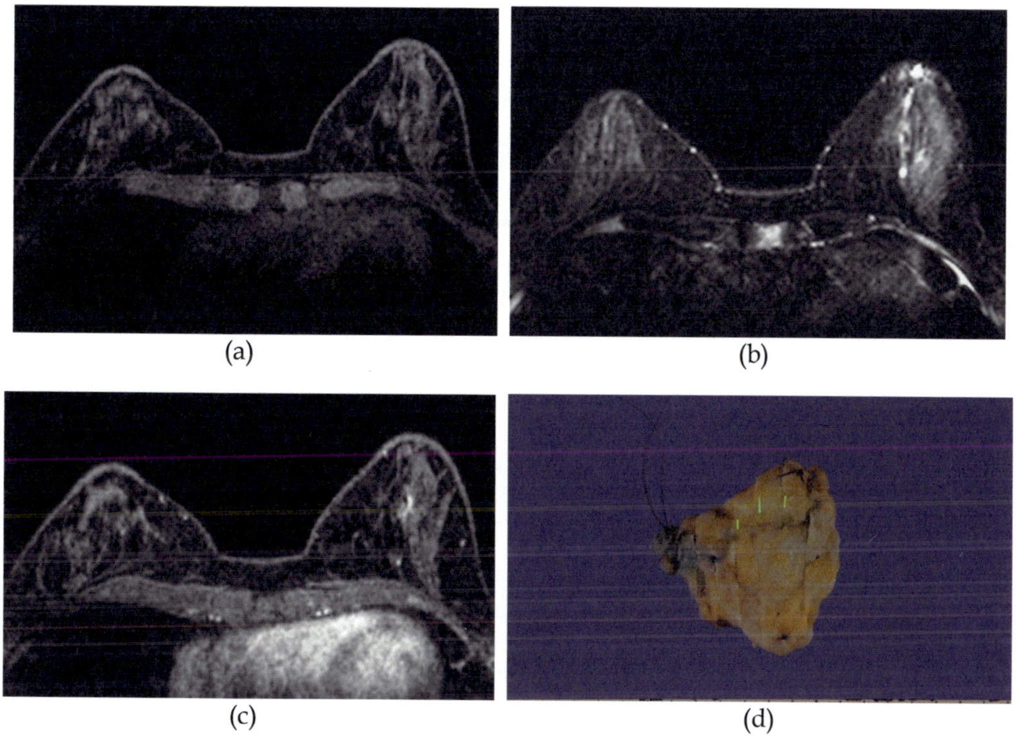

Fig. 6. Images of the breasts of a 49-year-old woman who presented with bloody discharge from the left nipple. (a) Pre-contrast fat-suppressed T1-weighted MR image showing no intraductal abnormal intensity. (b) STIR MR image showing duct ectasia and intraductal fluid accumulation. (c) A contrast-enhanced T1-weighted MR image showing homogeneous ductal enhancement. (d) Mapping of the lesion (green line area, intraductal papilloma.).

MRI findings may improve patient selection and treatment planning. However, MRI should not be used as an alternative for a breast biopsy to determine whether a given lesion is malignant, and it should not replace major duct excision as the gold standard for ruling out malignancy in patients with ND and a negative evaluation (Morrogh et al., 2007; Bluemke et al., 2004).

7.3 MR ductography (MRDG, also called MR galactography)

Several approaches to MRI of the secreting breast have been suggested, including direct (Schwab, 2008; Wenkel, 2011) and indirect MRDG and fusion MR imaging of contrast-enhanced and indirect ductography (Hirose et al., 2007).

7.3.1 Direct MRDG (direct MR galactography)

Direct MRDG is performed by filling the discharging duct with gadolinium-diethylene-triamine-pentaacetic acid (Gd-DTPA) diluted in saline, using a DG needle as for the conventional DG procedure, and obtaining 3D MRI sequences (Schwab et al., 2008). Schwab et al. (2008) reported findings in 23 patients with pathological discharge. Direct MRDG showed pathological findings in 82% of all findings, while indirect MRDG produced pathological findings in 33% of all findings with significant ($p < 0.01$) differences in the detection of ductal disease between indirect MRDG and all direct MRDG sequences. Wenkel et al. (2011) reported observations of 30 women who underwent conventional DG and direct MRDG. There was no significant difference in sector localization between conventional DG and direct MRDG. It was concluded that because direct MRDG is more effective in identifying the disease than indirect MRDG, conventional DG, direct MRDG may have the potential to become an alternative to conventional DG.

7.3.2 Indirect MRDG (indirect MR galactography)

Intraductal fluid accumulation and duct ectasia can be detected in 40–73% with patients with pathological ND (Daniel et al., 2003; Orel et al., 2000; Schwab et al., 2008), just as MR hydrography can noninvasively depict fluid-fluid tubular structures such as the bile and pancreatic ducts, the ureters, and the semicircular canals (Jara et al., 1998). This method, known as indirect MRDG, can demonstrate the peripheral part of the duct of the point obstructed by an intraductal lesion (Hirose et al., 2006). Advantages to this technique are that it is noninvasive; uses no radiation or contrast material; and causes none of the potential complications associated with cannulation of the duct and injection of contrast medium, including duct perforation, extravasation, and mastitis (Hirose et al., 2007).

The EUSOMA working group suggests that in countries where DG is considered a routine test for suspicious ND, non-contrast T2-weighted and CEMRI can be considered if DG fails for technical reasons or if the patient refuses the procedure.

Indirect MRDG does not identify ducts that are not dilated, although conventional DG may show an undilated duct after cannulation. In some cases, the fluid within the duct has a high signal intensity on T1-weighted images and a low signal intensity on heavily T2-weighted images. This suggests either hemorrhage or the presence of proteins (Hirose et al., 2007).

The single 3D fused image obtained by combining data from indirect MRDG and CEMRI not only demonstrates the existence of an intraductal abnormality but also reveals the shape, size, and extent of the lesion, and can clarify the relationship between the duct and the intraductal lesion (Hirose et al., 2006) (Fig.7).

8. Histopathological diagnosis

Most NDs are caused by benign lesions such as papillomas and duct ectasia. Microdochectomy or major duct excision is often performed on patients with ND to exclude the possibility of underlying ductal carcinoma. Morrogh et al. (2010) analyzed the histopathological findings in biopsies or surgical specimens obtained from patients with pathological ND and identified cancer in 65 of 287 (22%) cases. Among the 287 cases, 121 (42%) were papillomas (Morrogh et al., 2010). Another report identified cancer in 9 of 211 cases (4.3%). Among the 211 cases, 81 (38%) were papillomas (Dillon et al., 2006). A papilloma (Fig. 8a, b) consists of a proliferation of ductal epithelium supported by a fibrovascular stroma. The epithelium of the stromal supporting layer is composed of epithelial and myoepithelial cells. Many papillomas have a complex structure as a result of stromal overgrowth (Fig. 8c), epithelial hyperplasia, or a combination of both of these processes. Foci of apocrine metaplasia are often observed in papillomas (Fig. 8d). Ductal carcinoma (Fig. 9) shows various histopathological patterns.

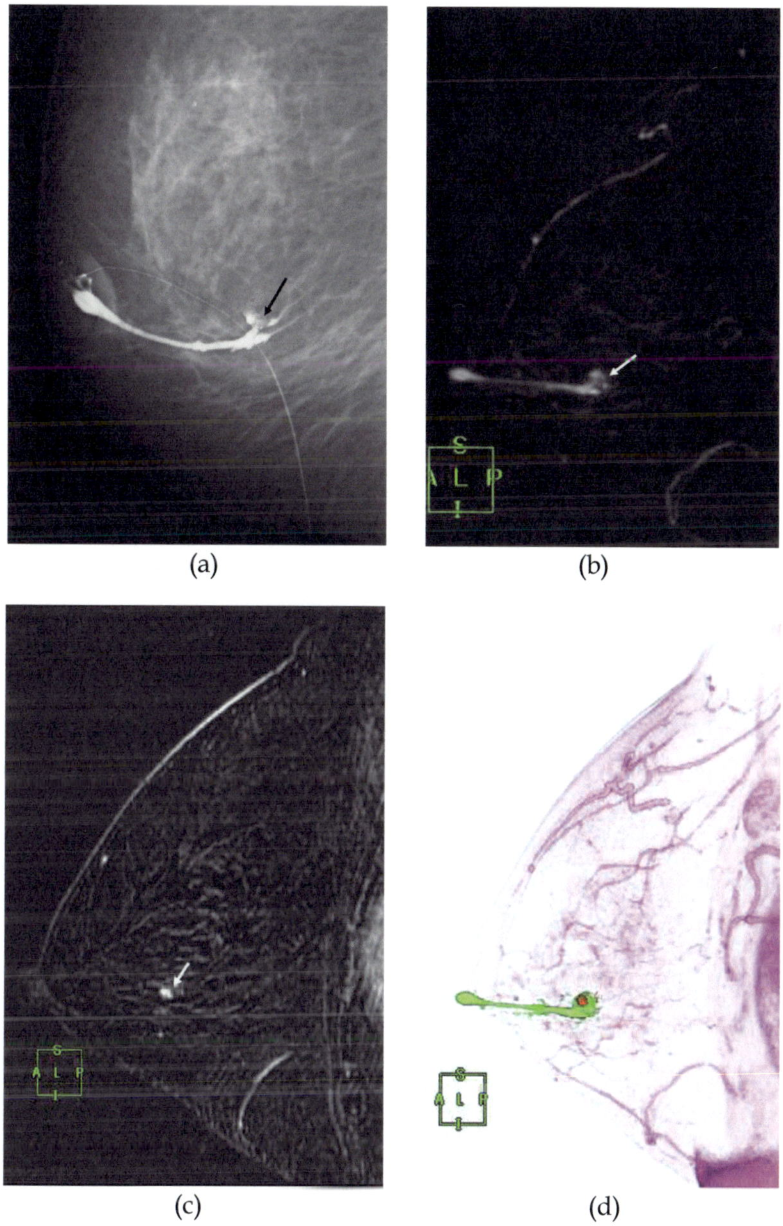

Fig. 7. Images of an intraductal papilloma in a 75-year-old woman. (a) The conventional ductogram and (b) indirect MR ductogram (MIP image) both show a dilated duct with a filling or signal defect (arrow), which represents an intraductal papilloma. (c) The MR mammogram (MIP image) shows a well-circumscribed enhanced lesion (arrow) that indicates the presence of a tiny papilloma. (d) The 3D fusion image shows the dilated duct (green) and the intraductal lesion (red). Reprinted from Hirose et al. (2006).

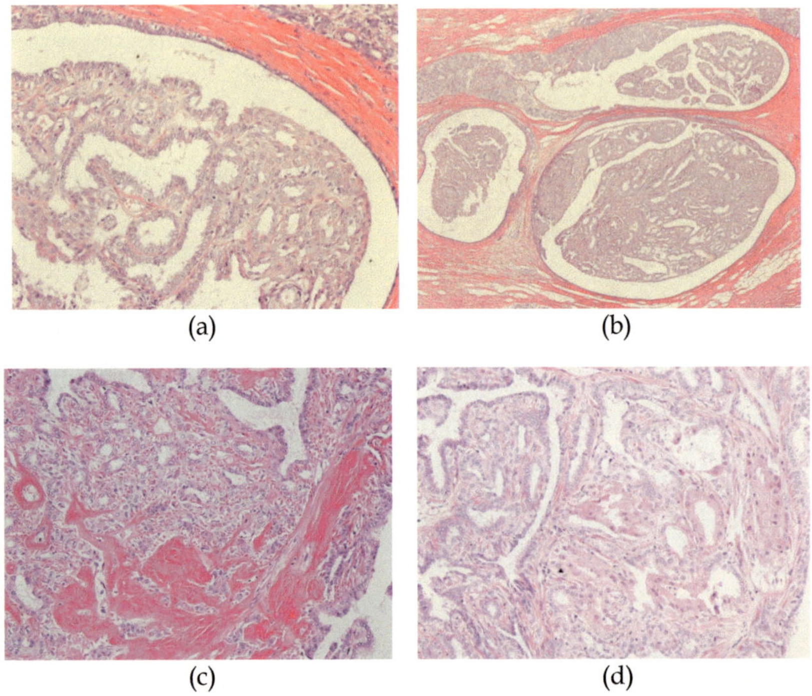

Fig. 8. Intraductal papilloma. (a) Low magnification. (b) Part of the papilloma in a cystically dilated duct. (c) Well-developed stromal sclerosis is present. (d) Apocrine metaplasia is observed.

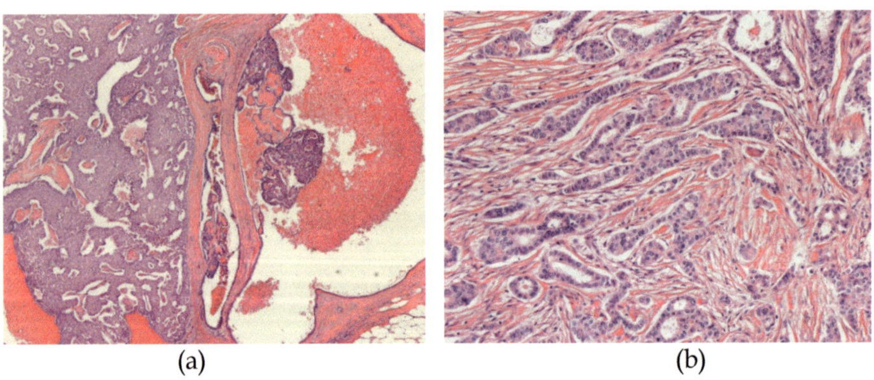

Fig. 9. Ductal carcinoma. (a) Ductal carcinoma in situ. Cystically dilated ducts contain hemorrhage. (b) Invasive ductal carcinoma.

9. Conclusion

MRI provides clinically useful information in patients with suspicious ND and negative standard evaluation. A larger prospective study to determine the use of MRI in the detection and differentiation of benign and malignant lesions causing ND is warranted.

10. Acknowledgments

The authors wish to thank the breast radiologists Tozaki M. and Hirose M. for offering the images from their papers, and the surgeon Masuda N. for providing many cases.

11. References

American College of Radiology. (2003) Breast imaging reporting and data system (BI-RADS), 4th ed. Reston, VA: American College of Radiology. ISBN-10: 0096505052, ISBN-13: 978-0096505054

Ballesio, L., Maggi, C., Savelli, S., Angeletti, M., De Felice, C., Meggiorini, M.L., Manganaro, L. & Porfiri, L.M. (2008). Role of breast magnetic resonance imaging (MRI) in patients with unilateral nipple discharge: preliminary study. *Radiology Medicine,* Vol. 113, No. 2, (March 2008), pp. 249-264. ISSN: 0033-8362 (Print), 1826-6983 (Electronic) 0033-8362 (Linking)

Berg, W.A. & Gilbreath, P.L. (2000). Multicentric and multifocal cancer: whole-breast US in preoperative evaluation. *Radiology,* Vol. 214, No. 1, (January 2000), pp. 59-66. ISSN: 0033-8419 (Print), 1527-1315 (Electronic), 0033-8419 (Linking)

Bluemke, D.A., Gatsonis, C.A., Chen, M.H., DeAngelis, G.A., DeBruhl, N., Harms, S., Heywang-Köbrunner, S.H., Hylton, N., Kuhl, C.K., Lehman, C., Pisano, E.D., Causer, P., Schnitt, S.J., Smazal, S.F., Stelling, C.B., Weatherall, P.T. & Schnall, M.D. (2004). Magnetic resonance imaging of the breast prior to biopsy. *JAMA*, Vol. 292, No. 22, (December 2004), pp. 2735-2742. ISSN: 0098-7484 (Print), 1538-3598 (Electronic), 0098-7484 (Linking)

Cardenosa, G., Doudna, C. & Eklund, G.W. (1994). Ductography of the breast; technique and findings. *American Journal of Roentgenology,* Vol. 162, No. 5, (May 1994), pp. 1081-1087. ISSN: 0361-803X (Print), 1546-3141 (Electronic), 0361-803X (Linking)

Chung, S.Y., Lee, K.W., Park, K.S., Lee, Y. & Bae, S.H. (1995). Breast tumors associated with nipple discharge. correlation of findings on galactography and sonography. *Clinical Imaging,* (July-September 1995) Vol. 19, No. 3, pp. 165-171. ISSN: 0899-7071 (Print), 1873-4499 (Electronic), 0899-7071 (Linking)

Ciatto, S., Bravette, P., Berni, D., Cararzi, S. & Bianchi, S. (1998). The role of galactography in the detection of breast cancer. *Tumori,* Vol. 74, No. 2, (April 1988), pp. 177-181. ISSN: 0300-8916 (Print), 2038-2529 (Electronic), 0300-8916 (Linking)

Daniel, B.L., Gardner, R.W., Birdwell, R.L., Nowels, K.W. & Johnson, D. (2003). Magnetic resonance imaging of intraductal papilloma of the breast. *Magnetic Resonance Imaging,* Vol. 21, No. 8, (October 2003), pp. 887-892. ISSN: 0730-725X (Print), 1873-5894 (Electronic), 0730-725X (Linking)

Das, D., Al-Ayadhy, B., Ajawi, M., Shaheen, A., Sheikh, Z., Mallik, M., Pathan, S., Ebrahim, B., Francis, I., Satar, S., Abdulla, M., Luthra, U. & Junaid, T. (2001). Cytodiagnosis of nipple discharge: a study of 602 samples from 484 cases. *Diagnostic Cytopathology,* Vol. 25, No. 1, (July 2001), pp. 25-37. ISSN: 8755-1039 (Print),1097-0339 (Electronic), 1097-0339 (Linking)

Dillon, M., Mohd, N., Nasir, S., McDermott, E., Evoy, D., Crotty, T., O'Higgins, N. & Hill, A. (2006). The role of major duct excision and microdochectomy in the detection of breast carcinoma. *BMC Cancer,* Vol. 6, (June 2006), p. 164. ISSN: 1471-2407 (Electronic), 1471-2407 (Linking)

Dinkel, H., Gassel, A., Müller, T., Lourens, S., Rominger, M. & Tschammler, A. (2001). Galactography and exfoliative cytology in women with abnormal nipple discharge.

Obstetrics & Gynecology, Vol. 97, No. 4, (April 2001), pp. 625-629. ISSN: 0029-7844 (Print), 1873-233X (Electronic), 0029-7844 (Linking)

El-Daly, H. & Gudi, M. (2010). Evaluation of nipple discharge cytology and diagnostic value of red blood cells in cases with negative cytology: a cytohistologic correlation. *Acta Cytologica*, Vol. 54, No. 4, (July-August 2010), pp. 560-562. ISSN: 0001-5547 (Print), 1938-2650 (Electronic), 0001-5547 (Linking)

Gupta, R., Gaskell, D., Dowle, C., Simpson, J., King, B., Naran, S., Lallu, S. & Fauck, R. (2004). The role of nipple discharge cytology in the diagnosis of breast disease: a study of 1948 nipple discharge smears from 1530 patients. *Cytopathology*, Vol. 15, No. 6, (December 2004), pp. 326-330. ISSN: 0956-5507 (Print), 1365-2303 (Electronic), 0956-5507 (Linking)

Hirose, M., Nobusawa, H. & Gokan, T. (2007). MR ductography: comparison with conventional ductography as a diagnostic method in patients with nipple discharge. *Radiographics*, Vol. 27, No. 1, (October 2007), pp. S183-196. ISSN: 0271-5333 (Print), 1527-1323 (Electronic), 0271-5333 (Linking)

Hirose, M., Otsuki, N., Hayano, D., Shinjo, H., Gokan, T., Kashiwase, T., Suzuki, K. & Sawada, T. (2006). Multi-volume fusion imaging of MR ductography and MR mammography for patients with nipple discharge. *Magnetic Resonance- Medical Science*, Vol. 5, No. 2, (July 2006), pp. 105-112. ISSN: 1347-3182 (Print), 1880-2206 (Electronic), 1347-3182 (Linking)

Hou, M.F., Huang, T.J. & Liu, G.C. (2001). The diagnostic value of galactography in patients with nipple discharge. *Clinical Imaging*, Vol. 25, No. 2 (March-April 2001), pp. 75-81. ISSN: 0899-7071 (Print), 1873-4499 (Electronic), 0899-7071 (Linking)

Hussain, A.N., Polocarpio, C. & Vincent, M.T. (2006). Evaluating nipple discharge. *Obstetrical & Gynecological Survey*, Vol. 61, No. 4, (April 2006), pp. 278-283. ISSN: 0029-7828 (Print), 1533-9866 (Electronic), 0029-7828 (Linking)

Jara, H., Barish, MA., Yucel, EK., Melhem, ER., Hussain, S., Ferrucci, JT. (1998). MR hydrography: theory and practice of static fluid imaging. *American Journal of Roentgenology*, Vol. 170, No. 4, (April 1998), pp. 873-882. ISSN: 0361-803X (Print), 1546-3141 (Electronic), 0361-803X (Linking)

Kuhl, C.K., Mielcareck, P., Klaschik, S., Leutner, C., Wardelmann, E., Gieseke, J. & Schild, H.H. (1999). Dynamic breast MR imaging: are signal intensity time course data useful for differential diagnosis of enhancing lesions? *Radiology*, Vol. 211, No. 1, (April 1999), pp. 101-110. ISSN: 0033-8419 (Print), 1527-1315 (Electronic), 0033-8419 (Linking)

Krishnamurthy, S., Sneige, N., Thompson, P.A., Marcy, S.M., Singletary, S.E., Cristofanilli, M., Hunt, K.K. & Kuerer, H.M. (2003). Nipple aspirate fluid cytology in breast carcinoma. *Cancer*, Vol. 99, No. 2, (April 2003), pp. 97-104. ISSN: 0008-543X (Print), 1097-0142 (Electronic), 0008-543X (Linking)

Lee, W. (2003). Cytology of abnormal nipple discharge: a cyto-histological correlation. *Cytopathology*, Vol. 14, No. 1, (February 2003), pp. 19-26. ISSN: 0956-5507 (Print), 1365-2303 (Electronic), 0956-5507 (Linking)

Liberman, L., Morris, E.A., Lee, M.J., Kaplan, J.B., LaTrenta, L.R., Menell, J.H., Abramson, A.F., Dashnaw, S.M., Ballon, D.J. & Dershaw, D.D. (2002). Breast lesions detected on MR imaging: features and positive predictive value. *American Journal of Roentgenology*, Vol. 179, No. 1, (July 2002), pp. 171-178. ISSN: 0361-803X (Print), 1546-3141 (Electronic), 0361-803X (Linking)

Lorenzon, M., Zuiani, C., Linda, A., Londero, V., Girometti, R. & Bazzocchi, M. (2011). Magnetic resonance imaging in patients with nipple discharge: should we recommend it? *European Radiology,* Vol. 21, No. 5, (May 2011), pp. 899-907. ISSN: 0938-7994 (Print), 1432-1084 (Electronic), 0938-7994 (Linking)

Morakkabati-Spitz, N., Leutner, C., Schild, H., Traeber, F. & Kuhl, C. (2005). Diagnostic usefulness of segmental and linear enhancement in dynamic breast MRI. *European Radiology,* Vol. 15, No. 9, (September 2005), pp. 2010-2017. ISSN: 0938-7994 (Print), 1432-1084 (Electronic), 0938-7994 (Linking)

Morrogh, M., Morris, E.A., Liberman, L., Borgen, P.I. & King, T.A. (2007) The predictive value of ductography and magnetic resonance imaging in the management of nipple discharge. *Annals of Surgical Oncology,* Vol. 14, No. 12, (December 2007), pp. 3369-3377. ISSN: 1068-9265 (Print), 1534-4681 (Electronic), 1068-9265 (Linking)

Morrogh, M., Morris, E.A., Liberman, L., Van Zee, K., Cody, H.S. III & King, T.A. (2008). MRI identifies otherwise occult disease in select patients with Paget disease of the nipple. *Jounal of the American College of Surgeons,* Vol. 206, No. 2, (February 2008), pp. 316-321. ISSN: 1072-7515 (Print), 1879-1190 (Electronic), 1072-7515 (Linking)

Morrogh, M., Park, A., Elkin, E.B. & King, T.A. (2010). Lessons learned from 416 cases of nipple discharge of the breast. *American Journal of Surgery.,* Vol. 200, No. 1, (July 2010), pp. 73-80. ISSN:0002-9610 (Print), 1879-1883 (Electronic), 0002-9610 (Linking)

Nakahara, H., Namba, K., Watanabe, R., Furusawa, H., Matsu, T., Akitama, F., Sakamoto, G. & Tamura, S. (2003). A comparison of MR imaging, galactography and ultrasonography in patients with nipple discharge. *Breast Cancer,* Vol. 10, No. 4, (October 2003), pp. 320-329. ISSN: 1340-6868 (Print), 1880-4233 (Electronic), 1340-6868 (Linking)

Orel, S.G., Dougherty, C.S., Reynolds, C., Reynolds, C., Czerniecki, B.J., Siegelman, E.S. & Schnall, M.D. (2000). MR Imaging in patients with nipple discharge: initial experience. *Radiology,* Vol. 216, No. 1, (July 2000), pp. 248-254. ISSN: 0033-8419 (Print), 1527-1315 (Electronic), 0033-8419 (Linking)

Pritt, B., Pang, Y., Kellogg, M., John, T. & Elhosseiny, A. (2004). Diagnostic value of nipple cytology: study of 466 cases. *Cancer Cytopathology,* Vol. 102, No. 4, (August 2004), pp. 233-238. ISSN: 0008-543X (Print), 1097-0142 (Electronic), 0008-543X (Linking)

Rissanen, T., Reinikainen, H. & Apaja-Sarkkinen, M. (2007). Breast sonography in localizing the cause of nipple discharge comparison with galactography in 52 patients. *Journal of Ultrasound in Medicine,* Vol. 26, No. 8, (August 2007), pp. 1031-1039. ISSN: 0278-4297 (Print), 1550-9613 (Electronic), 0278-4297 (Linking)

Rongione, A.J., Evans, B.D., Kling, K.M. & McFadden, D.W. (1996). Ductography is a useful technique in evaluation of abnormal nipple discharge. *The American Surgeon,* Vol. 62, No. 10, (October 1996), pp. 785-788. ISSN: 0003-1348 (Print), 1555-9823 (Electronic), 0003-1348 (Linking)

Sakorafas, G.H. (2001). Nipple discharge: current diagnostic and therapeutic approaches. *Cancer Treatment Reviews,* Vol. 27, No. 5, (October 2001), pp. 275-282. ISSN: 0305-7372 (Print), 1532-1967 (Electronic), 0305-7372 (Linking)

Sardanelli, F., Boetes, C., Borisch, B., Decker, T., Federico, M., Gilbert, F.J., Helbich, T., Heywang-Köbrunner, S.H., Kaiser, W.A., Kerin, M.J., Mansel, R.E., Marotti, L., Martincich, L., Mauriac, L., Meijers-Heijboer, H., Orecchia, R., Panizza, P., Ponti, A., Purushotham, A.D., Regitnig, P., Del Turco, M.R., Thibault, F. & Wilson, R. (2010). Magnetic resonance imaging of the breast: recommendations from the EUSOMA working group. *European Journal of Cancer,* Vol. 46, No. 8, (May 2010), pp. 1296-1316. ISSN: 0959-8049 (Print), 1879-0852 (Electronic), 0959-8049 (Linking)

Sardanelli, F., Giuseppetti, G.M., Canavese, G., Cataliotti, L., Corcione, S., Cossu, E., Federico, M., Marotti, L., Martincich, L., Panizza, P., Podo, F., Rosselli Del Turco,

M., Zuiani, C., Alfano, C., Bazzocchi, M., Belli, P., Bianchi, S., Cilotti, A., Calabrese, M., Carbonaro, L., Cortesi, L., Di Maggio, C., Del Maschio, A., Esseridou, A., Fausto, A., Gennaro, M., Girometti, R., Ienzi, R., Luini, A., Manoukian, S., Morassutt, S., Morrone, D., Nori, J., Orlacchio, A., Pane, F., Panzarola, P., Ponzone, R., Simonetti, G., Torricelli, P. & Valeri, G. (2008). Indications for breast magnetic resonance imaging. Consensus Document, "Attualita in Senologia," Florence 2007. *Radiology Medicine,* Vol. 113, No. 8, (December 2008), pp. 1085-1095. ISSN: 0033-8362 (Print), 1826-6983 (Electronic), 0033-8362 (Linking)

Schwab, S.A., Uder, M., Schulz-Wendtland, R., Bautz, W.A., Janka, R. & Wenkel, E. (2008). Direct MR galactography: feasibility study. *Radiology,* Vol. 249, No. 1, (October 2008), pp. 54-61. ISSN:0033-8419 (Print), 1527-1315 (Electronic), 0033-8419 (Linking)

Sickles, E.A. (2000). Galactography and other imaging investigations of nipple discharge. *Lancet,* Vol. 356, No. 9242, (November 11th 2000), pp. 1622-1623. ISSN: 0140-6736 (Print), 1474-547X (Electronic), 0140-6736 (Linking)

Simmons, R., Adamovich, T., Brennan, M., Christos, P., Schulz, M., Eisen, C. & Osborne, M. (2003). Nonsurgical evaluation of pathologic nipple discharge. *Annals of Surgical Oncology,* Vol. 10, No. 2, (March 2003), pp. 113-116. ISSN: 1068-9265 (Print), 1534-4681 (Electronic), 1068-9265 (Linking)

Tabar, L., Dean, P.B. & Pentek, Z. (1983). Galactography: the diagnostic procedure of choice for nipple discharge. *Radiology,* Vol. 149, No. 1, (October 1983), pp. 31-38. ISSN: 0033-8419 (Print), 1527-1315 (Electronic), 0033-8419 (Linking)

Tjalma, W.A. & Verslegers, I.O. (2004). Suspicious nipple discharge and breast magnetic resonance imaging. *Breast Journal,* Vol. 10, No.1, (January-February 2004), pp. 65-66. ISSN: 1075-122X (Print), 1524-4741 (Electronic), 1075-122X (Linking)

Tokuda, Y., Kuriyama, K., Nakamoto, A., Choi, S., Yutani, K., Kunitomi, Y., Haneda, T., Kawai, M., Masuda, N., Takeda, M. & Nakamura, H. (2009). Evaluation of suspicious nipple discharge by magnetic resonance mammography based on breast imaging reporting and data system magnetic resonance imaging descriptors. *Journal of Computer Assisted Tomography,* Vol. 33, No. 1, (January-February 2009), pp. 58-62. ISSN: 0363-8715 (Print), 1532-3145 (Electronic), 0363-8715 (Linking)

Tozaki, M., Igarashi, T. & Fukuda, K. (2006). Breast MRI using the VIBE sequence: clustered ring enhancement in the differential diagnosis of lesions showing non-masslike enhancement. *American Journal of Roentgenol*ogy, Vol. 187, No. 2, (August 2006), pp. 313-321. ISSN: 0361-803X (Print), 1546-3141 (Electronic), 0361-803X (Linking)

Van Goethem, M., Verslegers, I., Biltjes, I., Hufkens, G. & Parizel, P.M. (2009). Role of MRI of the breast in the evaluation of the symptomatic patient. *Current Opinion Obstetrics and Gynecology,* Vol. 21, No. 1, (February 2009), pp. 74-79. ISSN: 1040-872X (Print), 1473-656X (Electronic), 1040-872X (Linking)

Wenkel, E., Janka, R., Uder, M., Doellinger, M., Melzer, K., Schulz-Wendtland, R. & Schwab, S.A. (2011). Does direct MR galactography have the potential to become an alternative diagnostic tool in patients with pathological nipple discharge? *Clinical Imaging,* Vol. 35, No. 2, (March-April 2011), pp. 85-93. ISSN: 0899-7071 (Print), 1873-4499 (Electronic), 0899-7071 (Linking)

Yau, E.J., Bultierrez, R.L., DeMartini, W.B., Eby, P.R., Peacock, S. & Lehman, C.D. (2011). The utility of breast MRI as a problem-solving tool. *Breast Journal,* Vol. 17, No. 3, (May-June 2011), pp. 273-280. ISSN: 1075-122X (Print), 1524-4741 (Electronic), 1075-122X (Linking)

10

Radiotherapy After Surgery for Small Breast Cancers of Stellate Appearance

Laszlo Tabar[1], Nadja Lindhe[1], Amy M.F. Yen[2], Tony H.H. Chen[2,3], Sherry Y.H. Chiu[3], Jean C.Y. Fann[2], Sam L.S. Chen[4], Grace H.M. Wu[2], Rex C.C. Huang[2], Judith Offman[5], Fiona A. Dungey[6], Wendy Y.Y. Wu[2], Robert A. Smith[7] and Stephen W. Duffy[5*]

1. Introduction

Radiotherapy is widely used in breast cancer treatment, particularly in patients undergoing breast conserving surgery, principally in order to reduce risk of local recurrence (Liljegren et al. 1999; Fisher et al. 2002). Although radiation therapy has been observed in a major meta-analysis to confer a net survival benefit (Clarke et al. 2005), it is not without side-effects. It has been observed to confer increased risks of cardiovascular events and lung tumours (Clarke et al. 2005; Darby et al. 2005). The fact that radiation therapy confers both benefits and harms raises issues pertinent to all treatments, i.e., the importance of selecting patient populations for which the balance of benefits to harms is optimised, and of excluding those patients who will not benefit from the treatment, or at least not sufficiently to outweigh the risk of adverse effects. Given the current lack of confidence that the prognostic indicators for such selection exist, conservative therapy includes post-surgical radiotherapy as a standard of care.

It has been reported that patients with invasive breast tumours less than 15 mm in size have mammographic tumour features that are good indicators of prognosis, and in particular, good long term survival has been observed in stellate lesions of this size without accompanying calcifications or with only non-specific calcifications (Smith et al. 2004; Tabar et al. 2000). The large majority of these patients did not receive adjuvant therapy other than radiotherapy, and since long-term survival was very high, the potential for modern adjuvant therapies to further improve upon the survival of these cases is very small. However, the extent to which these patients benefited from radiotherapy, in terms of reduction of risk of local recurrence, is not known. In this paper, we review the treatment and tumour features of 425 stellate invasive breast cancers of

*1 *Mammography Department, Central Hospital, Sweden*
2 *College of Public Health, National Taiwan University, Taiwan*
3 *Tampere School of Public Health, Finland*
4 *Changhua Christian Hospital, Taiwan*
5 *Centre for Cancer Prevention, Queen Mary, University of London, UK*
6 *Cancer Research UK & UCL Cancer Trials Centre, UK*
7 *American Cancer Society, USA*

maximum diameter less than 15 mm, with a view to developing an index of risk of local recurrence and possibly of identifying patient populations suitable and unsuitable for radiotherapy. The research was approved by the Ethics Committee of Falun Central Hospital.

2. Patient data obtained for analysis

Mammograms were retrieved of all tumours of pathological size less than 15 mm, diagnosed in women aged 40-69 between 1977 and 1998 in Falun Central Hospital, Sweden. Of these, 425 were identified to have stellate appearance and either no calcifications or non-specific calcifications on the mammogram. Patient charts were retrieved and additional pathological information was obtained on exact tumor size in mm, node status, tumor grade and histological type. Treatment details with respect to surgery, adjuvant radiotherapy, chemotherapy and hormonal therapy were also retrieved. In addition, we recorded age, date of diagnosis, mode of detection (screening or symptomatic) and follow-up details including dates of local recurrence, death from breast cancer and death from other causes.

There was an average follow-up of 10.4 years to recurrence, death or last known date alive and disease-free, and a maximum follow-up of 27.9 years. The most recent date of follow-up was 20th March 2006. Local recurrence was defined as the occurrence of a histologically confirmed *in situ* or invasive carcinoma in the ipsilateral breast after treatment of the first breast cancer was completed.

3. Radiotherapy treatment regimens

For women who had breast conserving surgery for an invasive breast cancer, radiotherapy was regarded as standard treatment and computer dose-planned photon beam (6 and/or 15 MV) treatment was used. Care was taken not to treat the ipsilateral lung and, in the case of left-sided breast cancers, the heart. The whole breast parenchyma was defined as the target and 2 Gray per fraction times 25 was delivered over 5 weeks. If the patient was younger than age 45 yrs or if extensive DCIS (>25% of tumor) was present, additional photon-boost was used against the tumor bed. The boost-target was treated with 2 Gy per fraction to a total of 10 - 16 Gray. If one or more lymph nodes were engaged with cancer, separate fields were directed to the ipsilateral axilla and supraclavicular fossa, 2 Gray per fraction x 25 was used. Treatment of the intramammary lymph nodes was considered if 4 or more of the axillary nodes were metastasized.

Computer dose-planned radiotherapy was used also for some patients treated with a mastectomy. The thoracic wall was treated with opposed tangential photon fields if the tumor was > 30 mm or multifocal or N1. Regional lymph nodes were treated according the rules described above. Boost treatment was given only in the rare instances when surgical radicality could not be achieved.

4. Multifactor score of risk of recurrence

Data were analysed by stepwise Cox proportional hazards regression to build up a multifactor score of risk of recurrence. Analyses were adjusted for age and epoch of diagnosis, as radiotherapy practices depended on these factors. After exclusion of those factors that were not statistically significant when adjusted for other variables, we used the final Cox regression model to estimate the absolute reductions in 15-year risk of recurrence (only 22% of subjects had follow-up in excess of 15 years).

5. Recurrence rates in patients with small stellate breast cancers

Survival in this group was generally excellent. Figure 1 shows survival by size group (1-9 mm and 10-14 mm) and radiotherapy. In all four groups, long-term survival was 90% or greater. There was no significant effect of radiotherapy on survival.

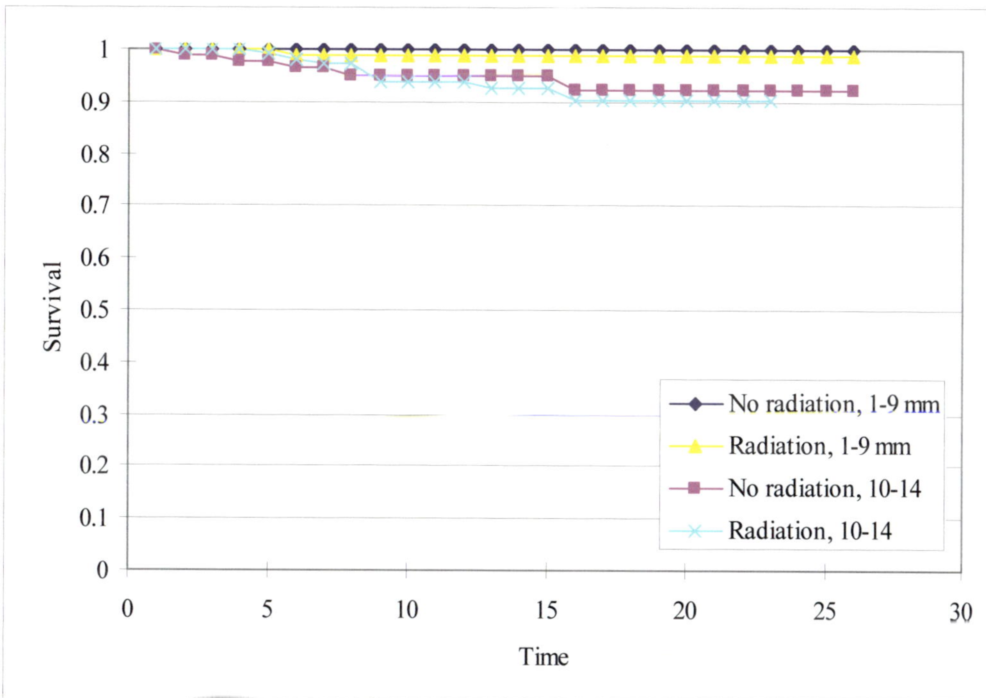

Fig. 1. Breast cancer specific survival of 425 1-14 mm stellate invasive breast cancers by size group and radiotherapy.

Table 1 shows the study subjects and recurrence rates by tumour, host, diagnostic and treatment features. There were 70 local recurrences in 425 patients. Overall, the average rate of recurrence was 1.6% per annum. Notably high recurrence rates were observed in grade 3 tumours and lobular carcinoma cases. Because 51% of the cases were diagnosed before 1990, the proportions of subjects treated with breast conserving surgery and with hormone therapy were considerably smaller than would be the case in tumours diagnosed at the present time.

Factor	Category	Cases (%)	Recurrences	Crude annual % recurrence rate
Epoch of diagnosis	1977-84	117 (28)	20	1.4
	1985-89	99 (23)	18	1.5
	1990-94	99 (23)	19	2.0
	1995-98	110 (26)	3	1.7
Age group	<55	142 (33)	26	1.5
	55+	283 (67)	44	1.6
Tumour size (mm)	1-9	156 (37)	25	1.6
	10-14	269 (63)	45	1.6
Node status	Negative	341 (80)	55	1.5
	Positive	45 (11)	10	2.0
	Not examined	39 (9)	5	1.7
Grade	1	204 (50)	24	1.1
	2	173 (42)	31	1.8
	3	34 (8)	10	2.9
	Unknown	14	5	4.1
Surgery	Mastectomy	136 (32)	21	1.3
	BCS*	289 (68)	49	1.7
Radiotherapy	No	168 (40)	31	1.7
	Yes	254 (60)	38	1.5
	Unknown	3	1	3.3
Chemotherapy	No	411 (97)	67	1.6
	Yes	12 (3)	3	2.9
	Unknown	2	0	0.0
Hormone therapy	No	391 (92)	64	1.5
	Yes	32 (8)	6	2.4
	Unknown	2	0	0.0
Histological type	Ductal	286 (67)	47	1.6
	Lobular	52 (12)	14	2.8
	Tubular	80 (19)	7	0.8
	Other	7 (2)	2	2.9
Detection mode	Symptomatic	102 (24)	22	2.0
	Screening	323 (76)	48	1.4

* BCS=breast conserving surgery

Table 1. Host, tumour and treatment characteristics, with the corresponding rates of local recurrence.

Table 2 shows the final model from the stepwise Cox regression for prediction of recurrence. Age and epoch of diagnosis were included regardless of significance. A highly significant increase in risk of recurrence was noted with grade (HR=1.93, 95% CI 1.31-2.85, p=0.001, trend test). Although the main effect of radiotherapy was not significant, it had a significant interaction with age (p=0.03), associated with lower rates of recurrence in patients aged 55 and over (HR=0.26, 95% CI 0.07-0.88), but not in patients aged less than 55. It also had a borderline significant interaction with histological type (p=0.07) with a high rate of recurrence in lobular carcinoma cases treated with radiotherapy (HR=3.58, 95%CI 0.90-14.13). The effects of BCS (p=0.01) and histological type (p=0.04) were significant before adjustment for these interactions, so these factors were retained in the model. No other variables had significant effects on risk of recurrence after adjustment for the factors in Table 2.

Factor	Category	Cox regression RR*	95% CI
Age group	<55	1.00	-
	55+	2.53	0.93-6.87
Epoch of diagnosis	1977-84	1.00	-
	1985-89	1.19	0.55-2.53
	1990-94	2.15	0.95-4.82
	1995-98	1.42	0.55-3.04
Surgery	Mastectomy	1.00	-
	BCS	1.81	0.93-3.51
Histology	Ductal, other	1.00	-
	Lobular	0.92	0.31-2.76
Grade	Trend	1.93	1.31-2.85
Radiotherapy	No	1.00	-
	Yes	1.21	0.40-3.62
Interaction	Lobular AND radiotherapy	3.58	0.90-14.13
Interaction	Age 55+ AND radiotherapy	0.26	0.07-0.88

* RR=rate ratio

Table 2. Relative hazards and 95% confidence intervals from the final Cox regression model after stepwise regression.

Table 3 shows the results from the final Cox regression model, in terms of estimated annual rates of recurrence in the absence of radiotherapy and absolute reductions in cumulative 15-year recurrence associated with radiotherapy. Overall, absolute effects were small. For example, for grade 1, non-lobular tumours, in women aged 55 or older, treated with mastectomy, the absolute reduction in risk of local recurrence associated with radiotherapy was 1.87%. Substantial reductions in recurrence rates were observed only for cases aged 55 or more at diagnosis, of grade 2 or 3 and of non-lobular histological type. For some combinations of factors, notably lobular carcinoma cases younger than age 55, the reductions were negative, i.e. showing increases in recurrence in those treated with radiotherapy. For lobular carcinoma cases age 55 or over, and for non-lobular cases younger than age 55, no substantial benefit of radiotherapy was observed.

6. Expert commentary

This study pertains to a very special subgroup of good prognosis tumours, i.e. stellate lesions less than 15 mm in size without calcifications. Within this group, our results suggest that radiotherapy was substantially beneficial only in terms of preventing local recurrence in women aged 55 and older diagnosed with non-lobular carcinoma grade 2 or 3, a subgroup constituting 31% of the subjects (131 out of 425). Of the remaining 294 cases, 183 (63%) received radiotherapy, and based on these results not only did not substantially benefit from it, but may indeed have had their risk of recurrence increased. It might be argued that in modern treatment practice, very few of the mastectomy cases would receive radiotherapy. Where margins are close, the NCCN recommends that radiotherapy should be considered (NCCN 2009). However, also in modern therapeutic practice, a large proportion of these cases, being smaller than 15 mm, would receive wide local excision.

Radiotherapy is primarily aimed at reducing the risk of local recurrence (Liljegren 2002). It has been suggested that radiotherapy might be dispensed with for low-risk patients (e.g.

Surgery	Age	Lobular histology	Grade	Estimated % annual recurrence rate without radiotherapy	Absolute reduction in 15-year probability of recurrence with radiotherapy
Mastectomy	<55	No	1	0.5	-0.0007
			2	0.9	-0.0026
			3	1.7	-0.0115
		Yes	1	0.4	-0.0114
			2	0.9	-0.0360
			3	1.7	-0.0748
	55+	No	1	1.2	0.0187
			2	2.3	0.0570
			3	4.5	0.1470
		Yes	1	1.1	-0.0030
			2	2.2	-0.0084
			3	4.2	-0.0235
Breast conserving surgery	<55	No	1	0.9	-0.0036
			2	1.7	-0.0088
			3	3.2	-0.0228
		Yes	1	0.8	-0.0319
			2	1.6	-0.0882
			3	3.0	-0.1800
	55+	No	1	2.2	0.0504
			2	4.2	0.1363
			3	8.3	0.2769
		Yes	1	2.0	-0.0078
			2	3.9	-0.0220
			3	7.6	-0.0340

Table 3. Estimated recurrence rates in the absence of radiotherapy and absolute reduction in 15-year risk of recurrence by surgery, age, histological type and grade of tumours, from the final Cox regression model.

older patients with lower stage non-lobular tumours) (Liljegren 2002; Liljegren et al. 1997). One study has found risk of recurrence to be particularly low in those with non-dense breast tissue (Cil et al. 2009). The results here suggest that a significant proportion of patients with small stellate lesions can be considered at low risk, and that some higher risk patients, such as lobular carcinoma cases, may have high local recurrence rates despite radiotherapy. These results are observational, and need to be validated.

Another observational study has found, contrary to our results, that radiotherapy is associated with substantially reduced risk of local recurrence in lobular carcinoma (Diepenmaat et al. 2009). There was, however, a comparatively shorter follow up time (median of 7.2 years). Issues such as this may be resolved by delineating the tumour populations in radiotherapy trials which have already been conducted, or by carrying out new prospective trials.

The point has already been made that small stellate lesions are a good candidate for less aggressive therapy (Smith et al. 2004; Alexander, Yankaskas, and Biesemier 2006). The potential to save almost 70% of patients in this group from the hazards of radiation therapy is a goal worth pursuing.

7. Five year view

The results of this observational study suggest that contrary to standard practice, post-operative radiotherapy may not be the ideal treatment for all breast cancers treated with breast conserving surgery, particularly those with good prognosis. This is not to deny the results of the randomised trials and meta-analyses. There is clear evidence from these that radiotherapy reduces local recurrence and improves survival. However, this does not necessarily imply that it is needed in all cases. There is potential for utilising patient and tumour information to assign treatment based on that which is appropriate for the subgroup. This tailored therapeutic approach uses simply obtained specifics, e.g patient age, radiological appearance and tumour histology/grade. It would enable a more accurate risk-benefit analysis to be calculated before prescription of therapies with adverse side-effects such as radiotherapy. It is therefore attractive in comparison with universal provision of radiotherapy to all patients. Before such policies can be implemented, it is essential that we are certain of the risks:benefit ratio for each patient subgroup and therefore these findings must be validated. This approach of investigating the level of benefit to different patient populations may be useful for other cancer therapies with adverse side-effects, with the objective of identifying other areas for improvement as medical oncology progresses to an era of individually tailored treatments.

8. Conclusion

Radiotherapy is widely used to reduce the risk of local recurrence of breast cancer, particularly after breast conserving surgery. However, radiotherapy to the breast has adverse long-term side effects (risk of heart disease, lung cancer, angiosarcoma, deformation), and therefore it would be useful to identify subsets of patients for whom this treatment is unnecessary. Patients with stellate tumours of 1-14mm have a good prognosis and a high proportion of them might benefit from omitting radiotherapy. A Cox regression was applied to follow up data from 425 such patients and a comparison of local recurrence rates made for different patient groups/tumour stages receiving or not receiving radiotherapy post surgery. These observations suggest that the only group of patients within the 1-14 mm stellate lesions to benefit from radiotherapy are those aged 55 or more, with high grade (2 or 3) disease and non-lobular histology. Radiotherapy may not be beneficial to certain groups with higher risk of recurrence (e.g. younger women or lobular carcinoma) and some groups with low risk of recurrence (e.g. low grade tumours). Further validation using subgroup analyses of trials already performed would be useful.

9. Acknowledgements

Fieldwork for this study was supported by Cancer Research UK. Analysis was supported by the American Cancer Society through a gift from the Longaberger Company.

10. References

Alexander, M. C., B. C. Yankaskas, and K. W. Biesemier. (2006). Association of stellate mammographic pattern with survival in small invasive breast tumors. *AJR. American journal of roentgenology* 187 (1):29-37.

Cil, T., E. Fishell, W. Hanna, P. Sun, E. Rawlinson, S. A. Narod, and D. R. McCready. (2009). Mammographic density and the risk of breast cancer recurrence after breast-conserving surgery. *Cancer* 115 (24):5780-7.

Clarke, M., R. Collins, S. Darby, C. Davies, P. Elphinstone, E. Evans, J. Godwin, R. Gray, C. Hicks, S. James, E. MacKinnon, P. McGale, T. McHugh, R. Peto, C. Taylor, and Y. Wang. (2005). Effects of radiotherapy and of differences in the extent of surgery for early breast cancer on local recurrence and 15-year survival: an overview of the randomised trials. *Lancet* 366 (9503):2087-106.

Darby, S. C., P. McGale, C. W. Taylor, and R. Peto. (2005). Long-term mortality from heart disease and lung cancer after radiotherapy for early breast cancer: prospective cohort study of about 300,000 women in US SEER cancer registries. *The lancet oncology* 6 (8):557-65.

Diepenmaat, L. A., M. J. van der Sangen, L. V. van de Poll-Franse, M. W. van Beek, C. L. van Berlo, E. J. Luiten, G. A. Nieuwenhuijzen, and A. C. Voogd. (2009). The impact of postmastectomy radiotherapy on local control in patients with invasive lobular breast cancer. *Radiotherapy and oncology : journal of the European Society for Therapeutic Radiology and Oncology* 91 (1):49-53.

Fisher, B., S. Anderson, J. Bryant, R. G. Margolese, M. Deutsch, E. R. Fisher, J. H. Jeong, and N. Wolmark. (2002). Twenty-year follow-up of a randomized trial comparing total mastectomy, lumpectomy, and lumpectomy plus irradiation for the treatment of invasive breast cancer. *The New England journal of medicine* 347 (16):1233-41.

Liljegren, G. (2002). Is postoperative radiotherapy after breast conserving surgery always mandatory? A review of randomised controlled trials. *Scandinavian journal of surgery : SJS : official organ for the Finnish Surgical Society and the Scandinavian Surgical Society* 91 (3):251-4.

Liljegren, G., L. Holmberg, J. Bergh, A. Lindgren, L. Tabar, H. Nordgren, and H. O. Adami. (1999). 10-Year results after sector resection with or without postoperative radiotherapy for stage I breast cancer: a randomized trial. *Journal of clinical oncology : official journal of the American Society of Clinical Oncology* 17 (8):2326-33.

Liljegren, G., A. Lindgren, J. Bergh, H. Nordgren, L. Tabar, and L. Holmberg. (1997). Risk factors for local recurrence after conservative treatment in stage I breast cancer. Definition of a subgroup not requiring radiotherapy. *Annals of Oncology* 8 (3):235-241.

National Comprehensive Cancer Network (NCCN). (2009). NCCN Clinical Practice Guidelines in Oncology: Breast Cancer. NCCN. Fort Washington, PA: 1-20

Smith, R. A., L. Tabar, H. H. T. Chen, M. F. A. Yen, T. Tot, T. H. Tung, L. S. Chen, Y. H. Chiu, and S. W. Duffy. (2004). Mammographic tumor features can predict long-term outcomes reliably in women with 1-14-mm invasive breast carcinoma - Suggestions for the reconsideration of current therapeutic practice and the TNM classification system. *Cancer* 101 (8):1745-1759.

Tabar, L., H. H. Chen, S. W. Duffy, M. F. Yen, C. F. Chiang, P. B. Dean, and R. A. Smith. (2000). A novel method for prediction of long-term outcome of women with T1a, T1b, and 10-14 mm invasive breast cancers: a prospective study. *Lancet* 355 (9202):429-433.